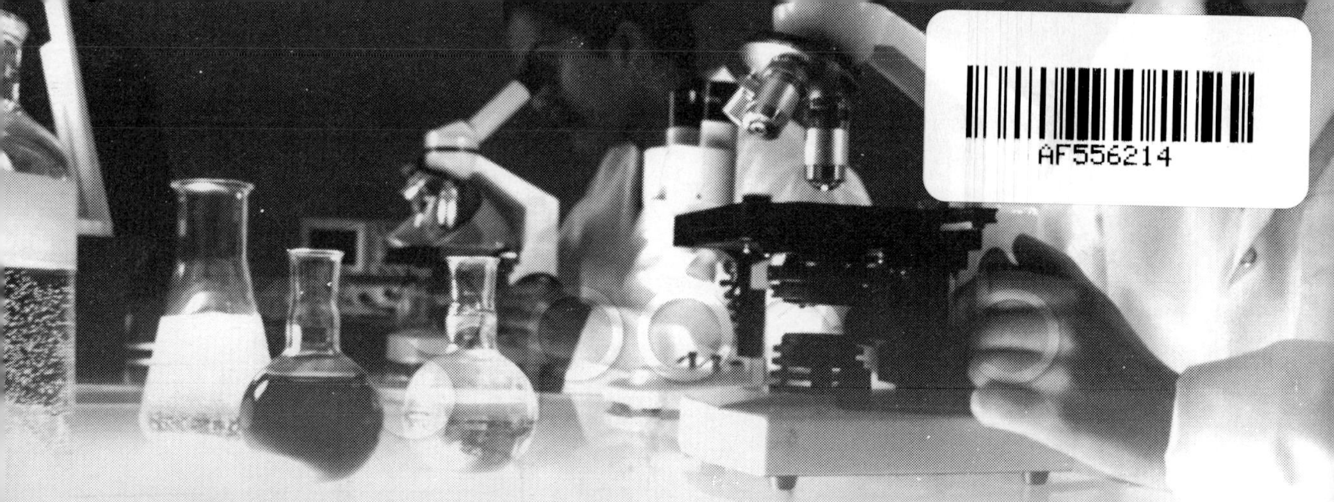

Basic Methods of Medical Research

Basic Methods of Medical Research

5th Edition

Abhaya Indrayan

Ph.D. (Ohio State University, U.S.A.), FAMS, FASc, FRSS
Ex-Head of the Department of Biostatistics and Medical Informatics,
Delhi University, College of Medical Sciences (UCMS), Delhi
Past Visiting Faculty at the Ohio State University, and
Past Visiting Research Scientist, University of Massachusetts.

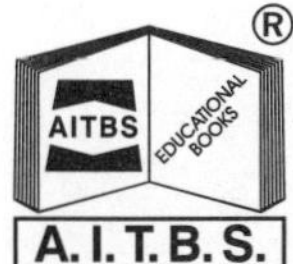

AITBS PUBLISHERS, INDIA
MEDICAL PUBLISHERS
J-5/6, Krishan Nagar, Delhi-110051 (INDIA)
Phone: 011-40167052, 49067602
E-mail: aitbsindia@gmail.com & aitbsindia@hotmail.com

First Edition : 2006
Second Edition : 2008
Third Edition : 2013
Fourth Edition : 2018
Fifth Edition : 2023
Fifth Edition Reprint : 2026

ISBN: 978-81-7473-335-1

Published by:
Virender Kumar Arya for
AITBS Publishers, India
MEDICAL PUBLISHERS
J-5/6, Krishan Nagar, Delhi-110051 (INDIA)
Phone: 011-40167052, 49067602
E-mail: aitbsindia@gmail.com & aitbsindia@hotmail.com

Printed by AITBS, Delhi

Preface to the Fifth Edition

With health awareness reaching to a zenith, the medical research is exponentially increasing. But a serious concern has been expressed time and again regarding the quality of this medical research now going on at an enormous pace around the word. This concern testifies that the basics of medical research are not clear to many researchers. The malaise perhaps starts from the theses done by the medical postgraduates (PGs). Many of these theses are done in a casual manner - perhaps providing a wrong training to the PGs in research methodology.

Methodology is the pillar on which a research stands. The results can't be predicted and may be positive or negative, but the methodology must be credible to command respect. The selection of an apt topic, comprehensive and unbiased review of the literature, correct identification of the lacunae, setting up of measurable and useful objectives that have bearing on health, choosing an appropriate design, selection of the right subjects, collection of truthful data, their proper collation and analysis by appropriate methods, valid interpretation, and to-the-point and a matter-of-fact writing are the steps that need to be strictly followed. Not just PGs, many who have been into research for quite some time need help in preparing their protocol, conducting the investigations, and drafting the paper or report. This book is aimed to impart this knowledge in a simple, medical friendly, language.

Devoid of polemics and equations, the text is designed for delightful reading with features such as key terms and concept at the beginning of each chapter that set the tone, and a crisp summary at the end that recapitulates the discussion. The intricacies of medical research are explained by clear and concise step-by-step procedure that appeals to conscience. Important concepts are repeatedly explained in different contexts. Thus, there is deliberate duplication. The text is supported by a large number of real-life examples to sustain the interest. A rich glossary of methodological terms is provided at the end. These pedagogical features may help in enhancing the learning.

This book has been extensively revised and updated at each edition. This is the fifth edition. I hope the readers will enjoy reading this and would be able to improve the quality of their research. I am grateful to those who have adopted this book for learning and have made it standard text on this topic.

I acknowledge the help I received from colleagues and critics who provided important inputs from time to time to my knowledge base and expertise. The material cited in this text is largely based on what I could collect from medical libraries at Yale and Harvard during my sabbaticals. My students on the hand, and the national and international agencies (WHO, World Bank, UNAIDS, DANPCB, IAVI, etc.) that I happened to work with on the other, have been a source of inspiration. I am also much obliged to Virender Kumar Arya of AITBS Publishers, India, for being always extremely helpful and accommodating.

—Abhaya Indrayan

Contents

CHAPTER 1

What is Medical Research and What are the Basic Methods

KEY TERMS AND CONCEPTS

- ✓ Medical Research and its Levels
- ✓ Epistemic Gaps and Medical Uncertainties
- ✓ Empiricism in Medical Research
- ✓ Research Ethics and Informed Consent
- ✓ Fruits and Frustrations of Medical Research

This book is a collection of ideas and advices to initiate a young mind into the fascinating world of medical research and provides complete details of the methods to carry out research with conviction and confidence. The rules given herein are both necessary and sufficient to produce results that would withstand the scientific scrutiny. The methods are explained in simple language and particularly geared to the level of a fresh graduate in medicine and the graduates in the related sciences such as health, dentistry, nursing and pharmacy.

1.1 THE FASCINATING WORLD OF MEDICAL RESEARCH

We all know that health is paramount in our daily life and almost everything else is secondary. Health maybe considered in its holistic sense to incorporate not just physical well-being but also social and mental and now spiritual aspects. However, we limit this book mostly to the physical component as mental and social aspects many times digress into abstract domain and defy measurement. Health is a homeostatic state that keeps balance between the needs of the body and available resources within the body by continuous adjustment.

Many people around us many times come across events that affect their health in unpredictable ways and they find themselves at the crossroads for dealing with these events. While mild conditions tend to vanish with time as the body defenses work effectively to produce the required counters, a consultation with doctor becomes necessary if the problem persists or becomes beyond the healing capacity of the natural process. In the case of serious illness, hospital admissions and surgery may be required. But do we have sufficiently effective treatments for all ailments? Patients and doctors like to have an instant cure – almost like a magic – but that magic wand eludes us. This is where medical research comes in. There are ailments for which no cure is available and there are so many others for which the efficacy of the treatment is not perfect. We give many examples of such conditions later on as we go along but we all like to have tools to replace the affected body parts and would expect that these replacements work as effectively as the original, if not better. We would also like that we are able to correctly diagnose the disease just by looking at the diseased person and to give a treatment that gives instant results. While that is utopian, a large number of advancements have been made in the recent past due to the research by dedicated scientists around the world that have helped in getting quicker results at less cost and less inconvenience. Humanity is grateful to them. Such is the fascinating world of medical research.

1.1.1 WHAT IS RESEARCH?

Medical research is a complex process and requires some explanation. Let us first understand what we mean by 'research' in general and then come to the specifics of medical research.

A **research** is a discovery of new truth that was either not known earlier or was in the realm of speculation. To state precisely, *research is either discovery of new facts, enunciation of new principles or fresh interpretations of the known facts or principles.* Propounding a new idea or method is also research, provided it is rooted in science. By science we mean the new proposal is based on evidence and can be replicated and verified. Confirmation and denial of the existing ideas and tools for a new setting also comes under the ambit of research when the need of confirmation is justified in the light of doubts of their application to the new setting. Sometimes research into researches is done to come up with a more reliable result. This can also refute the existing knowledge. The basic function of research is to answer why and how of a phenomenon, but searching answers to what, when, how much, etc., is also a part of research endeavours. The term 'research' has scientific overtones although colloquially people use this term for any enquiry. For example, children would say they were researching into the life of a footballer on internet or into the origin of the term radar. Indeed in many art forms such as literature and history, research can have an entirely different meaning. It could mean a detailed study of a phenomenon that may bring out some new features not sufficiently well known earlier. However, research in science has a very different meaning.

With another perspective, research is relentless search for truth. Howsoever strange it may sound, the truth changes from time to time. Ptolemy in the second century AD propounded that sun revolves around the earth. It remained truth for 14 centuries when Copernicus came up with a new truth in the 16th century that earth revolves around the sun. We will later give examples of medical discoveries that were later on found untrue – even harmful. Miscues do occur and the need to be extremely careful can hardly be overemphasized.

1.1.2 WHAT IS MEDICAL RESEARCH?

For those who are not clear, medicine is a science that provides tools and methods to put body systems back on track when they derail due to interference or disruptions such as infection, nutrition deficiency, injury, mental trauma, and frailty due to aging. These efforts to put system back on track come under classical **curative medicine** that alleviates suffering and requires steps such as diagnosis, treatment, and prognosis. Tools and methods to keep body, mind, and soul healthy so that the disruptors do not affect us or affect us minimally also come under the broad meaning of medicine when preventive and promotive steps are also included.

Epistemic Gaps

Despite enormous expansion of knowledge in the past two decades, the unknown segment of the medicine continues to be enormous. For example, no cure of cancer is yet available and we make-do with management of the condition to reduce the suffering and prolong life. We still do not know how to regenerate healthy cells in the body that can replace the aberrant cells. There are innumerable examples of such incomplete knowledge and called **epistemic gaps.** The irony is that the expansion of knowledge opens up new avenues and raises new questions that were not thought of earlier. Thus, research expands the avenues for more research. Scientific paradigm is that unknown segment of knowledge is far more than the known segment. The paradox of new knowledge creating more holes in knowledge propels science to go further and attain new heights.

With enormous epistemic gaps in our knowledge, it is imperative that we look for new ways to build up health and to minimize the suffering if and when an aberration occurs. Medical research is precisely this – finding new processes that can provide quick relief exactly of the type required by a patient, which are feasible in a variety of settings and can be implemented at a cost that is affordable by those who need it. This innocuously looking entity – called medical research – is not as simple as it looks. This requires that a comprehensive procedure is followed from conceiving and selecting a problem for research, to the methods adopted, and for communicating the results in a manner that can convince the scientific community that a new result has been obtained which deserves application for improving the health.

Whereas basic medical research is carried out at intracellular levels to understand how our genes mutate or interact with their environment within and outside the cells, and how can we modify this structure and behaviour when needed, most everyday medical research is carried out with a person as a unit. Our body is a systematic collection of almost innumerable interconnected nodes, each of which is a powerhouse by itself. Thus, it is natural that no two individuals have ever been exactly alike nor would be so in the future. They differ in their anatomical composition, physiological functions, mental capabilities, and their capacity to handle extraneous interrupters such as pollution and nutrition, and react differently to deliberate human interventions such as drugs and surgery. Whatever new tools and method one envisages, the response of the individuals to such new methods will almost surely vary from one person to another and this variation creates an environment of uncertainty.

Empiricism

This inter-individual variation just mentioned makes it necessary for us to study a group of people and count how many respond or what is the average response. Such a study is called **empirical** since it depends upon the observation and measurements. A pre-requisite is that a group of subjects is studied in a manner that their responses lead to a valid and reliable conclusion for the application to future subjects of the same type. Without future perspective, a research is devoid of its soul, but this also requires researchers to be extremely careful in drawing conclusions because a mistake can jeopardize life and health of many people. This happens when an erroneous result is used on thousands of cases. The same cannot be stated with similar emphasis for research in other disciplines such as Physics and Chemistry or History and politics, because they do not have direct and immediate consequences on the health of the people. Their effect is gradual and protracted although it could have far-reaching consequences in the long run.

The conventional medical research is relatively easy and can bring useful results for immediate application. Just conduct a trial or an observational study regarding the new method or tool and get the results. But this also heaps responsibility on the medical researchers that appropriate methodology is used that can provide valid and reliable results. For this, it is necessary that a researcher, such as a **postgraduate student**, has full and correct knowledge of at least the basic methods of medical research applicable to different levels of research.

1.2 TYPES AND LEVELS OF MEDICAL RESEARCH

Medical research is a vast subject, and the sphere is rapidly growing. It is in fact snowballing with time and quickly expanding its size and impact. A particular research gets its real face when binned into its types and levels.

1.2.1 TYPES OF MEDICAL RESEARCH

Medical research encompasses a whole gamut of endeavours that ultimately help to improve health of people. Functionally, it can be divided into basic and applied types. Basic, also termed as **'pure' research,** involves advancing the knowledge base without any specific focus on its application. The results of such research are utilized somewhere in future when that new knowledge is required. In medicine, basic research is generally done at the cellular level for studying various biological processes. This kind of research can provide a radical breakthrough. This book is not adequate for this kind of research. **Applied research,** on the other hand, is oriented to an existing problem. Applied medical research could be on the diagnostic and therapeutic modalities, agent-host-environment interactions, or health assessments. This book should be adequate to plan and conduct this kind of research when limited to the aspects mentioned next.

Most of what is stated in this chapter, indeed almost all this book, is about analysis of evidence. The objective of this analysis is to identify clear signals emanating from the varying and sometimes conflicting evidence from the study subjects. When these signals conform to one another, clear conclusions can be drawn.

There is another type of medical research that is very popular and very effective. This is collecting diverse evidence from various studies (not individual subjects) and synthesising it to get a holistic picture after resolving any conflicts. **Systematic reviews and meta-analyses** appearing in medical journals are of this type. The Discussion section of a Master's thesis, Doctoral dissertation, or a research paper also tries to do such synthesis although this is limited to fusion of your findings with the results of the others. Methods for research synthesis are not included in this text although we later present how Discussion section should be written.

Applied Research

Applied medical research can be classified into two major categories although this is not a universally accepted classification. First category can be called **primary research** that includes analytical studies such as case-control studies, laboratory experiments and clinical trials. It also includes descriptive studies such as surveys, case-series, and census (Figure 1-1). The second category is **secondary research**, which is quite common these days, that includes decision analysis (risk analysis and decision theory), operations research (prioritisation, optimisation, simulation, etc.), evaluation of health systems (assessment of achievements and shortcomings), economic analysis (cost-benefit, cost-effectiveness, etc.), qualitative research (focus group discussion), and research synthesis (reviews and meta-analyses). This text is designed to provide a holistic picture of methodology of primary medical research that still forms the bulk of modern research.

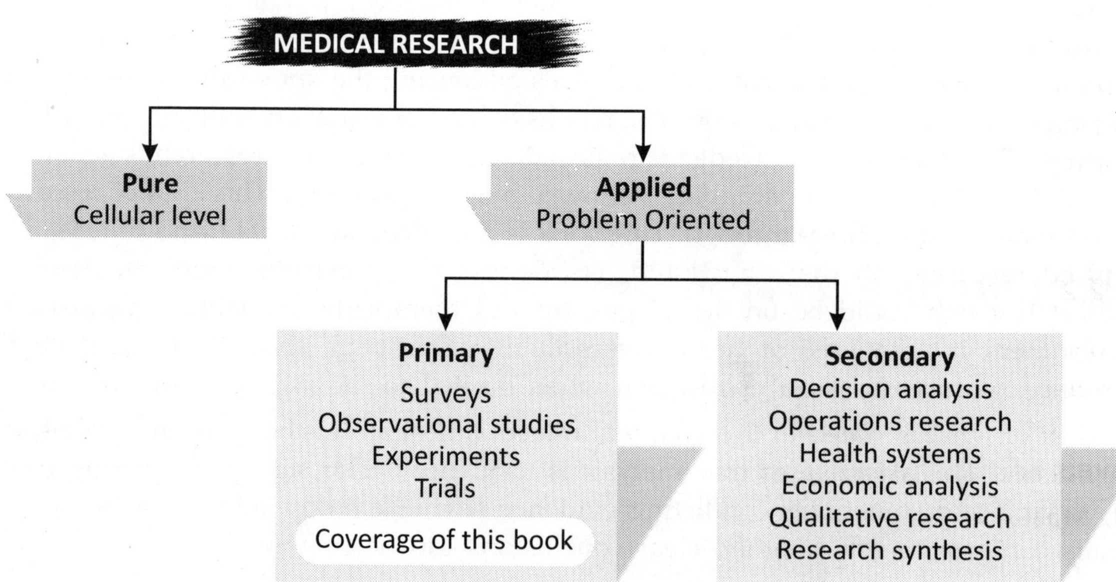

FIGURE 1-1: Types of medical research and the coverage of this book

The text is for basic methods only, and would be adequate for most research that is required to be collated as Master's thesis or Doctoral dissertation, and for such other small-scale endeavours. Advanced methods would be different for, say, cancer research than for tuberculosis research, and for drug trial than for behavioural research. For such focused research, particularly if it is on large scale, consult other relevant reference books and material. This book also does not contain methods required for pharmacokinetic and toxicological studies.

A new discipline of **translational research** is fast coming up that intends to serve as a bridge between pure and applied research. It promotes multi-disciplinary collaboration so that efficiency from bench to bedside increases and the applied process is accelerated. This has now become feasible as most research data are available online that can be quickly shared and immediately analysed. This book may not be sufficient to address this kind of research also.

Increasing number of medical postgraduates all over the world is opting for **inter-disciplinary research.** The need for such research in health and medicine indeed is urgent, and a positive attitude is required to be developed to encourage inter-disciplinary research. This kind of research can be highly relevant and can have immensely useful application. Remember that heart and soul of health care is inter-disciplinary. Such research provides unique opportunity for professional growth and can be very satisfying. But it has potential risks as well. Embracing relevance of multiple disciplines and to integrate this into focus for the problem in hand is not easy. An expanded frontier and increased breadth of knowledge of theory and practice is required for inter-disciplinary research to be successful. The process of bridging disciplines is challenging although it would be exciting as well. In case you plan to go inter-disciplinary, adopt abundant caution as there might be lack of respect for each other among basic, clinical, applied, and public health researchers. Teamwork is important for successful inter-disciplinary research, but individuals should also shine and flourish (Awasthi et al. 2005).

1.2.2 LEVELS OF MEDICAL RESEARCH

Levels vary from elementary research at Master's thesis level to advanced multicentric research. The details are as follows.

Levels of Medical Research

I. Master's Thesis:

- Generally a small-scale investigation that puts forward a *hypothesis* to be tested by further investigations.

- Student can rarely select a topic. It mostly depends on the Supervisor.
- Thesis must be completed strictly within a time frame not extending beyond 2 years. No time slot is provided to take courses on the topic of research.
- Duration of investigation is generally one year (part-time) and it is in part fulfillment of the degree.
- Objective is to provide training to the student in research methodology thus, process is more important than outcome.
- Seldom provides results that can be immediately implemented in health care.
- The guide is generally called Supervisor whose intellectual resources are extensively utilised.
- Supervisor is not chosen by the student but is assigned by the department
- Almost invariably based on institutional resources without support of any funding agency.
- There is no public defense of the findings.
- Volume is nearly 100 pages.

II. Doctoral Dissertation:

- A detailed discourse or treatise on a particular topic that provides a new result or new perspective must be capable of publication in a reputed journal.
- It must provide evidence of critical thinking of the candidate on the topic of research.
- Many times provides results that can be immediately implemented in health care.
- Duration is mostly three to four years (full-time) and dissertation itself is enough for the degree.
- Time is enough for a good research work that can provide satisfaction to the candidate and the advisor.
- Enough time is available to take short-term courses on the topic of research.
- Almost the entire time of the candidate is devoted to the research.
- Candidate can select a topic of his interest. Protocol can be revised and resubmitted.
- The guide is generally called Advisor and the work is mostly based on the candidate's own intellectual contribution. Advisor is generally chosen by the candidate based on his expertise in the area of research.
- Mostly based on institutional resources but can be part of a large-scale research funded by some agency.

- Required to be publicly defended.
- Volume is generally 200 pages or more.

III. Institutional Study:

- Generally conducted in only one location.
- A large-scale investigation that culminates into a full-fledged project report and mostly published in a reputed journal in concise form.
- Expected to provide a path-breaking result that can be immediately implemented in health care.
- Mostly based on specially marked funds.

IV. Multicentric Study:

- Conducted in several locations with common protocol to check replicability in a variety of settings.
- Necessarily a large-scale investigation for which a full-fledged report is prepared and almost invariably finds a place in a reputed journal in a concise form.
- Attracts attention because of its size but there is no evidence yet that this level of research produces path-breaking results more often than institutional level research
- Invariably based on specially marked funds

1.2.3 POSTGRADUATE (PG) THESIS

Almost all universities in India awarding Medicinae Doctor (MD) and Master of Surgery (MS) degrees require students to devote at least one year in conducting a small-scale research, involving planning, collecting, collating, and presenting results as a thesis. This is very different from a Doctoral dissertation. The primary purpose in MD/MS thesis is not frank research but only training of the students in research methodology. Both these are Master's degrees with similar requirements although MD is unnecessarily confused with Doctoral degree because of its name.

There are pros and cons of the provision of a thesis in the medical PG curriculum. When carried out as intended, PG thesis provides training and prepares the student for a research career. It helps in fine-tuning the thought process and inculcates the ability to critically evaluate the evidence, including those available in literature. If the students decide to go for teaching, they are better prepared to supervise MD/MS students. In Supervisor, PG students have a mentor who can give direction to their career and provide effective recommendations for a job. Your institution gets credit for research and sometimes the mankind is benefitted by discovery of improved procedures.

On the downside is one extra year needed to complete the education and sometimes being treated as assistant to the Supervisor. Sometimes the Supervisor is ill-equipped and adds to the confusion instead of clarity. She/He may lack time and the institution may not have necessary infrastructure.

There is another side of some PG theses. Some students tend to learn how to fudge the data and manipulate results. A new technology called 'copy-paste' has emerged as the computerology is spreading tentacles. There are examples when pages after pages in a PG thesis are traced to previous works. This malpractice tends to be replicated by your students when you become a supervisor. Ultimate loss is of the time and reputation. No wonder that Indian research is seen with microscopic eyes, sometimes with suspicion and sometimes with contempt, because of such malpractices.

1.3 WHAT IS THE NEED OF BASIC METHODS OF MEDICAL RESEARCH?

The methods of medical research depend on the type of medical research and its level as mentioned earlier. But the basic methods generally are the same and geared to meet the twin challenges of medical uncertainties as mentioned next, and the competence to handle these uncertainties in a manner that they do not affect our results. You will soon realize that the uncertainties would rarely allow to come to an infallible result but the science requires that we are able to state how the results would continue to hold in most cases despite the presence of these uncertainties, or why the results have not come up to the expectations.

Not many who undertake medical research are fully trained in research methodology. This tends to limit the quality of their effort. This limitation has lately attracted attention, but research methodology still is 'what is not taught in a medical school'. This book may fulfill the need of a text required to impart training in basics of medical research methods. These methods are equipped to handle challenges posed by medical uncertainties.

1.3.1 UNCERTAINTY CHALLENGES OF MEDICAL RESEARCH

All scientific results are susceptible to error, but uncertainty is an integral part of medical framework. The realisation of enormity of uncertainty in medicine may be recent but the fact is age-old. No two biological entities have ever been exactly alike; neither would they be so in future. Also, our knowledge about biological processes still is extremely limited. These two aspects—first variation, and second limitation of knowledge—throw an apparently indomitable challenge. Medical science has not only survived but is ticking with full vigour. The silver lining is the ability of some experts to learn quickly from their own and others' experience, and to discern signals from noise, waves from turbulence, trends from chaos. It is due to this learning that death rates have steeply declined in the past 50 years and life expectancy is showing a relentless rise in almost all nations around the world. Burden of disease is steadily but surely declining in most countries.

Categories of Uncertainties

Most uncertainties confronted in health and disease can possibly be categorized into diagnostic, treatment, and prognostic framework (see Example 1.1) and some could be called predictive uncertainties not related to prognosis (see Example 1.2). A prominent set remains that does not fit into this conventional framework (as in Example 1.3). However, all uncertainties can be classified into aleatory and epistemic types. This classification is new to medicine but is a big help in management and control uncertainties. These are described below.

EXAMPLE 1.1: Diagnostic, Therapeutic and Prognostic Uncertainties

Many examples are given in the text. Others are as follows:

Diagnostic uncertainties:
- Exercise stress test for coronary artery disease.
- FNAC, ultrasonography, and mammogram for breast in cancer.
- Extensive clinical evaluation, multiple sweat chloride test and genotype analysis for cystic fibrosis.

Therapeutic uncertainties:
- Surgical treatment for asymptomatic gland-confined prostate cancer.
- High-energy photon external beam treatment planning for cancers.
- Early stage of breast cancer.
- Management of ductal carcinoma in-situ because of possibility of recurrence after conservative surgery.

Prognostic uncertainties:
- Severe sudden illness.
- Early prediction of irreversible brain damage after ischaemic stroke.
- Terminally ill patients.

EXAMPLE 1.2: Predictive Uncertainties

Medicine is largely a science of prediction—prediction of diagnosis, prediction of outcome of treatment or surgery, prediction of prognosis. But there are many other types of predictions as cited below:

- Gender of a child immediately after conception.
- Number of years a person would live after onset of a particular chronic disease.
- Number of AIDS cases likely to come up every year for which the country has to prepare for providing care and support.
- The year when leprosy would be eradicated from the world.
- How many people will die by different causes in the year 2030 in any specific country.

EXAMPLE 1.3: Unclassifiable Uncertainties

There are other uncertainties that are not classifiable into diagnostic, treatment or prognostic framework nor as predictive uncertainties.

- Clinical significance of thromboembolic disease.
- Dynamics of infection, transmission, pathology, and control of schistosomiasis.
- Factors responsible for higher longevity in women.
- How to measure positive health.

We have several times mentioned about aleatory and epistemic uncertainties. **Aleatory** are those that have origin in variation – inter- and intra-individual, instrument to instrument, method to method, and such other sources. **Epistemic uncertainties** arise from our incomplete knowledge – how to treat a terminal condition, how to save a person in advance stage of cancer, and the like. Both these types of uncertainties can completely derail medical research results. For details, see Indrayan (2020).

Management of Uncertainty in any research requires a science that understands randomness, instability, and variation. Biostatistics is the subject that deals specifically with these aspects. This is the supportive science all through this book. Instead of relating it to conventional statistical methods such as test of hypothesis and regression, biostatistics is presented as an aid to solve problems of medical research. In doing so, we deliberately avoid mathematical intricacies. This text should be light and enjoyable for the medical fraternity so that medical research is perceived as a delightful experience, and not as a burden.

1.3.2 EPIDEMIOLOGY AND BIOSTATISTICS IN MEDICAL RESEARCH

Discourse on epidemiology and biostatistics methods in this book is restricted to the topics required for carrying out and reporting medical research in an effective manner.

Epidemiology *is the study of distribution and determinants of health and disease.* This is inherently a macro science that deals with groups rather than individuals. Much of modern medical research is also based on groups and not individuals. To show that a therapeutic regimen has more efficacy than the other, a trial is conducted on a *group* of patients. To show that spectrum of causes of deaths is changing, the data must be obtained for a group of persons. To show that a new diagnostic algorithm is better than the existing, comparison must be between groups using these two algorithms. To identify aetiological or risk factors, or to measure the risk, groups of patients are needed. To assess that one surgical procedure is better than the other, the trial must be conducted on groups of patients. Some kinds of groups of subjects are inbuilt in almost every type of applied medical research—thus, an epidemiological perspective remains prominent.

Biostatistics, otherwise perceived to be a desiccated science that crunches numbers, in fact *is the science that helps to manage medical uncertainties.* Uncertainties are omnipresent but they are especially prominent in medical situations. As a researcher, you need to be proactive to these uncertainties. The role of biostatistics knowledge is to help identify different sources of uncertainties, take steps for limiting their impact on decisions, provide procedures to measure uncertainties, and render help in taking those decisions that are likely to have least error. All this is a great help in medical research. Statistical reasoning using the laws of probability guides the entire inferential process in empirical research. Taking chance into account is critical. Biostatistics is increasingly becoming an integral part of medicine, particularly for medical research. This subject is one of the ways of finding the truth. Adopt whatever means you consider fit to get there. In addition to epidemiology and biostatistics, logic and critical thinking are natural domain that support evidence-based research.

1.3.3 BASIC METHODS OF MEDICAL RESEARCH

This book describes all steps of primary medical research in simple language. We hope that this will help emerging scientists to learn the concepts and principles of designing and conducting such a research project with precision.

The basic method of an empirical study comprises topics such as:

(i) identify the topic,

(ii) review of the literature to assess what is known and what is not known,

(iii) set the precise, aims and objectives of the study that will hone the topic and increase the focus,
(iv) identify the kind of subjects that will be studied,
(v) decide on the sample size and selection method,
(vi) specify what information will be obtained from different kind of subjects, and other sources such as records, and who will collect the information,
(vii) tools such as interview, examination and laboratory investigation required to collect the data,
(viii) how the data will be managed and analyzed,
(ix) how the conclusion will be drawn, and
(x) how the findings are proposed to be collated and communicated.

We discuss all of these in details in various chapters of this book so that you can carry out the research with confidence and conviction.

1.4 ETHICS OF MEDICAL RESEARCH

Almost all medical research is invasive in one sense or the other. Observational studies do not involve any biological intervention but are invasive to the time and privacy of the respondents. Experiments and trials in any case involve biological intervention. Thus, almost all types of primary medical research raise ethical issues. Beware of allegations that medical profession sometimes willingly inflicts unproven treatment on unsuspecting patients (Reddy 2003). Also, that research misconduct is a global problem (Smith 2006).

Laboratory experiments on chemicals or even biological products do not raise much concern but the individual well-being gets precedence over societal gains. There is some amount of consensus through globally accepted Helsinki Declaration (2013) on how research involving human subjects should be carried out about which we describe later, but there is not much consensus on animal experimentation.

1.4.1 ETHICS FOR ANIMAL EXPERIMENTATION

A clear dichotomy exists among scientists about the desirability of animal experimentation. One set considers it in the interest of science that a regimen is tried on a suitable animal model before it is passed for trials on human beings. The other asserts that experiment on animals takes undue advantage of their vulnerability. Moreover, many side-effects would not be correctly predicted by animal models. Just to make a point, note for example that strychnine is a deadly poison to humans but is harmless to monkeys, chickens, and guinea pigs. Some experiments do need animal sacrificing such as obtaining mitotic index and Proliferating Cell Nuclear Antigen (PCNA) in mice after giving them hormone replacement therapy. And almost all medical experiments on animals require exposing them to chemicals or procedures that could mean torture. This set of scientists and social activists feel that animal experiments are unnecessary for progress of medicine. However, the dominant view, particularly among medical professionals, is that learning on appropriate animal models is a great step forward in knowledge acquisition about pharmacokinetics, mechanism, functions, side effects, etc., of new formulations and procedures. Animals have become very important resource to learn about genetics also.

Some general rules for animal experimentation, particularly when their sacrifice is required, are as follows:

1. Researcher must first show that nonanimal alternative procedures cannot provide the required data.
2. Follow the national guidelines on care and use of laboratory animals. For example, in India, they must be bred within a laboratory specifically for research purposes. Experiments on smaller animals such as rats, mice, rabbits, guineapigs, and hamsters can be carried out with local permission. Use of larger animals is avoided, but if considered essential, permission of a designated national authority is obtained.
3. There are specific guidelines about care of animals, use of various painful procedures, disposal of carcasses after sacrifice, etc. Consult the incharge of the animal house of your institution to get full guidance on these aspects. For example, you may have to provide for after-care of used animals, and euthanasia may be permitted only under severe constraints. With such restrictions, animal experiments have become very costly.

1.4.2 ETHICS FOR RESEARCH INVOLVING HUMAN SUBJECTS

Whereas observational studies carry little risks to the subjects or society, interventions such as drugs, embedded devices, and procedures do entail risk of physical, psychological, social, or economic harms. Thus, all intervention studies must be done with utmost care. There must be sufficient reasons for starting such research on human subjects. Ask first that the research is justified or not to the subjects, to the institution, to the sponsor, and above all to yourself. Refrain from excessive zeal in experimenting with human subjects. Second, ask how you would like this intervention to be done on your loved ones—if at all. Some U.S. agencies in the past have been accused of conducting trials in developing countries since those trials would be unethical in the U.S.

Intense discussions go on all the time on how human beings can be involved in medical research endeavours without compromising their welfare. Much of the medical progress is based on human experimentation, and they are considered integral part of medical research endeavours. Without such trials how to know that a new modality is indeed beneficial or more beneficial than the existing one? Even the best proven modalities must be continuously challenged by competing new ones—and this would continue to require human experimentation.

Helsinki Declaration

World Medical Association in its General Assembly in Helsinki in 1964 adopted what is now popularly known as **Declaration of Helsinki** on Medical Ethics. This is periodically revised. The last revision occurred in 2013. Various countries have also drawn their guidelines. For example, Indian Council of Medical Research has prepared extensive ethical guidelines (ICMR 2017) for biomedical research on human participants. Salient features of Helsinki Declaration and such other guidelines are as follows:

1. For a physician "The health of my patient is my first consideration". Thus, considerations relating to the well-being of the human subjects should take precedence over the interest of the society or of science. A trial may have potential to provide immense benefit to others but cannot be conducted if the interest of experimental subject is compromised. This puts question mark on placebo-controlled trials. Wherever possible the control group should get existing treatment and not left on placebo if that can jeopardise his health.
2. No medical intervention is without risks and burdens. But the safety of the regimen should be established before the trial. The most successful regimen will never be 100 percent effective and all will produce some side effects of one kind or the other. It could be beneficial on one aspect but detrimental on the other. There should be a careful assessment of predictable risks and burdens compared to the foreseeable benefits. The assessment should establish that expected benefits exceed, in fact substantially exceed, the potential harm. Also, there must be a mechanism in place to manage risk if an adverse condition develops in some subjects.
3. The dignity of all human beings must be respected. Some disadvantaged sections of the society may need special protection. Consent must be taken after apprising the patient about entire spectrum of benefits and risks. This should be a volunteer consent and not under duress, and the patient should be fully informed about the implications. The details appear at the end of this section.

4. Researchers should have thorough knowledge of the topic of research. This can emanate from the literature, clinic, laboratory, and any other source. They should not have a-priori belief that one of the regimens under trial is superior, because that can introduce bias. The research objectives and methodology must be consistent and not conflicting with such knowledge unless there are valid reasons for adopting a conflicting posture. The validity of these reasons is judged by external experts and not by the researcher himself nor by the stakeholders.
5. The research protocol should be clearly formulated, and it should be reviewed and approved by a committee on ethical as well as on other aspects. This committee must be an independent body with no stakes in the research.
6. Only scientifically qualified persons should conduct medical research on human subjects. Health of human subjects should be the responsibility of a medically qualified person.
7. At the conclusion of the study, every patient entered the study should be given access to best proven prophylactic, diagnostic or therapeutic methods identified by the study.
8. When proven modalities are not available for a particular condition, unproven or new modalities can be used if in the physician's judgement it offers hope of saving life, re-establishing health, or alleviating suffering. But all efforts should be made to conduct proper research later to evaluate the efficacy and safety of such unproved procedures.
9. Negative as well as positive results should be published or otherwise publicly available. Sources of funding, institutional affiliation and any possible conflict of interest should be declared.
10. Privacy and confidentiality must be fully respected.

At the time of reporting of results, do not use patient's name, hospital case number, and such other identifiers, and in photographs suppress the features that could identify the patient. The participants can be provided compensation for their inconvenience, time and expenses incurred (such as on transport) but the payment should not be excessive that could be seen as inducement. Some general aspects of empirical research ethics are listed below.

Some General Aspects of Empirical Research Ethics

Research ethics require that:

(i) the protocol must be reviewed by those who do not have stakes in that research,

(ii) the researcher must be scientifically qualified to do that research,

(iii) the researcher must have adequate facilities to conduct that kind of research,
(iv) the accuracy of research results must be preserved,
(v) confidentiality of subjects must be maintained,
(vi) the methodology and results should be accurately reported, and
(vii) research should be based on adequate sample size – inordinately large sample is as unethical as a small sample.

1.4.3 INFORMED CONSENT

Informed consent is a sensitive issue in human research. It is an essential component but rarely strictly adhered in India. *Merely getting the signature on consent form is not enough.* Before the consent is obtained, the investigator much explain the following to the participant in the language she/he can understand.

1. The purpose of the research and how can it help the participant and the future subjects.
2. Methods to be followed and the role of the participant.
3. Foreseeable risk or discomfort that a subject might face during the course and after the participation.
4. Alternatives available to the participants of treatment and other procedure in case he wants to opt out.
5. Responsibility the investigations will assume in case a side-effect develops. Any compensation, reimbursement or insurance cover for the risks involved.
6. Any cost implications for the participant, and the time he needs to devote to the participation including investigations at repeat visits.
7. Freedom to participate and to withdraw at any time without penalty or loss of benefits.

The thrust of all this is that the participation is completely voluntary. No advantage should be taken of the patient's psychological or other weaknesses because she/he is sick. To rule out duress, sometimes a third party is involved who has no interest in this research. In case of minor children, very old, or unconscious, when indispensable for the research, legally authorised person can give consent. It should be written in local language and should not only be informed but also understood consent. If the patient is illiterate, ensure that the patient has really understood the implications, after explaining all the risks. The patient should be able to decide himself whether to participate or not. The process of informing is continuous throughout the study. Refusal by any patient at any time should not affect the patient-doctor relationship.

Onus is on the investigator to remain vigilant and conscious of his obligation towards the patients throughout the course of the study.

1.5 PLEASURES AND FRUSTRATIONS OF MEDICAL RESEARCH

Scientific enquiry is among the most challenging enterprises. Any research, more so medical research, is an occupation riddled with uncertainties. If successful in bringing out a path-breaking result, it may be idolized. If it fails to produce expected results, the consequent frustration could be disastrous. Nobody can predict. If the result is predictable, it is not research after all. The only thing one can do is to take full care of possible biases by developing a good design and use valid and reliable methods of measurement and analysis. Medical research is becoming increasingly complex and expensive, and the monitoring these days is very close. Since skepticism is accepted as an integral part of all scientific activity, make sure that the results stand upto third-party reviews. The key concern is credibility. The results can be positive or negative, but they must be reliable and valid.

1.5.1 FRUITS OF MEDICAL RESEARCH

Medical research can be enormously satisfying when conducted with conscience and dedication. You would be delighted to use your results on your patients, and their use by the fellow professionals can give ecstatic feeling. Sometimes the results can be so useful that they improve the well-being of a large segment of a population. Although a research that improves the quality of life of even one patient is worth the efforts but that can be very expensive to the society. Thus, efforts should concentrate more on aspects that benefit many persons. This rarely happens. The problems are generally pursued based on the researcher's interest instead of societal interest. Nevertheless, medical research, overall, has been very illuminating and has brought abundant cheers to the individuals and the society. With competition, the time lag between the research and its implementation has considerably reduced.

Considering major emphasis these days on methodological aspects, it is expected that the future research would be more efficient, and the benefits would be available to a larger segment of population at lower cost. You could be an important contributor to these efforts by following the simple rules described in this text.

Fruits include unexpected findings. It was a chance that Kune et al. (1988) found that aspirin may have protective effect on colorectal cancer. Nobody knew about it earlier. Subsequent research confirmed that use of 300 mg of aspirin a day for 5 years is effective in prevention of colorectal cancer. Had this accidental finding not published, further work and confirmation was unlikely.

1.5.2 FRUSTRATIONS OF MEDICAL RESEARCH

Research also requires owning up the responsibility. Few researchers realize that their result can benefit or imperil life of many people (Indrayan 2018). A mistake on operation table endangers life of just one patient but research results, when wrong and adopted for practice on millions of cases, can threaten hundreds of lives. For surgeries, a student is given rigorous training for years, but medical research seems to belong to everyone. No rigorous training is required. Ill-equipped researchers collect data, analyse and publish. The review process too is slippery in many cases. Thus, substandard research tends to guide the practitioners and lives of many are jeopardised.

Research results are unpredictable. Thus, a researcher must be prepared to accept negative result. The studies with negative results are being increasingly recognized as a contribution to science because they provide guidance on what not to do. Do not be discouraged if your research fails to give the expected results. Also, you may get a very encouraging result in your study, but some other researcher may not. Thus, refutations can also come in the course of time. Such adverse events are part of a researcher's life.

SUMMARY

Most medical research is empirical. It is based on evidence rather than hunches or preferences. It follows a series of steps that would be described in detail in this text. The research endeavours should be consistent with the accepted medical ethics. Most of the modern medical research requires epidemiological and biostatistical tools to reach to a valid and reliable conclusion. As a researcher, you must have an adequate knowledge and skill to effectively use these tools.

Medical research can provide immense pleasure when conducted on scientific lines and can be frustrating when years of efforts fail to produce expected results. Prepare to face the consequences either way if you are in this risky occupation.

REFERENCES

Awasthi S, Beardmore J, Clark J, et al. Five futures for academic medicine. PLoS Med 2005;2:e207.

Helsinki Declaration. World Medical Association Declaration of Helsinki Ethical Principles for Medical Research Involving Human Subjects. JAMA November 27, 2013;310(20):2191-2194.

ICMR. National Ethical Guidelines for Biomedical and Health Research involving Human Participants. Indian Council of Medical Research, 2017.

Indrayan A. Aleatory and epistemic uncertainties can completely derail medical research results. J Postgrad Med. 2020 Apr-Jun;66(2):94-98.

Indrayan A. Statistical fallacies & errors can also jeopardize life & health of many. Indian J Med Res. 2018;148(6):677-679.

Kune GA, Kune S, Watson LF. Colorectal cancer risk, chronic illnesses, operations and medications: case-control results from Melbourne Colorectal Cancer Study. Cancer Res. 1988;48:4399-4404.

Reddy KS. Commentary: Shaw's critique of health care is still valid. Int J Epidemiol. 2003;32:919-921.

Smith R. The Trouble with Medical Journals. Royal Society of Medicine Press, 2006.

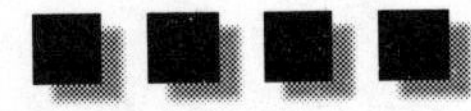

CHAPTER 2

What are the Broad Steps of Medical Research

KEY TERMS AND CONCEPTS

(Details of the following are given in the subsequent chapters)

- ✓ **Outline of the Preinvestigation Steps – The Problem, Objectives, Design, and Tools**
- ✓ **Outline of the Investigation Steps – Pretesting, Method of Data Collection, and Nonresponse**
- ✓ **Outline of the Postinvestigation Steps – Analysis, Interpretation, and Writing**

Science is known to be a systematic study that follows a discernible pattern and produces testable results. Thus, scientific research must follow a step-by-step pathway that fosters clarity and avoids the problem of multiplicity. These steps are much more elaborate for research in medicine than for other disciplines because of enormous uncertainties inherent in medical field and the implication is human health. Jenicek (2006) has provided a layout of modern argument in medical research. This involves processes that go on from what problem is in your mind to searching external evidence (e.g., literature) for or against, making a qualified claim, then conducting the study, leading to the results with limitations such as probabilities and applicability. Because of empirical base, investigations are sine-qua-non for a primary medical research. An outline of the preinvestigation, investigation and postinvestigation steps is given next. The details are in the following chapters.

2.1 PREINVESTIGATION STEPS

However, odd it may sound, the preparation and plan for the investigation would be more critical for sound research than possibly the actual investigation. Preinvestigation steps are as follows.

2.1.1 IDENTIFY THE PROBLEM

The first step in research is to identify a problem area to work on. One paradigm is that, notwithstanding knowledge explosion in the past century, the unknown segment of the universe is much larger than the known segment. An alert researcher will find a large number of issues floating around. You may have felt uneasy about how to handle a health problem, deficiency in evidence base, lack of clarity in implications of your actions, or any such bottleneck. For selection, match the research area to (i) the relevance and applicability for improving health in one way or the other, (ii) interest and expertise of yourself and your collaborators, and (iii) the feasibility of completing the work with available resources such as facilities, time, subjects, and tools. These three aspects should considerably narrow down the problem area. If the situation permits, select a topic that is in debate or meet a current demand. At PG level, do not think that your research will be grand. If it turns out to be so, thank the environment. For further details, see chapter 9 on Research Protocol.

Convert the problem to specific questions that require answer. The questions must pass the "so what?" test. Even when this is done with apparently sufficient specificity, the course of the investigation may reveal that those questions were not so specific after all. Further steps as given below may help to attain focus and clarity.

2.1.2 COLLECT AND EVALUATE THE EXISTING INFORMATION

The next step is to collect as much information on the identified problem as possible. We devote a full chapter (Chapter 3) on critically evaluating the existing information while discussing the literature search. But do not underestimate the potency of other sources. Secondary data might be available in various organisations that can enhance the focus of the problem. Thesis guide and the subject-experts can provide useful insight that they imbibe through years of experience of working in that area. Talk to them without inhibition. Do not think that your limited knowledge will be a hindrance. In fact, this limitation is propelling you to explore this problem. Experts might lead to the hitherto unexplored literature and, more importantly, to the work other agencies or institutions are doing in that area. Make sure that a reasonable answer to the proposed question is not already available. The objective of all this exercise should be to identify the specific information gaps, and to examine how the problem fits into the medical jigsaw puzzle. Assess if the problem is worth pursuing. If none or very little baseline information is available, consider carrying out an exploratory study as a first step.

2.1.3 FORMULATE RESEARCH OBJECTIVES AND HYPOTHESES

Critical evaluation of the literature and other data on the problem will greatly assist in focusing thoughts regarding what exactly to investigate. Translate these to the research objectives. The objectives must match with the perceived utility of the results. For example, for interventions, the objectives could be to find efficacy, effectiveness, affordability, efficiency, safety, acceptability, etc. Clearly identify the specific aspect to concentrate on and formulate the research objectives accordingly. They should be amenable to evaluation and should be realistic: clearly phrased and stated in logical sequence. The objectives should be consistent with meaningful decisions taken in actual practice. They should not focus on trivial issues that can be addressed without research.

Consider whether you expect to come up with entirely novel findings or just confirm previous work that left some doubt or would address the present conflict (Brand 2003).

From objectives emanate hypotheses. A hypothesis is a carefully worded statement regarding the anticipated status of a phenomenon. For example, one may hypothesise that recurrence of eclampsia in pregnant women is more common in those that have family history of hypertension. The hypothesis should be biologically plausible and supported by reasoning. It should be restricted to the research under plan. Further details about objectives and hypotheses are described in a later chapter.

2.1.4 IDENTIFY THE STUDY SUBJECTS AND SETTING

The definition of the subject of study and the target population should be clearly spelt out. Iodine deficiency can be diagnosed either based on the palpable or visible goiter, or now based on urine iodine concentration <100 mg/l. Borderline hypertension may be defined to start from 135/85 mmHg or from 140/90 mmHg. Choose a definition that is consistent with the objectives and can be justified. Besides inclusion criteria, the exclusion criteria should also be clearly stated so that the cases are not excluded mid-way through the study. For this, anticipate the type of cases that can become ineligible later after inclusion. For example, pregnant females may be ineligible. If there are two or more groups under research, define each with specifications as needed so that there is no overlap.

Also decide from where these subjects would come – from a clinic, admitted patients in a ward, undergoing specific surgery, emergency care, attendants or other relatives of the patients, follow-up of discharged patients, or from a community (and which one). Also, decide that whether you would use records of the patients previously admitted.

2.1.5 THINK OF A DESIGN

Now, think of a strategy to get valid and reliable answer to the research question, or to get a solution of the research problem. The strategy would be in terms of collection of data in a manner that inspires confidence. This requires identifying all sources of uncertainty and developing a design that can keep them under control (the details are in subsequent chapters). In effect, this means:

(i) sampling plan for a survey;

(ii) prospective, retrospective or cross-sectional strategy for observational study;

(iii) deciding on the specifics of intervention, if any;

(iv) determining the variables on which the data would be collected: the variables that are valid to provide the correct answer;

(v) the methods to obtain valid data on those variables—feasible yet robust methods that can stand scientific scrutiny – what information is to be collected by examination of the patients, what by interview, what by laboratory and radiological investigations, and what by inspecting the records;

(vi) tools such as questionnaire for easy recording of information;

(vii) the strategy to handle any ethical problem that might arise during the course of the investigation;

(viii) the number of cases or subjects that should be included in this kind of investigation;

(ix) the method of selection of the subjects of the study;

(x) the method of randomisation, blinding, matching, etc., and

(xi) the method of statistical analysis of data.

Most medical professionals do need expert advice from a biostatistician to develop an appropriate design. If needed, catch him or her at early phase of planning and seek collaboration for all phases of the study. Do not aim at methodological overkill. Marginally improved results at a substantially higher cost may not be worth.

2.1.6 WRITE THE PROTOCOL

All the hard work put into the preceding steps culminates into the draft of a research protocol. It incorporates all the information regarding the plan of research in a concise manner. Developing a protocol is just about the most important step in conducting a research. For this reason, we are devoting a full chapter on this aspect alone. When the thoughts are put together on a paper, they crystalise and concretise. Since protocol is a written commitment, further deliberations may be needed for example, to make the objectives and hypotheses more specific and to justify the strategy to be adopted. Protocol contains much more information than so far stated. For example, it also states the work plan and identifies the resources required for the project, including the timeline. The latter comprises the time point when each step is to be initiated and how much time this will take to complete. Work on two or more steps of research can go together, and this timeline will indicate this overlap also.

2.1.7 DEVELOP THE TOOLS

Tools for medical research are of two types. First is the recording questionnaire, schedule, or proforma that is uniformly followed throughout the investigation. Second are the measurement and investigation tools such as a scoring system and Holter test. Development of tools also encompasses arranging investigations such as for imaging and those to be done in a laboratory. In some situations, this may require procuring kits with the help of external facilities. Arrangements may also have to be made to procure drugs, including lifesaving drugs, to meet any contingency. Work out the modality for getting help from outside agencies when needed in case of exigency. For a large-scale investigation, instruction manual may be needed. The staff may have to be trained in interview, examination, or laboratory methods so that valid and uniform data are generated. The details are in a later chapter.

2.2 INVESTIGATION STEPS

Note that the preinvestigation steps are complex, and the major component is the thought process. After these steps comes the actual investigation. This also requires some preliminary steps before embarking upon the real study.

2.2.1 PRETEST AND DO PILOT STUDY

No matter how thoughtful you have been in developing the tools of the investigation, there is always a need to pretest them for their performance in actual conditions on the same kind of subjects as in the main study. Experience suggests that almost invariably some deficiency is detected, and the tools or their implementation are found to require some modification. Thus, do not shy away from this exercise. Similarly, a pilot study, which is a small forerunner of the actual investigation, also provides useful inputs regarding changes required in the measurements to be taken, in the interview or examination method, in the laboratory or imaging investigations, in the recording system, etc.

2.2.2 COLLECT THE DATA

Although the objective of this step is collection of the relevant data, but it actually entails administering the intervention such as a drug if any and observing the subjects. As always in a medical setup, the data are obtained by inspecting the records, by conducting interview, physical examination, or laboratory/imaging investigations, or by a combination of these data-eliciting methods. Continuous vigil is maintained to ensure that the data remain of good quality—that is they are correctly obtained for each subject without favour or fervour, and honestly recorded. The methods earlier decided in the protocol should be strictly followed. If the history is to be obtained by interview, do not replace it by records available with the patients. The data forms should be legibly filled, and they should be fully completed.

2.2.3 HANDLE THE NONRESPONSE AND ETHICAL ISSUES

In a science such as medicine, it is difficult to complete the investigation in all the planned subjects. Some subjects will invariably drop out during the investigation. Anticipate such nonresponse and keep it at the minimal level to avoid bias in the results. Make all efforts to extract at least the basic information that can help in adjusting for any bias.

Then there are ethical issues that need to be constantly monitored, particularly if the research involves an intervention such as a therapeutic maneuvre. Even when informed consent is taken, medical ethics requires that the intervention and data generation or collection should not subjugate the interest of the patient. We have discussed this in the previous chapter.

2.2.4 SCRUTINISE THE DATA

Despite all the care exercised at the time of taking history of patients, at the time of physical examination, and at the time of laboratory/imaging investigation, errors do occur. Most of these can be detected by scrutinising the data for internal consistency and external validity. For example, if a patient with hypertension has low cholesterol then sufficient reasons should be available within the record. A woman of age 23 years cannot possibly have six children. Such errors look odd, but they are practical occurrences, particularly in a large-scale research. Sometimes called data cleaning, this step of scrutiny is considered essential for quality research. The details are given in a later chapter.

2.3 POSTINVESTIGATION STEPS

After the data are collected, which should be adequate in terms of quality and quantity, they need to be exploited to their full potential to draw conclusions. This requires the following steps.

2.3.1 ANALYSE THE DATA

Analysis of data is an umbrella term that incorporates many mini steps. First is preparing a **master chart** by tabulating the data in a manner that all the information on one subject constitutes one record. In an Excel format, this really means that there is only one row of data for each person. Also, each field (column in Excel) must contain only one piece of information. If an AIDS patient has chronic peritonitis, toxoplasmosis, and kaposi sarcoma, with codes 7, 12, and 14 respectively, these three should be entered in separate fields, and not as 7,12,14 in one field.

Second step in data analysis is exploring the data for their pattern. Not many researchers appreciate the importance of this preliminary step. For example, pattern in geographical plot may reveal hidden mysteries in the medical phenomena you are studying. Outliers may reveal new relationships. Examine whether some selected variables are really following a Gaussian pattern or not. That will decide whether parametric tests of statistical significance should be used or nonparametric tests. For exploring relationship among various measurements, scatter plots can be immensely useful. These will indicate where and what type of relationship should be explored. Such data exploration methods are discussed in a later chapter.

Third step is to use the data for assessing the parameters of health and disease that were outlined in the protocol. Various indicators and indices of health and disease such as waist-hip ratio and scores may have to be calculated to assess risk factors and outcomes of interest. See a later chapter for details.

Fourth step is to summarise the data. This is done in terms of mean, standard deviation, proportion, rate, and more importantly in medicine in terms of odds ratio and relative risk. Such summaries tend to delineate the uncertainty levels in the results and help in grasping the essential features of data. The details are given later. This step sets the tone for statistical analysis.

The next step is grinding the data through the process of statistical analysis. This involves obtaining the confidence intervals, performing statistical tests to assess the significance of differences, obtaining the structure of relationships such as regression and their significance, assessing trends and agreement, etc. The details are provided later.

Wise researchers devote sufficient time to the examination of the data and to their analysis. Collecting quality data is important in itself, exploiting it fully is even more important. New results are sometimes missed despite availability of good data because the data are not properly exploited.

If your research involves intricate statistical analysis such as logistic regression, survival analysis and discriminant functions, enroll a statistician as your partner from the beginning. Statistical consultation after finishing a research is like postmortem. This can only conjecture what the research died of and cannot revive it.

2.3.2 INTERPRET THE RESULTS

Whereas statistical analysis is mostly computer-based, interpretation of the results requires critical thinking. A series of steps can be suggested.

(i) Examine the results in the context of the questions that prompted the research.

(ii) Verify that various results are consistent with one-another and a proper explanation is available for the inconsistent ones.

(iii) Check that all the potential biases have been either ruled out by design, or the results are properly adjusted for the biases.

(iv) Assess the reliability of the results.

(v) Confirm that a convincing biological explanation is available.

(vi) Show by sensitivity analysis and uncertainty analysis that the results are robust to the systematic variations.

(vii) Ensure that the final conclusions are indeed a further development and not repeat of previous knowledge.

In short, not only that you should be convinced about the correctness of the conclusions but also there should be enough reasons to convince others. Results should not be speculative, instead should be based on evidence as revealed by the data and other duly established facts.

2.3.3 WRITE AND DISSEMINATE THE REPORT

Report is a generic term that includes a thesis, a dissertation, an article, a paper, and a project report. It should contain all the details in a concise manner. Then disseminate it to the intended audience. Dissemination could be the most fruitful step in a research endeavour. The world is informed about the new conclusions, and a feedback is obtained regarding quality of the conclusions. A clear idea about the users of results will help to decide how to disseminate findings to the stakeholders.

We devote several chapters on how to present results effectively to an audience. In brief, the report should be sufficiently detailed that can remove any doubt a reader might have about any aspect of the results. The methodology should have complete details so that anyone can replicate the study and should be properly worded with a clear demarcation of the evidence-based results from opinions and comments. The report should be adequately illustrated by diagrams to enhance clarity. Numerical results can be summarized in the form of tables. Describe all the limitations candidly. No result has universal applicability, and the scientific community is fully aware of this fact. Thus, the limitations should be stated without inhibition.

The format of the report is geared to meet the expectation of the audience. A scientific paper would concisely state a particular aspect of the research in a paragraph that would take several pages in a thesis or a dissertation. The language for the press release would be very different than for a scientific paper. A report prepared for a funding agency may have a focus that fits their requirement.

2.3.4 MONITOR THE REACTIONS

Research is a continuous process. You might want to improve upon by learning from the reactions of the users of the research. It is necessary for this that all such reactions are systematically monitored. It is not uncommon in research journals to publish comments and the author's rejoinder. These help to crystalise thoughts and to improve in a subsequent endeavour. Also monitor whether the results are being utilised.

This book is written largely to address all these steps. Some steps are discussed at length and others quite briefly depending upon our perception about their relevance. The sequence of presentation in the book is broadly the same as the steps mentioned in the preceding paragraphs but there are minor alterations at places. We hope this text will help you to do quality research and to produce a credible report.

SUMMARY

Broad steps of medical research can be briefly stated as follows:

1. **Preinvestigation Steps:**
   (a) Identify the problem
   (b) Collect and evaluate the existing information to sharpen the focus
   (c) Formulate research objectives and hypotheses
   (d) Identify the study subjects and the setting from where the subjects of the study would come
   (e) Think of a design regarding who will be selected, how many, and whether it will be an observational study or a clinical trial, and what information will be collected in what manner to reduce the chance of bias and errors
   (f) Write the protocol containing all the details of the plan
   (g) Identify and develop the tools such as a questionnaire and scoring system
2. **Investigation Steps:**
   (a) Pretest the tools and do the pilot study to confirm the procedure you wish to adopt
   (b) Collect the data from all the sources (records, interview, examination, investigation) identified earlier
   (c) Handle the nonresponse and ethical issues
   (d) Scrutinise the data for errors and omissions
3. **Postinvestigation Steps:**
   (a) Analyse the data with statistical tools

(b) Interpret the results

(c) Write and disseminate the report (paper, thesis, or a full report)

(d) Monitor the reactions regarding peer review, feedback, application of the results, etc.

REFERENCES

Brand RA. Writing for clinical orthopaedics and related research. Clin Orthop Rel Res 2003;413:1-7.

Jenicek M. How to read, understand, and write 'Discussion' sections in medical articles: an exercise in critical thinking. Med Sci Monit 2006;12:SR28-SR36.

CHAPTER 3

How to Select a Problem for Research and the Literature Search

KEY TERMS AND CONCEPTS

- ✓ The Problem for Research
- ✓ Literature Search
- ✓ Quality of Journals and Articles
- ✓ Searching the Existing Data

The first problem faced by a researcher is the selection of an appropriate topic for research. When a broad area of research is identified, it is fine-tuned by a critical study of the existing literature and other evidence to find exactly what is known and what is not known. That finally determines the problem to be investigated. In this chapter, we list the parameters on which the selection of the topic of research can be made after review of literature and after examining the available resources, and then describe steps that sharpen the topic by precise statement of the objectives and hypothesis.

3.1 SELECTION OF THE PROBLEM

Successful research begins from selecting a right problem. It is colloquially said that a research is half done when the problem is clearly visualized. This assertion is not without truth. Thus, do not shy away from devoting time in the beginning on identifying the right problem, on understanding its various aspects thoroughly, and on choosing the specifics that you would like to investigate.

3.1.1 WHAT IS A PROBLEM?

A problem is a perceived difficulty, a feeling of discomfort about the way the things are, presence of a discrepancy between the existing situation and what it should be, a question about why a discrepancy is present, existence of two or more plausible answers to the same question, and such other aspects on which convincing answers are required (Brumback 2008).

Among countless problems, identifying the one that is suitable for research is not always easy. Researchability of course is a prime consideration but rationale, relevance, and feasibility are also important. The other consideration is your interest. Once these are established and the problem area filtered, the next important step is to determine the focus. For this, review the existing information to identify the parameters of the problem and use biological knowledge to refine its focus. Specify exactly what new the world is likely know through this research. This requires that the problem must be well-defined and focused. You should have full grip on the problem. Enormous efforts involving large sum of money and unaccountable hours of work are sometimes wasted in chasing the ill-defined concepts that fail to appreciate the nuances.

Choose a topic that needs development, verification, or refutation. You may have sufficient reasons to question even an established practice, but the topic should be ethically sound.

A postgraduate (PG) thesis can be on an extension of existing ideas, or replication with altered focus in a new environment. For example, you can strive to find if the strategy worked out in another country is applicable to your local setup where the underlying conditions can affect the outcome. Exact replication is also permissible if convincing reasons to doubt the existing result are present or if the earlier believable findings that have been questioned have to be confirmed. But do not try to re-invent the wheel. However, this does not apply to the frank research carried out beyond a PG thesis. A frank research must meet the criteria set out earlier in Chapter 1.

Sharpen the Focus

To sharpen the focus, go to a medical library and browse last few issues of a journal of your interest. Examine if the results can be extended to another relevant group of subjects, or whether the methods need improvement, or if another explanation is possible, or see the last paragraph of the articles published in various journals where authors generally identify new areas of research emerging from their study.

For a good research, examine whether the chosen topic has adequate theoretical backup. For example, if the role of a particular form of diet in a heart disease is to be investigated, consider why that diet can alter the risk of that heart disease. Biological plausibility gives a definite edge.

For a PG thesis, it is advisable to consider several topics and choose the one that suits your interest, caliber, and resources. Take guidance from your supervisor. Do not feel shy of selecting another topic if the one you earlier chose does not work out. Finally, believe in yourself, and remind yourself that human mind has unlimited potential.

3.1.2 STATEMENT OF THE PROBLEM

Statement of problem is not just wording the title. It is a comprehensive statement regarding the basis for selecting the problem, details of gaps in knowledge, a reflection on its importance, and comments on its applicability and relevance. The focus should be sharp. For example, if the problem area is dietary role in cancers, the focus may be on how consumption of meat affects occurrence of pancreatic cancer in males residing in a particular area. For further focus, the study may be restricted to only non-smoking males to eliminate the effect of smoking. For depth, meat can be specified as red or white. Further depth could be about how much red and how much white meat is consumed, and for how many years. Role of other correlates that promote or inhibit the effect of meat can also be studied. The actual depth would depend on the availability of relevant subjects on one hand and the availability of time, resources, and expertise on the other. Such sharp focus is very helpful in specifying the objectives and hypotheses, in developing an appropriate research design, and in conducting the right investigations.

Justification of the problem is crucial to get the support from faculty, institution, and other agencies. Explain rationale of the problem with convincing arguments. Juxtapose it in the context of local health care framework and convince others that the problem is important for health improvement. Include considerations such as timeliness, the segment of population affected, relationship with the ongoing health care activities or an ongoing research, kind of concern it generates among medical profession, etc. All this would require an extensive review of the available information on the chosen topic. The available information would be mostly in the literature and sometimes useful information is available in records of the hospital or at various websites such as of the universities, health organizations, and crowd-sourced databases. All these are described in detail later in this chapter.

3.2 LITERATURE SEARCH

Sound background knowledge of the topic is essential for research to succeed, although that by itself is not enough. You should be thoroughly convinced that the chosen topic requires further investigation then only you can hope to convince others. It is important to realise what you know and what you do not about that topic. Review of the existing information is a big help in

(i) confirming that the answers to the research questions are not already available and there are gaps that need to be plugged,

(ii) enhancing the understanding of the problem, including strengths and weaknesses of the established ideas,

(iii) identifying the relevant variables to be included in your study,

(iv) conceptualising the relationships that can be investigated,

(v) formulating the objectives and hypotheses,

(vi) improving methods that can be used in the investigation,

(vii) developing an appropriate design,

(viii) developing strategies for analysis of data,

(ix) learning how to effectively express the implications of your findings, and

(x) which journal would be appropriate to communicate your results.

The primary purpose is not just to get acquainted with the new developments but also to confirm that what you know is correct. The search for this information should obviously be undertaken at the time of planning the research and not afterwards. However, keep track of new developments during the investigations as well.

Your search should be wide enough to include all relevant material but also narrow to exclude irrelevant ones. Focus should be on recent findings and updated resources. Two major sources of existing information are literature and data. The present section in this chapter is on importance and methods for searching the literature and its critical evaluation. Section 3.4 is on searching the existing data.

3.2.1 SEARCHING MEDICAL LITERATURE

Literature is the best source of knowledge, and thus a very effective tool to reduce epistemic bottlenecks. Information explosion has resulted in a cloud with unclear signals. Thus, you should be smart to capture the relevant literature. Fortunately, medical literature is better organized with a host of indexing services, catalogues, and online resources.

The review of literature is done not only at the time of preparation of protocol but also as a regular surveillance during the research for tracking developments that can affect the course of the research. Readers of the research report would be tremendously impressed, and the users will feel great satisfaction if it is demonstrated that the research has considered the latest developments. They expect that the researcher has comprehensive information on the topic. A popular saying is that nobody knows more on the topic of research than the researcher himself. Others only evaluate. Live upto this saying by acquiring as much information on the topic of research as you can.

Consult the Experts

Among other ways to track the latest, easiest is to ask the subject matter expert. If he is really an expert, bet that he knows about new methodologies and new regimens. He may also know about **unpublished reports** and studies currently going on. Many useful studies are not published primarily because their findings are negative. Publications are biased towards positive findings and may provide a skewed picture. Beware of this risk while compiling various studies to get an overall picture. Expert's help in identifying and securing unpublished reports can reduce this risk.

A sapient expert will not give the information but will only refer to a source where that information is available. That is good for the research also because then the context and methodology with which the information is related can be examined. If the interest is in salt aetiology of hypertension, it would be nice to know what conflicting reports are available from different parts of the world, why they are not consistent with one another, what environmental factors are affecting this relationship, what the other confounding factors are, and how all these translate to the local setup. Experts can only help in leading to the relevant source, and not beyond. However, experts working with patients may have knowledge restricted to the severe cases that they see in the hospital, and this knowledge is not directly generalisable.

3.2.2 LIBRARY CONSULTATION AND LITERATURE DATABASES

Time spent in browsing through various titles in the stacks of the library never goes waste. If it is not used for current research, it can help in the next. Library consultation is a pleasure when the library is properly organized, user-friendly, and the library staff is supportive. Libraries of many institutions in India are yet to acquire these qualities. Many university libraries in Europe and the U.S. provide a cabin or a cubicle for research scholars so that they can concentrate without distraction. Libraries there are considered assets and revered. This culture is yet to catch up in India.

Always keep in mind that literature generally provides a lop-sided view. Negative findings are rarely published although the trend is changing. Thus, you get a biased positive view.

Authentic Information

Do not consider information provided in books and journals as authentic unless convinced. A lot of unsubstantiated impressionistic 'knowledge' goes into print. Rely on books of established publishers and reputed authors, and on landmark books that you can rely. Gray's Anatomy and Harrison's Medicine are examples of such landmark books. After several revisions in different editions, they have indeed become authentic sources of knowledge on their respective disciplines. Books are preferable source of general background knowledge such as how to diagnose a condition or how an intervention works. For questions pertaining to the research problem, journals are preferable.

Medical journals too have enormously proliferated in recent times, and many contain articles of dubious quality. Rely mostly on journals that publish articles after peer review by at least two experts. Contributor of articles to journals would know which journals maintain a good standard. Else, depend on the advice of your teacher or supervisor. Internationally reputed journals such as New England Journal of Medicine, British Medical Journal and Lancet can always be believed. It is helpful to consult specialty journals such as Pain if intention is to work on any aspect of pain, and AIDS if the plan is to work on this disease. If any lacuna is found in the articles published in these or any other journal, collect more information and send a letter to them for their 'Letters to the Editor' section. Do not be afraid to put across such views once convinced about the veracity of your assertions.

Case-reports are a good source to learn about exceptions such as a side effect of long-term use of a drug that was not known earlier. Then you can be alert about such occurrences—howsoever rare they might be. But do not rely on case-reports for choosing the management strategies. Haynes et al. (2005) have cited example of hundreds of case-reports and case-series about the virtues of extracranial-intracranial arterial anastomosis for preventing recurrence of stroke that was subsequently refuted by randomised trials. Case-reports are commonly used by the media to sensationalise an unusual finding. This is not science. Beware of being caught in such a web.

Review Articles

Full-length original articles are the best source of the happenings. Some review articles provide an excellent overview of research going on around the world that can provide very good lessons on a particular topic. These are the most frequently referred and quoted articles in research presentations. They also generally provide a big list of references of articles on the subject and discuss their merits and demerits. This makes it easier to select articles of your choice. But all review articles do not have the same quality. Sieve good articles from not so good. One extremely good source for health care interventions is Cochrane Reviews (details at *www.cochrane.org*). Reviews are published in almost all journals. In addition, there are dedicated journals such as 'Nutrition Reviews' and 'Nature Reviews Cardiology', which can be consulted.

Good reviews are those that efficiently integrate valid information. The reviews must be able to limit the bias that may be present in individual studies and reduce the effect of chance on conclusions. This is generally done with the help of **meta-analysis**—a very effective methodology to combine varying evidence in different reports. Reviews *synthesise* the research whereas individual studies *analyse* the data.

Editorials may not be peer-reviewed but are written with care and can be a good source for critical appraisal of the work. **Cross-references** at the end of each article can provide further information on specific items of interest. Make determined efforts to locate previous studies on the topic of research. Do not mind going back to several decades when required. But pay special attention to the recent developments.

Do not ignore the articles on methodology. Credibility of research depends to a large extent on the methodology adopted for the work. Methodological articles can provide important clues on how to improve quality of your research.

Important resources for recent developments are the conference abstracts and proceedings. Many of these are available on internet. Do not forget to consult previous theses on your topic. The ProQuest Dissertations & Theses Global provides details of many Ph.D. theses accepted in the universities in more than 100 countries.

Medical literature is expanding at an exponential rate. Luckily, we are in an era where tracking technology has expanded even at a faster rate. Manual search in libraries can be frustrating when it eludes the required information. Even if it provides little on the topic of interest, manual search can still be rewarding since it provides other information that broadens horizon. Nevertheless, electronic search is the best mechanism. This is now available almost universally.

Literature Databases

The best and the most used source to identify the articles of interest is MedLine. The National Library of Medicine (NLM) of the United States prepares this database, and the access is in public domain (no fee). It contains citations and abstracts of articles from nearly 8000 journals published around the world in different languages, and links to other data sources including full text in some cases. This database is generally updated every week. MedLine begins from the year 1966 but some articles published earlier are also available. **PubMed** is the larger database that includes MedLine. It now includes more than 30 million citations and increasing. Because of such huge collection, it is necessary to acquire skills for searching the relevant articles with minimal efforts. You may like to consult various on-line tutorials for PubMed search.

Another comprehensive literature database is EMBase containing more than 37 million records. This European database is updated daily and is an offshoot of Excerpta Medica (EM). It covers nearly 8100 journals from nearly 100 countries and nearly 4 million conference abstracts. It includes MedLine but many new articles can also be found. It requires subscription.

Cochrane Collaboration is an international organization with focus on systematic reviews of research on health care interventions. Their emphasis is on methodology and quality of research. They prepare, maintain, and disseminate a database of such reviews called Cochrane Library. These reviews are mostly for randomized trials, but the database includes some observational studies as well.

3.2.3 FREE MEDICAL JOURNALS AND OTHER ELECTRONIC RESOURCES

Strange as it may sound, there are about 3000 medical journals on the web that can be accessed free for full articles with download facility. Prominent among them are New England Journal of Medicine (NEJM) and Journal of Experimental Medicine both are free after 6 months. Among others are AIDS, Cardiology, Bulletin of the World Health Organization, Fertility and Sterility, Indian Pediatrics, and Journal of Infectious Diseases. Visit *www.FreeMedical Journals.com* for a partial list. An impressive addition is the series of journals published on internet by BioMed Central with full and free access. The other is a series published by Public Library of Science (PLoS). Some organizations are championing the cause of open access. They seem to be succeeding as more and more journals are moving to open access. Many journals restrict the free access to the articles published a while ago.

A big convenience with these and other electronic resources is the Find facility by Ctrl-F keys. Imagine how much time you would otherwise spend in browsing print counterparts. Electronic resources have indeed made access easy for scientists in developing countries as well, which otherwise was prohibitively expensive. For example, PubMed provides abstracts for free, and quite often these abstracts give sufficient information that obviates the need to locate the full article. Full text links are also provided, including free full texts. You can select Free full text articles while searching.

In addition, your institution may be subscribing to facilities such as **ERMed** (Electronic Resources in Medicine). This provides access to nearly 250 medical journals. But avoid mushrooming online journals that publish for money and are not indexed.

Other Electronic Resources

Citation and literature databases are just examples of many electronic resources that can be browsed. **Google Scholar** is a simple tool to broadly search scholarly literature. You can search across many disciplines and resources, peer-reviewed papers, theses, books, abstracts and articles, from academic publications, websites of professional societies, preprint repositories, university, and other scholarly organizations.

Engines such as Google and Bing and portals such as Yahoo provide link to a large number of web pages containing the specified terms or phrases. Click the link and get the concerned web page. See if it serves the purpose. The difficulty with this kind of search is that the matter may lack authenticity. Many companies tout a 'medical breakthrough' on the web to further their interest. Such less trustworthy sources can suppress less glamorous but solid studies. I am not a urologist, but I can put in a lot of information on this subject on my web page. Thus, carefully evaluate the utility and reliability of such information. Some of these, particularly those available on the website of the concerned societies or associations, government agencies, national institutes, or of the universities, may be authentic and useful. Many times, the concerned companies, such as pharmaceutical firms, give very authentic information on the drugs and tools they sell. You may be able to download several types of information on the same topic. If the information is contradictory, probe it thoroughly before accepting it.

E-Books

Books are extremely good source of knowledge that can help a research in several ways. Many medical books are available online with free access. One good website for this purpose is *Freebooks4doctors.com* that has 375 books on different topics. Among them are Gray's Anatomy (1918 edition), Maron's Cardiology and Baron's Medical Microbiology. Electronic books have tremendously useful facility of instantly reaching to a topic of interest through Ctrl-F keys. You can specify more than one term or a phrase to focus the search. The other obvious advantage is in storage space. You can browse them in your home. In contrast, the printed versions have the advantage that two or three books can be simultaneously opened on table, or two pages of a book can be seen together. Printed versions can travel with you such as in a flight. Electronic books require a computer, time to switching it on, inserting the CD or connecting it to an internet provider. All this may not be easily available at every place and takes at least a few minutes to setup even where access is available.

Among other electronic resources are medical dictionaries and encyclopedias. Websites such as MDConsult and Medscape are also useful for research endeavours. For medical research methodology, Concise Encyclopedia of Biostatistics for Medical Professionals by Indrayan and Holt (2016) may be very useful.

3.3 CRITIQUE OF MEDICAL LITERATURE

After identifying relevant literature comes the question of examining it critically. Whereas many reports and other material deserve attention, some are not worth the paper on which they are printed. You must be able to judge on some objective basis that a particular report—article, paper, document, letter, editorial, review—is valuable or not, or what part of it deserves cognisance.

3.3.1 ASSESS THE QUALITY OF PUBLICATIONS

All kinds of papers and reports are published, and you should be able to judge which ones to rely more than others. The following may help.

Quality of Journals

First aspect is the prestige of the journal. Good journals rarely publish unauthenticated information. For assessing international credibility of a journal, one index is the **Impact Factor** developed by ISI. This calculates the number of times an 'average' article in a journal is cited by others *in one year* in their report. Citations in the journals documented by ISI only are counted. This is calculated on the basis of articles published in previous two years. For 2016, cites in 2016 for articles published in 2014 and 2015 are counted and released in June-July next year. Good journals may have an Impact Factor of 3.0 or 4.0, possibly 30 or 40, and poor journals 0.1 or even 0.01. This can be understood as the scale on which usefulness of journals can be measured. Review journals generally have higher Impact Factor because these articles are frequently cited. Impact Factor of each journal covered by Science Citation Index (SCI) is provided by SCI.

Compared to the number of medical journals published around the world, the coverage of SCI is extremely limited. Also, there are serious question about how impact factor is calculated (Brumback 2008). The concerned company will not provide access or sell their data, raising concerns about their methodology, particularly the denominator (Rossner et al. 2007). If the denominator is small, the impact factor would be large. An alternative to impact factor is the number of citations as counted by Google Scholar and freely available. This may have wider reach although restricted to electronic media, mostly from the year 2000. Thus, other parameters are needed to evaluate the quality of published research findings. In any case, there are well-known or reputed journals in almost every branch of medical science. They publish articles after rigorous peer review. Almost all journals indexed in databases such as MedLine and EMBase are peer reviewed. Most research reported in these journals is believable but note that reviewers have access only to the manuscript and not the data. Thus, publications in some cases can provide false reassurance about the quality. Nevertheless, increased impact of research is not only beneficial to the profession but also helps the researcher in getting the recognition and encouragement to do better. Thus, there is all-round thrust for publishing in a good journal. Although general journals such as JAMA and BMJ have wide circulation, speciality journals have definite impact on the audience they serve.

Open Access Journals

In this age of information technology, open access journals have gained prominence. Many researchers believe that availability of information is fundamental to quality research. Consequently, the public domain is expanding. Empowered by technology, open access allows instant sharing of knowledge, Thus, journals such as published by BioMed Central can have tremendous impact at a quick pace. This has given rise to **immediacy index,** which is the average number of times an article in a journal is cited within a year of its publication. These journals and other open access sites such as of universities and of academic societies are respected for quality information. A new trend may come up if academic bodies start developing repository of research articles on their respective websites. Some researchers may self-archive their work. Some journals allow such archiving after the publication in their journal.

Before going to the main body of the paper under these headings, critically look at the summary or the abstract that almost invariably precedes the text of the paper in all good journals. Many journals give key messages in short that very succinctly describe the contents of the paper. Guidelines for evaluating quality of a document are summarised below.

Guidelines for Evaluating Quality of a Research Document

Quality can be assessed on the following parameters:

- Is research question sufficiently specific and clearly worded without ambiguity?
- Is the problem worth investigating – how the answers from the study would advance the knowledge, and help in improving the health?
- Did it require setting up a hypothesis – was it stated in a measurable format?
- Is there any assumption made, and is it sufficiently justified?

- Is the study material (e.g., type of subjects) appropriate to answer the question posed?
- Whether the number of subjects adequate to give enough confidence in the results?
- Whether the ethical questions resolved?
- Are the measurements valid to answer the questions?
- Is the design appropriate to take care of all the confounders and other sources of bias?
- If nonresponse is substantial, whether appropriate adjustment to the results made.
- Are the statistical methods appropriate and the interpretation correct?
- Are the results based on evidence provided within the document, focused on the initial question, and meaningful?
- Are the incidental findings and comments distinctly stated?
- Whether the limitations adequately stated?
- Do the conclusions really emanate from the results and coincide with the research questions?

Quality of Authors

Two other indices have been recently devised that purport to measure the worth of publications of a scholar. The first is called **h-index** (Hirsch index) that counts the number r of papers of that scholar with at least r citations in other publications. If you have 4 papers each with 4 or more citations, your h-index is 4. You can see that it tends to improve with time as your publications increase and increasingly cited. The second is **g-index**. This index is r if top r articles of a scholar are cited together at least r^2 times. If you have 12 publications and the most cited 3 articles have been cited as least 9 times, your g-index is 3. These 9 citations could be distributed as 5 for first article, 3 for second and 1 for the third. The others could simply be the number of citations (say, in the last 5 years), or number of publications with at least 10 citations (called **i10-index**).

3.3.2 ASSESS THE CONTENTS

Some good quality journals may carry articles of dubious validity. Validity of contents can be assessed as follows:

Validity of the Findings

Caution is required in assessing the validity of the findings reported in a document. The findings must be internally valid within the confines of the study in the sense that they appear consistent with the other findings, methods, and analysis used in the study. They must also be externally valid in the sense that they are generalisable to the target population and consistent with the existing proven knowledge. Try to detect fallacious reasoning that some authors can cleverly camaflouge. Exceptions must also be stated. Assess next that target population matches to your setup. Look at any literature with initial suspicion and leave it to the document to remove that suspicion. Reserve the right of final judgment to yourself. For further details see Gehlbach (2006). All articles, even when published in a reputed journal, may not be telling you the whole truth. Some may be even empty rhetoric.

Quite often various articles and reports on the same topic give varying findings. It may be difficult to comprehend the final message from such diverse evidence. Easy way out is to say that the evidence is not uniform. In most situations however it is imperative to come to some conclusion. For this, give more credence to better quality studies. Small-scale studies and those not written with sufficient clarity deserve low priority. If three out of five studies give consistent results, it may be more acceptable. Best resources are published reviews and meta-analyses in reputed journals since they tend to give a holistic picture. For medical interventions, consulting Cochrane Reviews can be very rewarding. These have been discussed earlier in this chapter. Also consider that the articles you are reviewing are giving just results or giving holistic answer to a question. An answer requires much more detailed consideration of the evidence in the literature and biological relevance.

3.4 SEARCHING THE EXISTING DATA

Search for information on a topic of research is incomplete without peeking into the other existing resources. Important among them are data, either as disparate records or organised as a database in a predefined structured format. Much of this information will be numerical rather than textual.

A research does not command respect unless all existing avenues of information are explored. Besides the literature, all existing data should be thoroughly searched and examined to avoid duplication, to get clues for research, and to assess the worth of the proposed research. Relevant data for a research might exist in:

- Clinic and hospital records,
- Disease registries,
- Computerised databases on the web,

- Reports of the national and international health agencies,
- Reports of various health surveys.

Before using such data for the purpose of research, examine them for uniformity of procedures, completeness, and their relevance to the topic. Sift relevant data from the available mass.

3.4.1 RECORDS OF PATIENTS

Besides the patient's own records, perhaps the most useful source of clinical data for research is the records of previous patients of the similar types in a clinic, hospital, or a health centre. Quite often these are computerised. If so, the selected records can be quickly retrieved and analysed. Electronic records of patients provide a unique opportunity to select large sample sizes and, in many cases, more complete information can be obtained by linkages with other related databases. However, exercise abundant caution in using such data because they may be biased for specific types of cases. Yet they can provide useful leads. Merits and demerits of various sources are as follows.

Clinic Records

The focus in a clinic is on patient care and not on data generation. The purpose generally is to keep the history of each patient at hand when the patient visits next time. But availability of serial measurements on a group of cases can provide useful information on the baseline characteristics of the cases, how the disease progressed, and how the patients responded to the therapeutic maneuvers. They can also indicate why and what type of patients leave mid-way, possibly for treatment elsewhere. All this can provide useful inputs to plan a research with minimum selection bias.

Hospital Records

Hospital records are straight extension of the clinic records, but they can be more elaborate because a full-fledged section is generally available in a hospital to maintain medical records of in-patients. Among the responsibilities of this section is to ensure that the records are accurate and complete. If this is indeed done, the records are fairly reliable. They are readily accessible and perhaps most relevant because patients or study subjects for research may come from this milieu.

An advantage of hospital records is that the records of various laboratory and imaging investigations, various examinations from time to time, the schedule of drug intake, discharge slip, etc., are available together so that a comprehensive picture can be woven. This can give an idea of what complications to expect in patients of that type, what possibly can be done to handle emergencies, what is the rate of mortality, etc. If the topic of research is on intestinal perforations, take out records of previous patients of this condition, and get a very good feeling about the clinical profile, response to various surgical interventions, post-operative care and morbidity, and the kind of cases who could not be saved and died. Such information can be useful input to the proposed research. There is one rider though. Different physicians/surgeons in the same hospital may be using different definitions, different terminology, different diagnostic aids, and different treatment strategies. Specialty hospital cases would be severely biased for specific type of cases. Consider all these variations before coming to a conclusion. Also, hospital records may consider repeated arrival of cases as new cases and count them repeatedly, causing another kind of bias.

Disease Registers

Disease registry is a special database that contains longitudinal information on the patients of specific type. Cancer registries are very popular. There may be a registry of congenital malformations, for genetic diseases (e.g., thalassaemia), for multiple births, for diabetes, for epilepsy, even for tuberculosis. Registries are for chronic disorders rather than for acute conditions. If they are really population based, as they ought to be, in the sense that all clinics, hospitals and health centres, are reporting cases then such a registry can be a very useful resource to find incidence, prevalence and distribution of the disease in different segments of population. In the case of cancer, for example, the registry can tell what percentages are breast, pancreatic, lung or blood cancer cases, and what the trends are. If age and gender are also available, then the role of these antecedents can also be studied. Examine how, if at all, such registries can help to get some background information on the type of patients you intend to include in the research.

Web-based Databases

Several databases are available that collate numerical data. Many have facility to select the indicator, time, and geographical area of your choice. Among these are:

(i) Global Health Observatory of the World Health Organization (WHO) on morbidity and mortality due to various diseases in different countries of the world,

(ii) GLOBOCAN of International Agency for Research on Cancer on incidence and mortality due to various cancers around the world,

(iii) Diabetes atlas of the International Diabetes Federation, and

(iv) Global InfoBase of WHO on noncommunicable diseases and risk factors.

These provide tremendous help in assessing the magnitude of the problem and the pattern around the globe.

Some other databases available on the web are on diseases such as HIV infection and AIDS, STDs, and heart diseases. These databases may or may not be in conventional format but contain enormous amount of information on that disease that could be useful for your research. The website of National Institutes of Health of the US lists a large number of resources for information on various diseases. MedLine Plus has segments devoted to various diseases. In addition, there are many websites that contain medical dictionaries and encyclopaedias that could be useful to develop precise definitions of the cases, and to plan the research.

3.4.2 REPORTS

Reports of various agencies of the government and of nongovernment organisations and institutions are extremely good source of the existing data on a health problem. First, the government reports may provide an official view that you might like to comment on in your research. Second, government reports might be oriented to population issues rather than to the clinic patients. For a community-oriented research, such reports are a definite plus. For clinical research also, these reports sometimes provide a good insight on the kind of patients of different diseases, effectiveness of treatment strategies in the field, morbidity, mortality rates, etc.

Survey Reports

Many countries undertake population surveys for various diseases and health conditions. United States carries out National Health and Nutrition Examination Survey every few years. This survey includes physical and laboratory examination, and collects useful information on various diseases and other conditions inflicting that country. India carries out a cause of death survey each year in rural areas of the country. Many developing countries, including India, now undertake demographic and family health survey every five years or so. UNICEF is promoting a multi-indicator survey in developing countries to collect data on child development and maternal health. Reports of these surveys may contain useful information to develop better plan of a research and to enhance its focus.

Reports of Various Agencies

Various national and international agencies collect data in a routine manner on different aspects of health and incorporate them in their annual or special reports. Annual

World Health Reports of the World Health Organization are a useful resource to get international data on aspects such as life expectancy, incidence and prevalence of various diseases, cause of death distribution, etc. Their 2002 report lists 10 leading health risks globally which may still be valid. If your research is on any of these, you can emphasise the importance of these risks by citing this report. UNICEF reports contain data on under-five mortality, neonatal tetanus, immunization coverage, low birthweight, etc. Agencies such as Population Council, US Agency for International Development (USAID), Danish International Development Agency (DANIDA) are also interested on health aspects, and publish reports that can be useful for your research.

In addition, annual reports of various nongovernmental organisations (NGOs) and government departments, particularly health department, sometimes also contain useful medical data. Programmes such as National Family Welfare in India and Medicaid in the US also publish periodic reports. Examine whether such publications can help in planning your research.

3.4.3 Cautions in Using Secondary Data

Caution has been already advised regarding using secondary data. Bias, incompleteness, lack of comparability, and relevance must be considered before using such data. Examine how those agencies collect the data, and how is it used by them. Selecting the 'right data' from the 'available data', or collating available data into the right data, is a challenging task. Assess whether these data adequately supplement the literature information or that they are in conflict. If in conflict, more in-depth investigation into the quality of secondary data may be required. Use judgement where necessary. In particular, assess

(i) representativeness of the data,
(ii) any relevant group of cases not excluded,
(iii) response rate is adequate, and
(iv) method of assessment is valid and reliable.

SUMMARY

Literature is the best-known source to learn from the experience of others. Thus, it is important to scan all the literature that one can to understand the present state of knowledge on the topic of research, and to identify the lacunae in knowledge.

Library consultation is an art that requires judicious mix of judgement and instrumentation. Identify important journals and books on the topic of the interest.

Electronic resources such as PubMed, and websites of reputed associations, societies and institutions can provide wealth of information. Check cross-references of the articles to add to the search.

Even more important is that the literature is critically evaluated. All that goes in print, or on the web, cannot be taken on face value. Review articles, particularly those emanating for Cochrane Collaboration, can provide very useful information. Also consider aspects such as Impact Factor of journals. Methodology is a major factor in deciding whether to believe the reported findings or not.

Other important avenues are the databases that are regularly built up for specific diseases, and during clinical practice. Scan them to get a feeling of what is currently available, and how can they supplement the literature findings.

REFERENCES

Brumback RA. Worshiping false idols: The impact factor dilemma. J Child Neurol 2008;23:365-367.

Gehlbach SH. Interpreting the Medical Literature: Practical Epidemiology for Clinicians, 5th ed. McGraw Hill Medical, 2006.

Haynes RB, Sackett DL, Guyatt GH, Tugwell P. Clinical Epidemiology: How to do Clinical Practice Research, 3rd ed. Lippincott Williams & Wilkins, 2005.

Indrayan A, Holt M. Concise Encyclopedia of Biostatistics for Medical Professionals. CRC Press, 2016.

Rossner M, van Epps H, Hill E. Show me the data. J Cell Biol 2007;179:1091-1092.

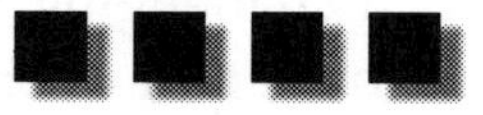

CHAPTER 4

How to do Quality Research

KEY TERMS AND CONCEPTS

- ✓ Quality of Medical Research
- ✓ Aleatory and Epistemic Uncertainties in Medical Research
- ✓ Assessment and Control of Medical Uncertainties
- ✓ Scoring System
- ✓ Reliability and Validity

After selecting a topic and working out the details of what is to be studied and what is to be left out, you may like to understand the nuances of quality of research so that you can accordingly plan and conduct the study. Quality of research primarily pertains to controlling and delineating medical uncertainties which can completely derail the findings (Indrayan 2020). We mentioned in Chapter 1 regarding the challenges of uncertainties – now provide more details. This chapter is in advanced mode for those who are keen for conducting quality research and can be skipped by others.

Introspection can provide answers to some questions in moments but can also take endless years in some situations. A quick method to find reasonable answers is to collect evidence from whatever source, collate it, analyse it, and come to a conclusion. Many times, this evidence is in terms of numbers — number of subjects with and without disease, number of subjects with different levels of cholesterol, number with different signs-symptoms, etc. The purpose of these numbers is to get a handle on underlying uncertainties and help in reaching to an objective decision. Dealing with vitalities of life, medical research requires that these uncertainties be precisely identified, their magnitude properly assessed, and their impact on medical decisions minimised.

Section 4.1 gives details of what we mean by quality of research. Section 4.2 is on various kinds of uncertainties and their sources in medical research that severely affects quality. In Section 4.3, we present methods to control some of these uncertainties—a topic that also is unwittingly pursued in subsequent chapters. Section 4.4 is on the tools for assessing the magnitude of the uncertainties, particularly the reliability and validity. These two concepts are confused by many.

4.1 QUALITY OF MEDICAL RESEARCH

4.1.1 WHAT IS A QUALIY OF RESEARCH

Many endeavors around the world do not succeed in reaching to a new result, but most leave a lesson for us. Failure to get anticipated results does not render the research useless. If we know the result already, there is no need for research. But there are several other "research" that do not contribute anything to our knowledge. This can happen because their research questions are hazy, the methodology is sloppy, the results are vague, or the reporting is unclear. Perhaps "such space-occupying lesions" have proliferated more in medical research quagmire than any other discipline. Quality has taken a back seat amidst rush for quantity.

Unsuccessful Research

Unsuccessful research that fails to come up with a positive finding is not a waste so long as a useful hypothesis was examined with appropriate methodology. It generates lessons for us and gives the direction for future research. Miscues, such as finding that arthroscopic surgery for osteoarthritis of the knee is not better than placebo (Moseley 2002), are also not a waste as they add to our knowledge. Wasteful research has one or more of the following ingredients:

- Irrelevant questions that do not need an answer or whose answers are already known.
- Unclear research question and tardy objectives that cannot be directly measured.

- Inappropriate design, such as using an observational study to assess cause–effect relationship and studying an unrepresentative sample.
- Inaccurate data either due to use of unstandardized instruments (questionnaire, laboratory investigations, clinical assessment, scoring system, etc.) or due to ignoring fallacies and errors, sometimes even cooked up data.
- Superficial or wrong analysis such as using arbitrary categories of quantitative measurements, doing logistic regression where Cox's regression should be done, or ignoring confounders.
- Subjective or wrong interpretation of the results due to incomplete understanding or to serve a preconceived notion. Mixing of opinion with evidence-based results in reaching to a conclusion also compromises the integrity of research.
- Insufficient or unclear reporting of either the methods or results or conclusions.

The basic ingredient of quality medical research is that it should be well intentioned and should be performed with care and sincerity it deserves, done by using an appropriate methodology, and is honestly reported. The details are given next.

4.1.2 WHAT IS A GOOD-QUALITY MEDICAL RESEARCH?

Quality is a subjective term that takes varying meaning with different professionals and in different situations. Yet, the quality of a medical research can be assessed using the points listed in Table 4-1. These have been briefly presented by Indrayan (2020) and Ioannidis (2016) but a much more comprehensive list in a language conducive for medical researchers of all hues from postgraduate students to university professors is presented in Table 4-1. Those who have conducted research and published their findings may like to introspect and reexamine their papers in the light of these criteria and assess the quality of their research. The most important aspect that defines quality is not the result but the methodology. When a relevant question is examined with appropriate methodology, the research is likely to have a good quality irrespective of the result. However, a research that reaches to an unexpected result has wide ramifications or the one that contradicts the current understanding has much more impact than a research with a routine result. But, for this too, the methodology must be appropriate because only then the result can be believed.

TABLE 4-1: Steps to conduct research of good quality

Steps	Details
Step 1: The problem under research	Clear specification of the research question. Justify the research question and consider how it will contribute to improved health in real-life situation. Assess the feasibility after considering the available resources such as time, expertise, and material. Review all the relevant literature without leaving out the opposite view and underscore the lacunae in the existing knowledge. State the hypothesis, if any, and list the objectives in measurable format with a specification of the outcome and antecedents under investigation.
Step 2: Complete specification of the methodology	Choose the appropriate setting (clinic, laboratory, and community) that can elicit the correct answer to the research question. Include the right type of subjects or patients, adopt a procedure for their unbiased selection, and determine the sample size in consideration of the reliability of the estimates or power to detect a medically important effect. Devise a suitable design for selection/allocation of the patients keeping in view of the possible confounding factors. Use data collection tools (questionnaire, clinical assessments, investigations with their units expressed clearly and correctly, scoring systems, etc.) with established validity and reliability. Ensure that the data obtained are correct and complete as much as possible. Use the appropriate method of statistical analysis considering the type of data and the research objectives.
Step 3: Obtain evidence-based results	Obtain the results exclusively from the data obtained in the study without imputing any opinion and keep the focus on the research question. Take care of the missing values, outliers, confounders, and inter- actions, and do the required analysis to minimize their impact on the results. Prepare the right type of the tables and illustrations that can improve understanding of the results. Assess internal and external validity of the findings and try to detect possible fallacies that can affect the findings.
Step 4: Study the implication of the results	Evaluate the results in view of the current knowledge as available in the literature and take inputs from colleagues and experts. Explain the rationale of any variation from the existing knowledge and resolve any conflict with other internal findings or external knowledge. Explore the possible alternative explanation of the results and provide sufficient arguments against it. Consider how the associated uncertainties (in the data) and the limitations of the methodology can affect the results.
Step 5: Draw modest conclusion	Draw conclusions based on the results and other corroborative or conflicting evidence. Be modest in conclusions because of the all-pervasive uncertainties in a medical setup.

4.1.3 QUALITY OF REPORTING

There may be instances where a research is performed with utmost care as provided in the rule books (Ray et al. 2016) but it fails to be noticed because of sloppy presentation. This is not just language deficiency but some of us are not able to prepare a draft in a manner that can make an impression. We will present this in a later chapter where writing of thesis and papers are discussed in detail.

Medical research is on cross-roads and is being intensively scrutinized for validity and reproducibility. Errors and fallacies are common that can jeopardize the health of many people when such results are applied to millions (Indrayan 2018). Sloppy research is a wastage of resources.

Researchers have the responsibility to produce research of high quality that can be believed and can be applied to improve health. Clear reporting is necessary to achieve this goal.

4.2 VARIETY OF UNCERTAINTIES IN MEDICAL RESEARCH

Medical uncertainties can be considered as the greatest challenge for quality research. We have discussed diagnostic, prognostic, and other uncertainties earlier. Uncertainty is an endemic affliction to all human activities. Science too is immersed in uncertainty even though it works and flourishes. Science is distinguished from other forms of knowledge by its reproducibility. A worker on sequence of genomes is likely to reach to nearly same conclusion as another if they follow the same scientific principles. However, two workers researching on thought process of Socrates may reach to very different conclusions. This should not occur with science. Medicine is especially vulnerable, more so research, since uncertainties in medical research arise from a large variety of sources.

4.2.1 SOURCES OF UNCERTAINTIES

Most apparent reason for enormous uncertainties in medicine is the profound variation in this setup. The other is limitation of knowledge that hampers medical research despite immense advances in recent times. We discuss both types of uncertainties to make you aware of them and alert you to keep a close watch. Keeping an effective control of these uncertainties is the key to quality research that will give believable and practically useful results.

Variation

Major source of variation in medicine is biological differences among individuals. This includes host factors such as genetic make-up, age, gender, birth-order, height/weight, and blood group. However, the most important contributor, particularly for pathological conditions, is the environment with which biological factors interact in an intricate manner. Details are given later.

Laboratories vary with respect to equipments, appliances, reagents, and methods; and the quality and quantity of technicians. This also contributes to uncertainty. Diagnostic tools are never perfect even in most ideal conditions, and they do give false negative and false positive results in some cases. Observer variation, such as in measurement of blood pressure, is quite common. Physicians would differ in managing a borderline case such as with intra-ocular pressure 22 mmHg. Effectiveness of a therapy depends on the expertise of the medical attendant, on the quality of prescriptions, availability of drugs, laboratory investigation results, compliance of the regimen, etc. All these vary from situation to situation.

Incomplete Knowledge

Two types of deficiencies in knowledge are common. First is lack of full information on a patient either because the patient has forgotten, is not able to explain, the records not available, the investigation required such as CT scan is prohibitively expensive, or because of lack of time as in an emergency. Thus, the patient management has to start with incomplete information. All these aggravate uncertainty in research as much as in medical practice.

Second important contributor to the spectrum of uncertainty in medicine is the limitation of knowledge. Medical science is incomplete in many respects. Nobody knows yet a useful protocol to treat a leukaemia case, how to revert essential hypertension that could obviate dependence on drugs, or how to treat a patient for urinary tract infections when the patient has impaired renal functions. In addition, there are limitations of recall. A clinician might know all that is known for a health condition but the ability to recall everything at the time when a patient is confronted is rare. Physicians and surgeons, just as anybody else, have biases, and the memory storage and recall is always selective. Furthermore, the expertise of medical professionals is not uniform. Some are good, and the others are not so good.

4.2.2 ALEATORY UNCERTAINTIES

Aleatory uncertainties can be understood as those arising from factors internal to the system. They are inherent, unpredictable, and stochastic in nature. Sources of such uncertainties were briefly mentioned earlier while explaining variation but now we divide them into the following categories for effective control. The other type of uncertainty is epistemic that arises from limitation of knowledge. The details of epistemic uncertainties are also given in the next section.

Variation Due to Host Factors

Most prominent contributor to aleatory uncertainty in the context of medicine is biological variation among the subjects. This could be both in terms of factors such as age, gender, heredity, and parity that cannot be manipulated, and in terms of anthropometric, physiological, and biochemical parameters that can be manipulated to a degree. Different signs-symptoms can emerge in different patients of the same disease because of these variations.

Other factors at individual level include socio-economic factors such as income, education, and occupation. They can work through lifestyle, personal hygiene, and nutrition on one hand, and knowledge-attitude-practice regarding health on the other. Cultural and behavioural factors also cause a lot of variation. Psychological factors such as personality traits and tension-anxiety-stress can cause independent variation or can operate through addictions such as smoking and drug abuse, altered sexual and other behaviour, as also through self-esteem and confidence level that could be dominant factors for some health conditions. All these can affect the susceptibility or vulnerability, and the response to a stimulus such as a drug can vary. We have presented these variations in a simplistic format – they all work in a web affecting each other in an intricate manner.

Other Natural Variation and Environmental Factors

Natural variation among observers, instruments, and laboratories is also aleatory. This includes inadvertent measurement errors. Human reliability is not uniform as each person performs differently on different occasions—perhaps interacting with the nature of the occasion. Thus, there is inter-observer variability and there is intra-observer variability. Only the chance component of these is aleatory. Biases, preferences, and inadequacies are epistemic about which we discuss later.

The last level of aleatory factors is environment. This comprises factors such as water supply, pollution levels, infection load, weather conditions, population and vehicular density, and communication facilities. In addition, accessibility and affordability of health care services, their timeliness, and quality can make a substantial difference. Family and societal support also are prominent contributors.

Obviously, all the above mentioned factors cannot be simultaneously observed in any practical set up. At the same time, interaction cannot be studied without observing them simultaneously. Unobserved factors can cause substantial uncertainty. Even among observed factors, unobserved values also generate certain amount of uncertainty.

Whereas these two aspects are basically epistemic, they have chance component that is aleatory.

Sampling Fluctuation

A product of one or more of the above factors is the sampling fluctuation. However, the *term sampling fluctuation applies to the estimates of the characteristics of the target population and not to the individual values*. One group of subjects tends to give results different from the other groups despite being chosen from the same target population. Medicine is an empirical science that invariably depends on the evidence provided by samples. Uncertainty remains a prominent component of the decision in this set-up.

Another aleatory uncertainty arises from applying group results to individual cases. Even if the study is perfectly executed on a representative group, the results are in terms of probabilities. These results hold in certain percentage of cases in the long run but can desperately fail in some individual cases.

A summary of sources of aleatory and epistemic uncertainties is as follows and the details are in the next section.

Sources of Medical Uncertainties

Aleatory Uncertainties (Inherent)

- Biological – nonmodifiable (age, gender, heredity or genetic make-up, birth-order, height, etc.).
- Biological – modifiable (anthropological, physiological, biochemical).
- Socio-economic (income, education, and occupation) that can affect personal hygiene, nutrition, and self-esteem.
- Cultural, behavioural, and psychological (mental status, family system, faith in prayers, sexual practices, addictions, personality traits, tension-anxiety-stress, etc.).
- Observers, instruments, and laboratories—inherent variation in measurements.
- Environmental (climate, dust, mosquitoes, flies, pollution, sanitation, water supply, infection load, quality and quantity of health facilities, family and societal support, communication, traffic, laws and their enforcement, etc.).
- Multifactorial (lifestyle, hygiene, nutrition, knowledge-attitude-practices, susceptibility, utilisation of health services, etc.; importantly, sampling fluctuations).

Epistemic Uncertainties (External)

- Universal ignorance about appropriate treatment, cause-effect, etc., for certain ailments, or lack of consensus among experts.
- Nonavailability of data, inadequate knowledge.
- Individual (patient and physician) and societal biases, including biased samples, and suppression of facts.
- Not being able to consider all the factors because they are far too many, or because they are not correctly stipulated.
- Chance that cannot be explained, other than inherent variation.
- Nonavailability of appropriate instrument or facility for any particular measurement because it is too expensive or for some other reason, and thus inability to obtain the required information.
- Incompetency, memory lapse, biasedness, carelessness, lack of validity of observers, instruments, and laboratories, etc.
- Inadequate design, wrong analysis, or sloppy data interpretation.
- Noncompliance of the regimen or nonresponse.

4.2.3 EPISTEMIC UNCERTAINTIES

Unfamiliarity breeds uncertainty. Epistemic uncertainties are subjective in nature and arise primarily from limited knowledge. They can take several forms. First is the universal ignorance such as for cure of advance-stage cancer—for that matter even diabetes—that nobody knows how to reverse; or could be data gaps such as unavailability of the information on risk of leukaemia in males with low ferritin level, or cause attribution of deaths in India. The former requires a long-term research whereas the latter is just a question of carrying out a survey in the relevant groups of people.

Another aspect of ignorance is that two or more treatment strategies may be equally good, or equally bad, and nobody knows yet which one to adopt and when. For example, amoxicillin and cotrimaxazole could be equally effective in nonsevere pneumonia. Mortality risk reduction in coronary artery disease by behavioural changes such as yoga, exercise, diet, lipid modification, and smoking may be similar to the other medical therapies such as aspirin, beta-blockers, and bypass surgery. Adoption of one or the other would depend on the personal preference rather than scientific considerations.

Knowledge Gaps

Ignorance permeates across all biological phenomena although degree varies. This includes parameter uncertainty regarding the factors causing or contributing to a particular outcome. Experts tend to differ, such as for aetiological factors of vaginal and vulvar cancer. Inadequate knowledge can also be for the role of values that have not been observed. That lung functions are affected by pollution exposure is well known but what happens if NO2 level reaches extreme level of 100 mg/m^3 is not fully known. Nobody has observed this yet. In many situations the only knowledge is that the health is adversely affected by a specified exposure but exactly how much is the effect is uncertain. In fact, quantitation of the effects has remained a major epistemic bottleneck in evidence-based decisions. Also, many times it is not clear why some factors cause disease in one person and not the others. An everyday example is exposure to iodine deficient water and soil that cause goitre in some people – that too of varying degrees – and not in the others residing in the same area. All such unknown factors are sometimes called **chance**.

There are instances when medical science has been practiced on a wrong premise. A recent example is peptic ulcer that was thought to be caused by excess acid produced by stress but now it has been discovered that *Helicobacter pylori* is the culprit in many cases. A similar scenario of infection origin seems to be emerging for coronary artery disease. Intake of tamoxifen for long duration is now being implicated for endometrial cancer.

Another aspect of inadequate knowledge is the **model uncertainty** that pertains to functional form of relationship between aetiologic factors and outcome. *Model, by definition, is a simplistic version of the relationship.* Thus, it is never perfect. Modifications that improve the model can always be suggested but the practical gain with such modification can be debated.

Rarely acknowledged aspect of inadequate knowledge is the confusion about definition of various health conditions. For example, there is so much debate on the definition of an apparently simple-looking condition such as hypertension with the Blood Pressure (BP) cut-off starting from 130/80 mmHg and reaching to 160/95 mmHg. Isolated systolic hypertensions (sysBP ≥140 mmHg and diasBP < 90 mmHg) is no longer considered a benign condition but is considered a cardiovascular risk factor. Definition of diabetes now includes the concept of pre-mellitus stage such as obesity that requires prophylactic weight control. Many such examples can be cited that illustrate epistemic insufficiency.

Individual Ignorance

Whereas the preceding discussion refers to collective ignorance, the second source of epistemic uncertainty is at individual level, either at the level of the clinician or at the level of the patient or the family. Physician's lack of awareness about new developments and their implications come under this category. Human fallibility is not uncommon. Even the most responsible researcher can make an honest mistake. The possibility of incomplete or wrong analysis of the data or interpretation also causes this type of uncertainty.

Patients also quite often do not know how to describe their complaints. Depending upon their education and knowledge, they adopt different styles with varying emphasis. It is not uncommon that vital information is missed. Incomplete information due to memory lapse or for any other reason also causes epistemic uncertainty that can affect research findings.

Limitation of Instruments

Third type of epistemic uncertainty arises from non-availability of appropriate instruments for some conditions. Perhaps no instrument is perfect but what causes specific concern is difficulty in measuring some characteristics such as psychological stress and positive health. How do you measure blood loss during a surgery with unstandardised swabs and spilling occurring in some cases? Surrogates are used that work only as a stopgap till such time that a more valid tool is developed. Non-availability of instruments could be at the micro level also such as of the facility of CT scan that might be strongly indicated in a particular case, or the lack of a right laboratory facility for evaluating specific enzyme level. These facilities may not be locally available or might be too expensive for the patient.

Biases and Errors

Fourth are the biases, perceptions, and preferences. For the physician, they can intensely affect the choice of investigations and their interpretation, treatment strategies, prognostic assessment, etc. For prostate enlargement, one may give more importance to prostatic specific antigen test over the ultrasound image when they are discordant. Value judgments and errors are always epistemic. For the patient and the family, these judgments can affect their acceptability and adoption of an advice or a procedure. At the macro level, these can take the form of publication bias of the journals, and the bias present in trials.

Errors of judgement or otherwise in medical care can result in perforation, laceration, or injury to an organ during an invasive procedure, unplanned return to operation theatre, infection developing after the admission, and transfer of patients from general care to special care. The level of competence and expertise of the clinician is always of concern. Some are meticulous in piecing together the history, examination, laboratory, imaging, and other evidence into a solid framework for management but some lack this knack. Not all are equally good in extracting relevant information from the patient. Distinguish such individual incompetence from the inherent weaknesses in universal knowledge while planning a medical research.

Faith of the patient on the care-provider and on the system can also be a significant determinant of the outcome. A related parameter is compliance. Directly Observed Therapy Short course has been devised precisely for the problem of compliance in tuberculosis treatment, and this problem persists in many other settings such as anaemia prophylaxis. Noncompliance and nonadherance may occur with regimens for cardiovascular risk reduction programs and such other prophylactic and treatment modalities. Uncertainties arising from such inadequacies are epistemic and not aleatory.

We have used some statistical terms in the Examples 4.1. Do not worry if you are not able to make full sense. The purpose of this example is to give an idea of aleatory and epistemic uncertainties. To understand them fully, return to them later after going through the book.

EXAMPLE 4.1: Aleatory and epistemic uncertainties in predicting systolic blood pressure by age and BMI

Consider the possibility of predicting the normal level of Systolic Blood Pressure (SysBP) in healthy male adult obese residents of hypothetical Townsland. Two important correlates of SysBP are age and obesity. A survey was conducted on a random sample of 200 apparently healthy male adult (age 30 to 49 years) overweight (BMI ≥ 25) residents. No other factor was considered in the selection of subjects. Suppose the regression (Chapter 11) obtained is as follows:

SysBP = 96.6 + 0.72 (Age) + 0.26 (BMI); $30 \le \text{Age} < 49$ years; $\text{BMI} \ge 25$.

Confidence Interval (CI) (Chapter 11) for *mean* SysBP for specific age and BMI can be straightaway obtained by using this equation and by using the properties of Gaussian distribution in view of a fairly large sample size. For age = 45 years and BMI = 26, suppose 95% CI for mean SysBP is 135.1 to 136.2 mmHg. Prediction interval for an *individual* of this age and BMI would be relatively large, say, 133.1 to 138.2. Statistical theory tells us that CI would be relatively narrow when age and BMI are close to the respective averages of the group. The regression coefficients are estimates and subject to sampling fluctuation themselves. Simultaneous 95% CI for age coefficient, which is 0.72 in this equation, could be 0.65 to 0.78, and for BMI coefficient, which is 0.26, it could be 0.16 to 0.36. The latter is really large in this example that can happen due to collinearity between age and BMI. When these lower and upper ends are used, the prediction interval for SysBP becomes 128.5 to 142.8 mmHg for an individual of age = 45 years and BMI = 26. Note how quickly the interval has enlarged in this case when errors in estimates of regression coefficients are considered. This would further enlarge if the possibilities of inadvertent random errors in measurement of age and BMI are admitted. Both may be correctly assessed but if age is measured as on last birthday and BMI to nearest integer, the implied range already is 45.0 to 45.9 for age and 25.5 to 26.4 for BMI. These apparently small looking variations can also make a difference of 1 mmHg in the predicted SysBP. If inherent variation in measuring SysBP is also admitted, the range could finally be something like 126 to 145 mmHg. This interval delineates the **aleatory uncertainties**. But such a large interval in a way shows a limitation of the conventional CI as well as inadequacy of the statistical model used in this example.

Now consider **epistemic uncertainties** associated with such prediction. The question at the outset is whether normal level is person specific, or there is some absolute normal valid for all adults. Already we have referred to the debate on what is hypertension (see, e.g., O'Brien and Staessen 1999). If various body functions indeed work in synchronisation with each other to attain dynamic homeostasis, is it specific to the person? The next question is whether age and BMI are the adequate determinants of physiological levels of BP in adult males. Rise in SysBP with age and BMI can partly transgress into pathological domain. If these two are not adequate, what variables should be considered? These simple looking questions do not have simple answers and point to the limitation of knowledge on this aspect. Depending on how these questions are answered, the normal SysBP would change.

Even if age and BMI are considered as the appropriate determinants, epistemic uncertainties arise because BMI is used as a surrogate for obesity. There are suggestions that waist-hip ratio, skin-fold thickness, waist circumference, index of conicity, and weight-height ratio can also be used. There is no universally accepted criterion to measure obesity. On the outcome side, SysBP can be just one reading or can be average of three readings. Accordingly, the results could vary, although the variation may not be large in these instances.

The regression model in this example is linear. This is the most common and most preferred form because of its simplicity. But it is not known what functional form best expresses normal level of systolic blood pressure in terms of age and BMI. Various other forms such as quadratic and inverse can be tried and the one that provides best empirical fit can be adopted. A very large number of options are available, and it may not be possible to try all of them. Then it needs to be externally validated. Each model may give different values of normal level of SysBP and different uncertainty interval.

Because of diurnal variation in SysBP, all measurements have to be taken on specific time of the day for all the subjects and in a similar posture and surrounding. It is sometimes not possible to adhere to this strictly. Some subjects may not be fully relaxed when measured. There might also be some 'white-coat effect' (Parati et al. 1996) that occurs while facing a doctor.

This survey was intended on a random sample of subjects from an area. If the design actually adopted were different from simple random, an adjustment in the CI would be required. The selection process should be examined to assess that the sample was indeed random or not. Then is the question of cooperation of the subjects. Nonresponse, if any, would also affect the results.

There would be other nonsampling errors. Digit preference in blood pressure readings is known. Hopefully, the instruments used for measuring SysBP, height and weight are standardized and accurate. Errors in recording and in data entry to the computer also have to be ruled out. If a sphygmomanometer is used, hearing acuity of the observer and the care adopted in deflating the cuff can affect the reading. If there are more than one observer, the inter-observer differences may not be negligible. Thus, a large variety of sources of uncertainties exist that put a question mark on the results.

Extrapolation of the results requires that the subjects included in the trial are truly representative of the target population and the new patients are from this target population. Also, that there is no dropout, or else the dropout effect is properly adjusted. Possibility of bias in the sample introduces another component to the epistemic uncertainty. The method of analysis of data and their interpretation should be complete and free from bias. In this particular example, the possibilities of these positives are bright, but the situation may not so nice in other setups.

Basic message from the Example 4.1 is that the uncertainty around an estimate is much more than what is made out by the conventional statistical confidence interval. Consideration of aleatory uncertainties may provide an enormously large uncertainty interval, and epistemic uncertainties put a further question mark on the validity of this interval. Many of such uncertainties go unnoticed and uncared for, leading to unexpected results in some cases.

4.3 CONTROLLING SOME EPISTEMIC UNCERTAINTIES

Whereas aleatory uncertainties are controlled by using appropriate statistical methods for designing, sampling, collecting and collating the data, and for their analysis, epistemic uncertainties are difficult to handle. Howsoever, contradictory it may sound, tools are available that can help in reducing epistemic uncertainties in certain situations. Primary among them are clinimetrics, aetiology diagram, expert system, and decision tree. For others, lateral thinking is required so that a new explanation can be conjectured and tested.

4.3.1 CLINIMETRICS

It is now fashionable in health and disease to use scores to measure a multivariate entity. This methodology is generally identified as clinimetrics. This reduces a multivariate entity to univariate—thus, increasing the comprehension and utility. A simple example is body-mass index that integrates height and weight. We discuss two types of scoring system that are used in medicine to reduce epistemic uncertainties. One is for diagnosis and the other is for gradation of severity.

Scoring System for Diagnosis

Attempts have been made from time to time to quantify medicine and develop scoring systems that can help in diagnosis.

Similar scoring system is available for diagnosis of acute appendicitis (Kanumba et al. 2011), to differentiate between lateral neck node metastasis from papillary thyroid cancer (Jeong et al. 2011), for assessing pulmonary disease in premature infants (Boechat et al. 2010), and to predict outcome of intrauterine pregnancies of uncertain viability (Bottomley et al. 2011). See Example 4.2 for scoring for diagnosis of catheter related infections. These are just some examples of various scoring systems available for diagnosis and prognosis purposes that can help in reducing epistemic uncertainties. You may like to review literature and find a scoring system that is suitable for your research in case considered useful.

EXAMPLE 4.2: Scores for diagnosis of catheter related infections

Clinical diagnosis of catheter-related infections is difficult. Lugauer et al. (1999) show that it can be done with relative ease with the help of a **scoring system** comprising: Magnitude and rate of rise of body temperature, attendant shivering, identification of pathogens in blood and/or catheter tip cultures, improvement in the clinical course after catheter removal, signs of catheter exit site inflammation, and results of diagnostic tests for other possible sources of infection. These criteria were graded using points and weighted according to their specificity. The patients were also diagnosed using the existing but complex clinical criteria. The agreement of scoring system with the clinical diagnosis was 85 percent in a group of 65 cases. There was no false-negative and 10 were false-positive. It turned out that 9 of these 10 were not false when additional findings are considered (clinical diagnosis criteria was expanded). Thus, the scoring system appears to be more sensitive than existing diagnostic criteria without loss of specificity.

Almost all such scoring systems are based on data from developed countries. Because of nutrition and environmental factors, they may not directly apply to the subjects in developing countries. Consider modifications before using them for patients in such countries. Such system should be used only when a valid diagnosis otherwise is difficult to establish. Or when the diagnosis depends upon the physician's preferences, his expertise, or on results of laboratory or radiological investigations that lack reliability. Such inadequacies in the diagnostic process are more common than are otherwise apparent. A useful strategy is to use these scores as just one more evidence in addition to the clinical and laboratory evidence and take a decision in the holistic manner.

Scoring for Gradation of Severity

Prognostic assessment and the management of a patient depend to some extent on the severity of the disease. There is considerable epistemic uncertainty about how to assess severity of a disease. Different physicians use different methods. For uniformity and exactitude, at times scoring is considered desirable.

The Glasgow Coma Scale (Jennett et al. 1979) is used to grade coma patients by using numeric scale for eye, motor, and verbal response. Acute Physiology and Chronic Health Evaluation (APACHE) is used to assess critically ill hospitalised adults (Knaus et al. 1991). Various variations of this score are available. Scoring system to predict the outcome of patients with acute liver failure (Naiki et al. 2011), and for prediction of prognosis in acute paraquat poisoning (Min et al. 2011) are the recent examples. Indrayan's smoking index (Indrayan 2008) measures the life-long burden of smoking. Apgar score is used to assess the prognosis in a neonate. These are just few examples. In case you are stuck with a problem of grading the severity of patients under research, see if a scoring system is available. If not, try to devise a scoring system.

As already stated, all scoring systems try to convert multiple measurement into a unified single but meaningful index. They transform multivariate data into a univariate score. Applicability of scoring systems however depends on their validity and reliability (see Example 4.3). Sometimes several scoring systems are available for the same condition and it would be difficult to choose the right system. For example, severity in peritonitis cases can be assessed by APACHE score, Peritonitis Severity Score (PSS), Mannheim Peritonitis Index (MPI), Hacettepe Score, American Society of Anesthesiologists (ASA) Score, etc. Choose a scoring system that looks appropriate for your patients.

EXAMPLE 4.3: Reliability of scores for severity of rickets

Severity of nutritional rickets can be assessed by the degree of metaphyseal fraying and cupping, and the proportion of the growth plate affected, based on radiographs of wrists and knees. Thacher et al. (2000) evaluated the utility and reproducibility of a 10-point scoring system that progresses in half-point increments from zero (normal) to 10 points (most severe). They found that inter-observer correlation of the score was 0.84 or greater for all observer pairs used by them, and intra-observer correlation was 0.89 or greater for each observer. Thus, there is a fair amount of consistency. The authors conclude that the score should be useful to objectively assess the severity of rickets.

4.3.2 OTHER TOOLS TO CONTROL EPISTEMIC UNCERTAINTIES

Other tools that can help in controlling epistemic uncertainties are based on arranging and documenting experts' knowledge in a manner that a person lacking expertise can utilise to reduce opportunities of error. Popular among them are aetiology diagram, expert system, and decision tree.

Aetiology Diagram

Epistemic uncertainties regarding aetiological factors and their interdependence can be sometimes minimised by using or developing an aetiology diagram of the type shown for Myocardial Infarction (MI) in Figure 4-1. The postulated independent factors are encircled, and the others are shown as a consequence of these factors.

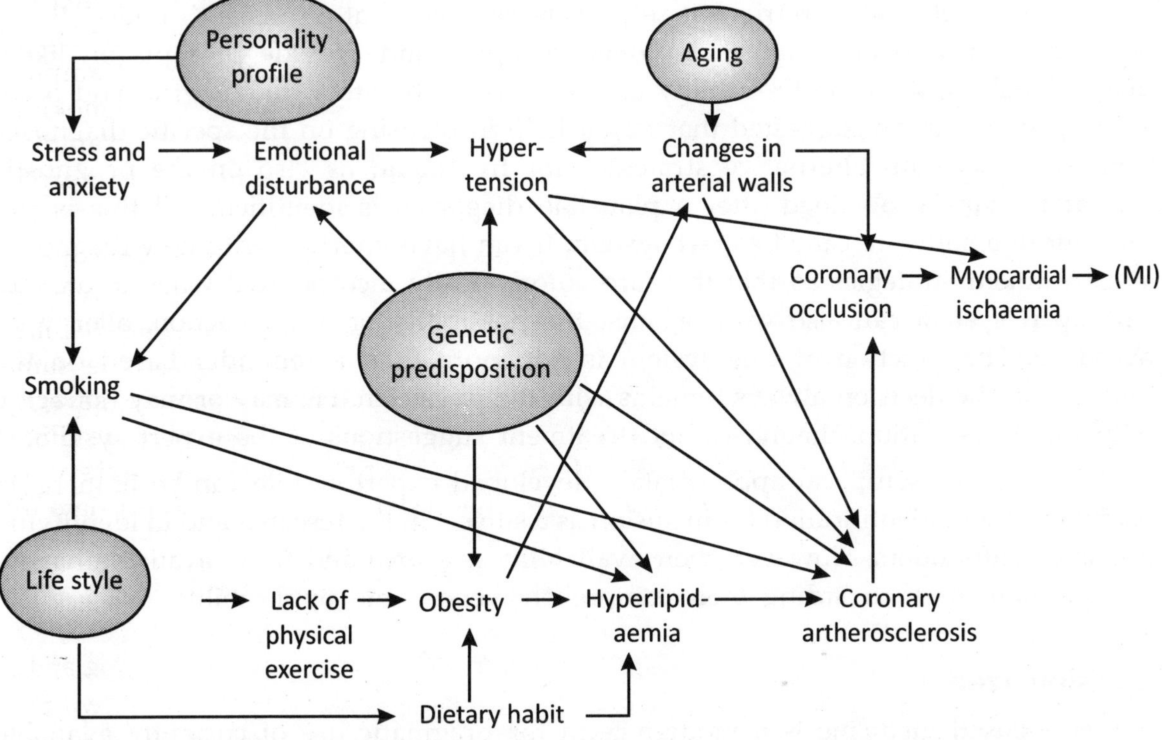

FIGURE 4-1: Suggested aetiology diagram for myocardial infarction

The process leading to MI is intricate, and the representation in Figure 4-1 is simple. In a way, this is a hypothesis that postulates various ways that an MI can occur. Yet an aetiology diagram such as this has tremendous potential in helping in clinical assessment of a patient, and in proposing strategy for its prevention. The diagram reminds a physician about what to assess in which context, and what intervention can be most effective in a particular case. This knowledge is easily transformed to a research setup where the interest is in working out MI cases, or in control of MI in a community. Thus, some of the epistemic gaps can be plugged. Similar diagram can be devised for many diseases. You may like to devise one for the condition you are studying so that epistemic gaps in your research are minimised.

Expert System

Epistemic uncertainties arise not only because of universal ignorance about some biological processes, but also substantially from the failure to judiciously apply the available knowledge. The base of medical knowledge is enormous, and it is rapidly increasing. It is becoming difficult for a physician to remember and recall everything about a disease at the time of confronting a patient. Medication errors are not uncommon. Computers have tremendous capacity to store the information in a systemic manner, and to retrieve it selectively as needed at an instant's notice. It can be programmed to take signs-symptoms as inputs and provide prompts on likely diagnoses along with the probability of each. Also, laboratory, radiological and other investigations can be suggested that might help in focusing on the specific diagnosis. Computer alerts on alternative strategies for treatment, as also on the prognostic indicators, can be obtained after a plausible diagnosis is identified. All this is put together in a software called **expert system.** It can have interface with new diagnostic and treatment strategies so that they are automatically incorporated when approved. An expert system can also warn against the possibility of drug reaction, allergy, or overdose. The function of this system is not more than a reminder based on the inputs, and the decision always remains with the physician. He may or may not agree with the investigation, diagnosis, and treatment suggestions of the expert system.

In a research setup, an appropriately developed expert system can be immensely useful in patient identification for inclusion as a subject in the research and in identifying possible confounders. However, their availability is scarce and those available have a big question mark regarding their comprehensiveness and applicability.

Decision Tree

Evidence-based medicine is a modern term for pragmatic use of currently available best evidence for management of individual patients with full awareness of the inherent uncertainties. Two basic components of this process are probabilities of various outcomes as available in the literature, and value judgement regarding action to be taken at different stages. The probabilities are assessed in terms of prevalence, incidence, risk, sensitivity, specificity, predictivity, etc. All these are discussed in a later chapter. They must have an effective interface with clinical acumen so that they are examined in the context of actual condition of a patient. Judgement regarding advising a test or not, treating or not treating, treating by medication or by surgery, discharging from the hospital or not discharging, etc., are subjective assessments based on experience and knowledge of the physician. The final outcome depends on judicious mix of the probabilities and the judgments. A **decision tree** helps to visualise various possibilities, and act accordingly. Value of a decision tree substantially enhances when 'utility' is assigned to each possible outcome. This utility can be either to the patient such as 0 for death and 1 for full recovery, or to the society such as the chance of recovery is 0.75.

When resources permit, examine if such a diagram can help in minimising the role of chance in decision and in assessing the outcome for various options on objective basis. In some research setups, decision tree can provide deep insights and greatly reduce epistemic uncertainties.- For details of decision trees, see Pardeshi (2019).

4.4 ASSESSING UNCERTAINTIES

Solar eclipse can be predicted centuries in advance. This is a deterministic phenomenon. Medicine is not so fortunate. Never enough is known about biological systems to predict with that accuracy. Reasoning is the tool of choice in an uncertain environment. Going from qualitative notions such as possibility of presence or absence of disease, to quantitative notions such as 0.7 probability of disease, statistics is extremely useful in considering the in-between notions of plausibility. This is based on various logics of reasoning about uncertainty that seeks to detect order out of chaos. Amidst wide fluctuation in cholesterol level from person to person and time to time, it is still known for healthy individuals of age 40-49 years that it varies between 150 and 200 mg/dl, and any level beyond 250 mg/dl is a risk for coronary disease.

4.4.1 BIOSTATISTICS FOR CONTROLLING THE EFECT OF UNCERTAINIES

It is generally believed that statistics is the science that crunches numbers. But the fact is that *statistics is the science concerned with variations and uncertainties.* In fact, it helps in managing uncertainties to a great extent. It would be surprising to some that random variations too follow a pattern, namely the Gaussian. Thus, predictions are possible based on the random fluctuations also. Isn't it irony that chance events can be used to make strong predictions in some situations? Stochastic variability of nature after all is not that bad!

Although the statistical philosophy and theme remain same in all branches yet 'bio' part of biostatistics makes it very different from, say, economic statistics. Most part of this section is devoted to the explanation of this basic theme that permeates in all dimensions of statistical thought but is distinctly biased for medical disciplines.

What is Biostatistics?

Several sources of medical uncertainties were listed earlier. Yet this is not a comprehensive list. Medical profession has a tall order to deliver quality care in the face of indomitable variations and uncertainties. Uncertainties are omni-present, and no decision in any science, least in medical science, can be infallible. The science is becoming complex by the day, and the need to control and evaluate uncertainties is increasing. *Biostatistical methods help in controlling medical uncertainties and in taking decisions that are least likely to be in error.* It would not be hyperbolic to say that biostatistics is the science of management of medical uncertainties, particularly those arise from empirical observation. This premise is rarely accepted but the centrality of statistical thinking in the medical decision process is gradually gaining ground. More important is that this management is based on evidence rather than on opinions.

Most important function of statistical methods is to transform the data into a degree of belief in a particular phenomenon so that a decision can be taken with a certain level of confidence. Biostatistical methods help to separate real effects from random patterns, signals from noise, patterns from turbulence, order from chaos, and trends from variations. Explosive growth in statistical reasoning in the study of human health is among the important scientific developments of the twentieth century. It is not a revolutionary strategy, but only common sense laced with enhanced rationality applicable to medical and health sciences. Mere availability of good data is not enough: proper exploitation of data is more important. Biostatistical methods tend to minimise speculation and increase the credence by providing methods to improve quality of medical data and to exploit them properly.

Medical research steps in Chapter 2 show that statistical methods are essential ingredients for primary research. If you have aptitude, acquire statistical skills yourself. If not, find a biostatistician who is interested and willing to collaborate. Expert collaboration will surely be needed for a large scale or complex research. Statistical advice should be sought before the research is undertaken and not after collection of data. In any case basic knowledge about statistical methods is essential to be able to effectively communicate with a biostatistician.

Aleatory and Epistemic Uncertainties and Biostatistics

Aleatory uncertainties may look statistical but conventional statistical methods are designed primarily to handle sampling fluctuations, that too if the sampling is random. For example, statistical confidence intervals are built to delineate uncertainties arising from sampling fluctuations in the estimates. They assume that the inputs to the model are known or fixed. If the input values are changed, the results could be very different. We have tried to illustrate this in Examples 4.1 earlier in this chapter. Under the aleatory category is not only confidence interval but also how this interval changes when the input values and the model coefficients change within the plausible range. This gives rise to **uncertainty intervals**. Increasing the sample size can narrow down confidence interval but uncertainty interval is not so much affected by sample size. This can be reduced by narrowing down the plausible choices of the input values by collecting evidence against values that deviate too much from those observed.

Statistical methods also help, albeit in a limited way, in managing some types of epistemic uncertainties also. Scoring system is essentially a statistical tool. Evolving a scoring system requires data reasoning and data collation. Expert system also uses the probability paradigm. Aetiology diagram is not statistical although in this case also the interdependence is evaluated through statistical methods before depicting it in the form of a diagram. An important component of decision tree is statistical probability of various intermediary outcomes.

Let us also not overemphasize the role of biostatistics. It deals mostly with aleatory uncertainties: particularly those arising from sampling fluctuations, which themselves are by-products of different source of variations. Although known biases can be adjusted by using biostatistical methods but realise that most epistemics are to be prevented or dealt with before the collection of evidence, and practically nothing can be done afterwards to minimise their impact on a research decision except using ifs and buts in the conclusion. Wide knowledge, expertise in piecing the information together, and clinical acumen are required to control most epistemic uncertainties rather than biostatistical methods.

4.4.2 THE CONCEPTS OF RELIABILITY AND VALIDITY

Reliability and validity delineate uncertainties in a variety of settings. *Reliability is reproducibility in identical situations.* The other term for this is **precision**. *Validity is the ability to correctly measure the phenomenon that is intended to be measured.*

The difference between validity and reliability is illustrated in Figure 4-2. When you measure BP of an individual as 132/72 mmHg, how confident are you that this really is the level? Variations can occur from a variety of sources. External sources such as non-standardized instrument and patient under stress are one component and the other is inherent reproducibility. In the case of sphygmomanometer, not being careful in gradual deflation of cuff, in making the reading at the right moment, and in missing Korotkoff sounds, are among the aspects that would certainly vary from observer to observer.

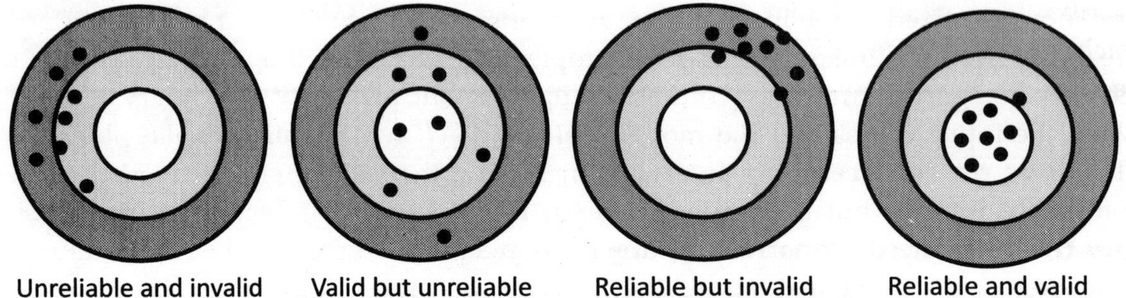

FIGURE 4-2: Dart game illustrating validity and reliability.

Reliability in Research

Other things being equal, a study based on 400 patients is more reliable than the one based on 60 patients. As explained in a later chapter, summary measures such as mean and proportion are more reliable when based on large *n*. Confidence interval becomes narrow, and statistical test of hypothesis procedure attains more power to detect a given difference. Thus, a reasonably large sample size is necessary to provide confident results. Such results are reliable in the sense that another study based on similar subjects is likely to give nearly the same result when both are based on equally large sample from the same target population.

A measurement is considered reliable if it can be reproduced under identical conditions. The variation would always be there, but it must be minimal. This variation is measured in terms of standard deviation and coefficient of variation that we discuss later. Efforts in acquiring expertise and in putting precision into the task can increase the reliability. Perhaps the most important component in all such efforts is the human being. Even when the measurements are machine-based, proper maintenance of machines and their correct operation determine the reliability.

Body temperature is considered reliable because it depends only on proper application of clinical thermometer. The reading comes out almost without human intervention. It is univariate in this sense. Opposed to this, measurement of T_4 level is multivariate as it depends on several interactive factors. Even BP measurement is multivariate because it depends on various other factors—listed earlier. Thus, it is less reliable.

The other question is whether mercury sphygmomanometer is a reliable instrument for measuring BP. This reliability can be evaluated only if it is assumed that there is practically no variation in BP itself. Ideally, use of the same instrument for measuring the same level should give the same answer. In a mannequin with known BP of 126/75mmHg, the instrument should be able to give nearly the same level when repeatedly used with proper care.

Practical situations for assessing reliability of instruments are not as ideal. We describe three methods to evaluate instrument reliability. One is test-retest reliability, which should be used for an instrument such as blood gas analyser but is generally used for an instrument such as a questionnaire, the second is split-half consistency which is specifically for a tool such as questionnaire, and the third is Cronbach's alpha that has somewhat more general applicability.

How to Check Instrument Reliability?

The reliability of a questionnaire can be examined by evaluating agreement between two sets of answers when it is administered twice to the same group of subjects. The questionnaire should not provide any learning, i.e., the second set of answers should not improve by the first set of answers. Such agreement is called **test-retest reliability**. This can be used for an instrument such as mercury sphygmomanometer. The extent of agreement is measured by intra-class correlation coefficient or Cohen's kappa.

A tool such as questionnaire can possibly be split into ostensible equal halves by randomly dividing the questions into two parts. The correlation between the scores obtained by subjects in the two halves gives an indication of, what is called, **split-half consistency**. Such consistency is also considered part of reliability.

The other method to measure internal consistency is **Cronbach's alpha**. This is based on the correlations between various pairs of items in a tool. For details see Carmines and Zeller (1979).

Validity of Research of Tools

Epistemic uncertainties relating to the research tools such as a questionnaire, laboratory test, and diagnostic criterion are assessed in terms of their validity. Pain is measured in several ways, yet they fail to describe it fully. Thus, no measure of pain is fully valid. Such uncertainties remain a concern in most research situations. Validity assumes slightly different meaning in different contexts.

In the context of a single measurement, validity is its ability to be close to the reality. This depends on the care adopted in measurement. For example, the validity of liver function test results depends on the quality of reagents, analysis method, care in recording, etc. With such care, the value recorded can be believed to be true.

Similar concern can be expressed for validity of a response. When a patient is asked about duration of complaints, how correctly is he able to report? A person of age 73 years may not report vision problem considering that it is natural at his age. A smoker may not report about cough, and a VDRL positive man may intentionally suppress sexual history. Such instances adversely affect the validity and increase the uncertainty level in research.

There is some confusion in medical literature about the difference between validity and accuracy. The term **accuracy** is used for closeness of the measurement to the reality. A BP reading 132.3 is more accurate than 132 mmHg and a cholesterol level 223 is more accurate than 220–229 mg/dl category provided correctly measured. However, such accuracy can be redundant for valid application of the measurement for patient management.

Would you prefer visual analogue scale or verbal rating scale to assess intensity of pain? Two such devices may not give same results—thus, choice is important. One is more 'appropriate' than the other in a given situation. If two devices are equally valid, the one that is more convenient to implement can be adopted.

Validity of a device is obtained in terms of its predictive value for positive outcome and negative outcome, respectively. A gold standard is necessary against which this kind of validity is evaluated. Sensitivity and specificity are also indicators of validity.

In a clinical trial setup, initial equivalence of two groups of subjects, one of which is put to a drug and the other on placebo, indicates **internal validity**. Then the difference arising in the outcome can be safely ascribed to the drug. Treatment effect is correctly portrayed. Imbalance and biases such as paying more attention to the cases than controls are threats to validity. Even when no such hiccup is present, the conclusion could still be valid only for the groups of subjects actually studied. Generalisability is achieved when those groups are adequate representative of the target population. Random sampling that we discuss later as a strategy to achieve representative sample affords **external validity**. But this is just one aspect. The setting of the study, eligibility criteria for inclusion of subjects, applicability of the test regimen to the patients available in normal clinical practice, suitability of outcome measure, occurrence of side-effects, balanced approach, all contribute to external validity. In short, judge that the results would be applicable to the next eligible patient you encounter. For details of criteria of external validity of trials, see Julian and Pocock (1997).

Types of Validity

Validity is an intricate concept that changes according to the set-up. Important types of validity for the purpose of medical research are face, criterion, concurrent, content, and construct validity.

Face validity is apparent correspondence between what is intended and what is actually obtained. Grossly speaking, ovarian cancer cannot be in males and prostate cancer cannot be in females. Cleft lip, deafness, dental caries cannot be causes of death. If any data show such inconsistency, they are not face-valid. Face validity is violated also when a patient is shown discharged alive from a hospital and cause of death within the hospital is also recorded. Current age cannot be less than the age at first childbirth. Thus, face validity is achieved when the observations look just about right. If a man tells his age 20 years but looks like 40 years, the response is not face-valid. If a family reports consuming food amounting to 2800 calories per unit per day, but the children are grossly undernourished then, again, the response or the assessment is not face-valid.

An instrument or a method is called **criterion-valid** if it gives nearly the same information as a criterion with established validity. Carter et al. (2002) report criterion validity of Duke Activity Status Index with respect to standard pathologic work capacity indices in patients of chronic obstructive pulmonary disease. Whenever a new index or a score or any other method is developed, it is customary that its criterion validity is established by comparing its performance with a standard. Our review of literature suggests that the statistical method generally used is correlation whereas the right method for establishing criterion validity is showing high predictivity.

It is not uncommon in medical setup that no validated standard is available. For example, no valid measure is available to assess characteristics of balance in people with vestibular dysfunction. The Berg Balance Scale is often used but is not considered a fully valid measure. A relatively new tool is Dynamic Gait Index. The two can be investigated for agreement. Again, this is different from correlation. If agreement is good, the two methods can be called **concurrently valid**. That is both are equally good (or, equally bad). This however, does not establish superiority of one over the other. The superiority can be inferred only when two methods under evaluation are compared with a known gold standard.

Fourth type is **content validity**. This is based on the domain of the content of the measurement or the device. Fever by itself is not content-valid for infection. Would you consider kidney function tests such as urea clearance and diodrast clearance content valid for assessing health of kidneys? Such tests restrict to specific aspects and do not provide a complete picture. Content validity is often established through qualitative expert reviews. Wynd and Schaefer (2002) report content validity of osteoporosis risk assessment tool established through a panel of experts.

The last is the **construct validity** that seeks agreement of a device with its theoretical concept. Body-mass index is construct-valid for overall obesity but not for central obesity, whereas waist-hip ratio is construct-valid for central obesity and not for overall obesity. Construct validity is sometimes assessed by the statistical method of factor analysis that reveals 'constructs'. If such constructs correspond well with the ones that are otherwise theoretically expected, the tool is considered construct-valid.

SUMMARY

Medical research has mushroomed, and concerns are expressed regarding the quality of this voluminous research output for improving the health care. Among several factors, quality of research is affected by effective control of aleatory and epistemic uncertainties that afflict al empirical research.

Uncertainty is an endemic affliction of human activity, and medical research is particularly susceptible. Two primary types of medical uncertainties are aleatory and epistemic. The former is inherent due to biological, environmental, and other natural variations, and the latter arises mostly from lack of knowledge.

Biostatistical methods are equipped to handle sampling fluctuations that are a source of major part of the aleatory uncertainties. Inherent variations manifest in terms of sampling fluctuations. Tools such as scoring systems, aetiology diagram, and expert system can help to reduce some types of epistemic uncertainties. For most epistemics, however, steps should be taken before the collection of evidence by proper choice of research material.

Uncertainties are assessed by calculating probabilities. Biostatistical methods are extremely helpful in controlling and assessing uncertainties. Reliability and validity considerations help reduce uncertainty levels in research results.

REFERENCES

Boechat MC, Mello RR, Silva KS, et al. A computed tomography scoring system to assess pulmonary disease among premature infants. Sao Paulo Med J 2010;128:328-335.

Bottomley C, Van Belle V, Pexsters A, et al. A model and scoring system to predict outcome of intrauterine pregnancies of uncertain viability. Ultrasound Obstet Gynecol 2011;35:588-595.

Carmines EG, Zeller RA. Reliability and Validity Assessment. Sage Publications, 1979.

Carter R, Holiday DB, Grothues C, Nwasuruba C, Stocks J, Tiep B. Criterion validity of the Duke Activity Status Index for assessing functional capacity in patients with chronic obstructive pulmonary disease. J Cardiopulm Rehabil 2002;22:298-308.

Indrayan A, Kumar R, Dwivedi S. A simple index of smoking. COBRA Preprint Series 2008:40.

Indrayan A, Malhotra RK. Medical Biostatistics, 4th ed. CRC Press, 2018.

Indrayan A. Statistical fallacies & errors can also jeopardize life & health of many. Indian J Med Res 2018;148(6):677–679.

Indrayan A. Improving the quality of medical research. Annals National Acad Med Sciences (India) 2020;56(01):6-8.

Ioannidis JP. Why most clinical research is not useful. PLoS Med 2016;13(6):e1002049.

Jennett B, Teasdale G, Braakman R, Minderhoud J, Heiden J, Kurze T. Prognosis of patients with severe head injury. Neurosurgery 1979;4:283-289.

Jeong JJ, Lee YS, Lee SC, et al. A scoring system for prediction of lateral neck node metastasis from papillary thyroid cancer. J Korean Med Sci 2011;26:996-1000.

Julian DG, Pocock SJ. Interpreting a trial report. In: Clinical Trials in Cardiology. Pitt B, Julian D, Pocock S (eds.). WB Saunders 1997:pp 33-42.

Kanumba ES, Mabula JB, Rambau P, Chalya PL. Modified Alvarado Scoring System as a diagnostic tool for acute appendicities at Bugardo Medical Centre, Mwanza, Tanzania. BMC Surg 2011;11:4.

Knaus WA, Wagner DP, Draper EA, et al. The APACHE III prognostic system: risk prediction of hospital mortality for critically ill hospitalized adults. Chest 1991;100:1619-1636.

Lugauer S, Regenfus A, Boswald M, et al. A new scoring system for the clinical diagnosis of catheter-related infections. Infection 1999;27 (Suppl 1):S49-S53.

Min YG, Ahn JH, Chan YC, et al. Prediction of prognosis in acute paraquat poisoning using severity scoring system in emergency department. Clin Toxicol (Phila) 2011; 49:840-845.

Moseley JB, O'Malley K, Petersen NJ, et al. A controlled trial of arthroscopic surgery for osteoarthritis of the knee. N Engl J Med 2002;347(2):81:88

Naiki T, Nakayama N, Mochida S, et al. Novel scoring system as a useful model to predict the outcome of patients with acute liver failure: application to indication criteria for liver transplantation. Hepatol Res 2011; Nov. 2 [Epub ahead of print].

O'Brien E, Staessen JA. What is "hypertension"? Lancet 1999;353:1541-1543.

Parati G, Ulian L, Santucciu C, Mancia G. Reproducibility of blood pressure measurements. Blood Press Monit 1996;1:205-209.

Pardeshi R. Decision Tree Modeling: Decision Science Series – A Practical Handbook For Decision Tree Analysis. Pardeshi, 2019.

Ray S, Fitzpatrick S, Golubic R, Fisher S, Eds. Oxford Handbook of Clinical and Healthcare Research. Oxford, United Kingdom: Oxford University Press; 2016.

Thacher TD, Fischer PR, Pettifor JM, Lawson JO, Manaster BJ, Reading JC. Radiographic scoring method for the assessment of the severity of nutritional rickets. J Trop Pediatr 2000;46:132-139.

Wynd CA, Schaefer MA. The osteoporosis risk assessment tool: establishing content validity through a panel of experts. Appl Nurs Res 2002;15:184-188.

CHAPTER 5

How to Design a Medical Study

KEY TERMS AND CONCEPTS

- ✓ What is a Design?
- ✓ Descriptive Studies
- ✓ Level of Evidence
- ✓ Observational Studies – Prospective, Retrospective, and Cross-sectional
- ✓ Interaction and Confounding
- ✓ Animal Experiments
- ✓ Phases of Clinical Trials
- ✓ Randomisation, Masking, and Blinding
- ✓ Equivalence, Superiority and Noninferiority Trials
- ✓ CONSORT Statement
- ✓ Biases and their Control

Medicine is an empirical science and the decisions are based on evidence. They must also stand upto the reasoning. Hunches or personal preferences have no role. The nature of evidence is important but credence to this is acquired by the soundness of the methodology of collecting such evidence. ***Design** is the pattern, scheme, or plan to collect evidence.* It is the road map by which credibility of research findings is assessed. The function of a design is to permit valid conclusion which should be justified and unbiased. The details of design bring in clarify and permit conclusions in the face of the confounding and such other complications that could interfere with the interpretation. Thus, the design should be able to provide correct answers to the research questions. The objective of a design is to get best out of the efforts. Design is in your hands a – you decide what design is to be used. Findings and results are not in your hands – they come from the responses over which you have no control. It is mostly due to the holes in design that allegations such as some treatments reported effective actually cause more harm than good come up. Various elements of design are listed below.

Elements of a Design

A design contains the following elements:

- Definition of the target population: Inclusion and exclusion criteria, area to which the subjects would belong, and their background information.
- Specification of various groups to be included with their relevance.
- Source and number of subjects to be included in each group with justification including statistical power or precision considerations as applicable.
- Method of selection of subjects out of those who meet the inclusion and exclusion criteria.
- Strategy for eliciting data—animal experiment or human trial, or observational study (prospective, retrospective, or cross-sectional).
- Method of allocation of subjects to different groups if applicable or matching criteria with justification.
- Method of blinding if applicable and other strategies to reduce bias.
- Specification of intervention, if any.
- Definition of the antecedent, outcome, and cross-sectional characteristics to be assessed alongwith their relevance for the study objectives.
- Identification of various confounders and the method proposed for their control.
- Method of administering various data-collecting devices such as questionnaire, laboratory investigation, and clinical assessment; and the method of various qualitative and quantitative measurements including scoring.
- Validity and reliability of different devices and measurements.
- Time-sequence of collecting observations and their frequency (once a day, once a month, etc.), duration of follow-up, and duration of study, with justification.
- Methods for assessment of compliance and strategy to tackle ethical problems.

Broad Types of Study Designs

We will discuss various types in detail but note the broad types for the time being.

Descriptive Study

For establishing the existing status of a disease or any other condition in a segment of population, and associations without cause-effect implications.

Analytical Study

For establishing relationship between two or more factors—generally antecedents and outcomes:

By observing natural course of events (observational study)

- Prospective is from antecedent to outcome
- Retrospective is from outcome to antecedent
- Cross-sectional when antecedent and outcome are studied together

By human intervention

- Experiments on animals and biological material
- Trials on human beings

5.1 DESCRIPTIVE AND ANALYTICAL STUDIES

The design depends on the objectives of the proposed study. Broadly, a primary medical research can have two types of objectives. One is **descriptive** that seeks to delineate the hitherto unknown levels of one or more parameters in different kinds of subjects, and the other is **analytical** that seeks explanation of a phenomenon.

5.1.1 DESCRIPTIVE STUDY

This covers the distribution part of epidemiology of a disease or a health condition, such as what is common and what is rare, and what is the trend. It helps to assess the type of diseases prevalent in various groups and their load in a community. But a descriptive study does not seek explanation or causes, nor tries to find which group is 'better' relative to the other. Evaluation of the level of β_2 microglobulin in cases of HIV/AIDS is this kind of study. A study on growth parameters of children, or for estimating prevalence of blindness in cataract cases is also a descriptive study. Unless the existing status is known, how can one find the cause? Unfortunately, even the body temperature among healthy subjects is not known with precision for many populations. Thus, there is a considerable scope for carrying out descriptive studies.

Such studies can provide baseline data to launch a programme such as of control of breast cancer and can measure the achievements made when the study is repeated after some time.

A descriptive study can also generate hypotheses regarding aetiology of the health condition under review when the disease is found more common in one group than the other. In some situations, a descriptive study can be designed to test a hypothesis regarding status of a parameter such as whether at least 80 percent patients of abdominal tuberculosis come with the complaints of pain in abdomen, vomiting, and constipation of long duration, or whether the prevalence of noninsulin dependent diabetes is at least 10 percent among married females of age 50 years or more whose husband is diabetic. A descriptive study can also be used to study relationships such as between systolic and diastolic Blood Pressure (BP), or between haemoglobin (Hb) and retinol level, so long as they are viewed as mere associations and not cause-effect.

Case-study, which generally describes features of an unusual disease entity, is also descriptive. Case-study (or case-report) presents unusual and unexpected findings for one or a few cases. For guidelines on how to write a case-report for publication, see Green and Johnson (2006). A series of such cases forms **case-series**. This too can generate a new hypothesis. Case-series of HIV positives in San Francisco, which was found almost exclusively among homosexual men, led to the suspicion that sexual behaviour could be a cause. **Surveys** too are descriptive studies although this term is generally used for community-based investigations. This is the primary format of descriptive studies. When repeatedly done, surveys can reveal time-trends. Complete enumeration such as population **census** is also descriptive. A descriptive study generally has only one group since no comparison group is needed for this kind of study, although strata may be present. Its design mainly is in terms of sampling plan that we discuss in the next chapter.

5.1.2 ANALYTICAL STUDY

The other kind of medical studies is **analytical** that tries to investigate aetiology or cause-effect type of relationship. Determinants of a disease or of a health condition are obtained by this kind of study. Differences between two or more groups are also evaluated by analytical studies. Although the conclusions are associational, the overtones are cause-effect. A properly designed analytical study indeed can provide a conclusion regarding cause-effect relationship. Two types of strategy are available for analytical studies—observation and experiment. Observational studies are based on naturally occurring events. There is no human intervention. Record-based studies are also placed in this group. Observational studies can be further subdivided as explained in Section

5.2. Experimental studies require deliberate human intervention to change the course of events. These include clinical trials. They are discussed later in this chapter.

Choice of the Strategy for Analytical Studies

A good research strategy provides conclusions with minimal error within the constraints of funds, time, personnel, and equipment. A useful strategy that works in some situations is comparison of characteristics of population with high incidence with those of population with low incidence. Thus, the factors contributing to the difference can be identified. This is called an **ecological study**. For example, Korkeila et al. (2007) compared frequency of use of anti-depressants and the suicide rate in Finland and found an inverse relationship in the two. You can see that an ecological study compares the group characteristics, and individuals as such have no role. If you study correlation between Infant Mortality Rate (IMR) and per capita income in 27 major states of India, you are doing an ecological study. The data in this study pertain to the states and not individuals. Results of an ecological study cannot be automatically applied to individuals. Many researchers unknowingly do this and give rise to, what is called, an **ecological fallacy.**

Although many strategies exist on paper, in some situations choice for intervention is not available. For investigating relationship between smoking and colon cancer, intervention in terms of exposing some people to smoke is not an option. Observation of those who are already smoking is the only choice. For establishing efficacy and safety of a drug, intervention in terms administering the drug is a must. In this case observational strategy is not an option. Role of potentially harmful factors is generally studied by observations, but potentially beneficial factors can be studied by either strategy. Effect of garlic on cholesterol level can be evaluated by studying people naturally ingesting garlic in various quantities; and also by asking people who almost never took garlic to consume it for a while in specified quantity. Experiments have the edge in providing convincing results. Also, they can be carried out in controlled conditions—thus, a relatively small sample could be enough. But they raise questions of ethics and feasibility. Guidelines for choosing a strategy for analytical studies can be listed as follows:

1. The strategy should be ethically sound, causing least interference in the routine life of the subjects.
2. Generally, it should be consistent with the approach of other workers in the field. If not, the new approach should be fully justified.
3. The strategy should clearly isolate the effect of the factor under investigation from the effect of other factors in operation.
4. It should be easy to implement and acceptable to the system within which the research is being planned.

5. Confirm that the subjects would sufficiently cooperate during the entire course of the study and would provide correct responses.
6. The strategy should be sustainable so that it can be replicated in case required.

Different strategies provide different levels of evidence of cause-effect relationship. The hierarchy is represented in Figure 5-1. Expert opinion and case-reports can be highly biased. A double blind RCT has the least bias although this also does not eliminate bias. This is explained later in this chapter where experiments and clinical trials are discussed.

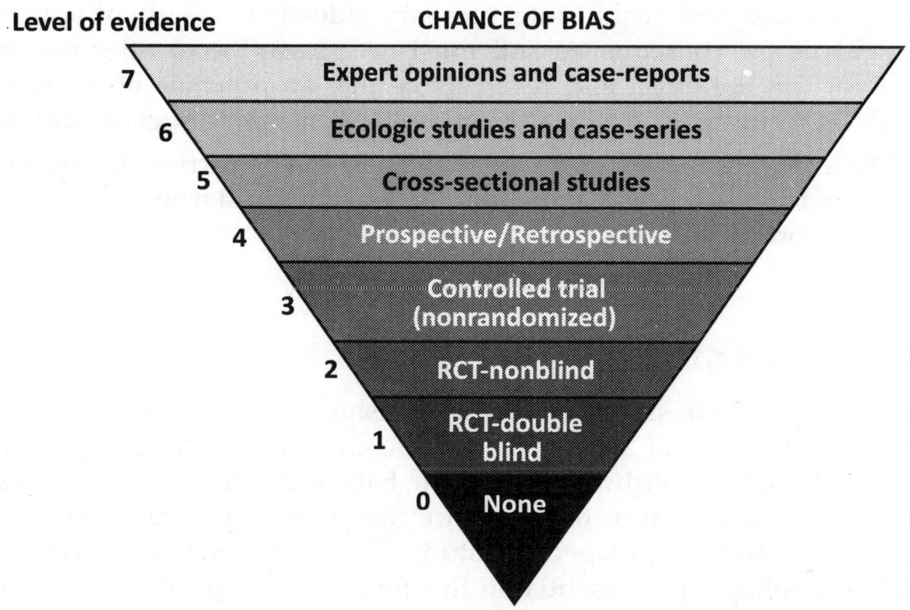

FIGURE 5-1: Level of evidence of cause-effect provided by different designs

5.2 OBSERVATIONAL STUDIES

Nature is a great experimenter. Many interventions or changes occur naturally that require no human intervention. Some people are naturally exposed to iodine deficiency in water, and some women naturally have low Haemoglobin (Hb) level. Study of such naturally occurring events can provide invaluable help in studying cause-effect relationship with conviction. Such a study can be based on records or on actual observations, or a combination of both. This is generally categorized as an **observational study**: sometimes also referred to as an **epidemiological study.** Since there is no deliberate human intervention (such as a drug) in this setup, such studies carry little risk of harm to the subjects or the society. However, such a study is generally conducted for specific groups such as those with high disease prevalence—thus, extrapolation to the general population is not immediate. Many observational studies are done in hospital setup rather than in a community.

Antecedent and Outcome

An observational study of the effect of pre-existing maternal anaemia on birthweight of their babies can be done in various ways. To understand these, note first that maternal anaemia is an antecedent factor in this example and birthweight is the outcome. An antecedent is a precursor such as an exposure (e.g., sex with a subject with sexually transmitted disease) or a risk factor (e.g., high cholesterol) suspected to affect the disease. The other names for antecedent are cause, predisposing factor, and determinant.

An outcome could be a health state, recovery, side-effect, death, or any other event of interest. This is the consequence and must necessarily occur after the antecedent. Other terms for this are effect and result. Note that an outcome of interest could be positive such as recovery to full health or could be negative such as death.

Three different ways that an observational study can be carried out are prospective, retrospective, and cross-sectional, depending upon that the starting point is antecedent or outcome, or none at all.

5.2.1 PROSPECTIVE STUDY

Most desirable format for studying the relationship between maternal anaemia and birthweight is that antenatal women with different levels of Haemoglobin (Hb) are selected and followed for birthweight of their babies. Antecedents are assessed prior to the outcome in this format in the sequence they naturally occur. A study following such a format is called a prospective study. Since any outcome occurs after the antecedent, some follow-up is essential in this format, although it can be short in some situations. Thus, this is also called a **follow-up study.**

Cohort Study

If a fixed group of subjects is followed, all beginning with a common baseline, it is called a **cohort**. In case of a usual prospective study, the subjects can continue to be enrolled whereas in the case of cohort this is rarely admissible. There could be a cohort of children born in a particular year followed for growth pattern, or a cohort of adults residing in an area at a particular time who are followed for diet-exercise and occurrence of coronary events. There could be a cohort of smokers and a matched cohort of nonsmokers followed for 20 years for development of Chronic Obstructive Pulmonary Disease (COPD). If the group identified for the study is the one that has been recently exposed to a risk factor, it is called an **inception cohort**. For example, an inception cohort of early rheumatoid arthritis can be studied for assessing predictive factors of orthopaedic surgery.

Historical cohort or **retrospective cohort** is the group of subjects with exposure in the past, which is investigated for development of an outcome. Terms such as

retrospective follow-up and **historical prospective** are also used for this kind of method. For example, in the year 2020, live births occurring in an area between 2000 and 2019 can be investigated for early life factors such as birthweight, nutrition, and overcrowding in the household, and subsequently noted for occurrence of childhood acute lymphoblastic leukaemia. This requires that past records are fully available. Despite being based on past records, it is not a retrospective study since the direction of investigation is from antecedent to outcome.

Longitudinal Study

Another version of prospective study is **longitudinal** when observations or measurements are repeatedly made at several points of time, particularly over a long period. When a cohort of low birthweight children born in the year 2018 is followed-up *every year* for growth, development, anthropometry, biochemical profile, pathological conditions, etc., it is a longitudinal study. Framingham Heart Study is among the most popular longitudinal studies, now going on for more than 50 years. In a longitudinal study, different subjects can be observed at different points of time. When each subject is observed at same fixed time, it is generally called a **repeated measures** study.

Prospective, cohort, and longitudinal are not mutually exclusive terms. Prospective study is an umbrella term that includes cohort and longitudinal studies, as well as other types of follow-up studies. Cohort study can be longitudinal comprising observations at several points of time or can have only two assessments – one at the beginning and the other at the end.

EXAMPLE 5.1: A cohort study on relation of level of cognition with birth weight parameters

Richards et al. (2002) report findings of a 53-year follow-up of 1946 birth cohort, initially consisting of 5,362 children of nonmanual and agricultural workers, and a random sample of one-in-four of manual workers selected from all single and legitimate births that occurred in England, Scotland and Wales during one week in March 1946. (Note the rigorousness with which the specifications are stated.) The cohort was studied on 21 occasions between birth and age 53 years, when information about socio-demographic factors and medical, cognitive, and psychological function was obtained by interview and examination at each point of contact. They concluded that birthweight and postnatal growth are independently associated with level of cognition at different ages. In this case the main outcome of interest was level of cognition and the antecedents are birthweight and postnatal growth. The former was repeatedly measured over the period so that the cognition achieved at different ages could be studied.

Side note: Postnatal growth may be a function of birthweight but as far as cognition was concerned, this study found that the two act independently.

Comparison Group in a Prospective Study

Quite often the comparison group (the group of subjects who do not develop the outcome) come from within the prospective study. During the process of follow-up in such a study, some develop the outcome who become cases, and those not developing the outcome become controls. Subjects with different exposure levels can be chosen for follow-up that could provide multiple groups for comparison of the outcome. You can have one group with exposure and the other without exposure. However, in some situations, an external group can be used for comparison. Adequate number of nondiabetics may not be available in a diabetes clinic for studying kidney diseases. External controls can be included in such a situation although they should come from the same milieu. In a rare situation when an appropriate external group is also not available, comparison can be done with the outcome rates in the general population. For example, incidence of preterm deliveries in women of age 45 years or more can be compared with the incidence in the general population of women. The actual control group in this setup should be women of age less than 45 years but separate incidence of preterm in them may not be easily available. The incidence in less than 45 years may not be much different from that in the general population since births after that age are rare. However, in many situations, the rate in the general population is not comparable and a great degree of precaution is required.

Nonresponse and Other Nonsampling Errors in a Prospective Setup

One problem with any follow-up is the nonresponse in the subsequent contacts. The person may migrate, may die due to an unrelated cause, may refuse to cooperate, etc. In a clinic-based follow-up, when the patients are advised to report at periodic intervals, some may not come on the required day, and one or two follow-ups may be missed. If such nonresponse were substantial (but not major), an adjustment in the results would be required at the time of analysis because the dropouts are typically different type of subjects and their exclusion can introduce bias.

Nonresponse is one source of nonsampling error that researchers disdain; others arise due to insufficient accounting of confounders and epistemic bottlenecks. The latter is discussed at length in one of the previous chapters, and the former is explained later in this chapter.

5.2.2 RETROSPECTIVE STUDY

The second format for examining birthweight in relation to maternal anaemia is that babies with different birthweights are chosen and anaemia status of their mother during antenatal period is retrieved from records. First assessment in this format is outcome and antecedents are subsequently assessed for each type of known outcome. This is a **retrospective study**, which moves from outcome to the antecedent. Note the quickness with which a study in this format can be carried out. There is no need to wait for the outcome to develop or not develop. Outcome is already known, and the antecedent is obtained either from records or enquiry. The cases and in most studies controls are assembled, and information regarding their past exposure or risk factors is collected. The cases can arise or can be recruited in future such as of breast cancer coming to a clinic now on, yet the study is technically retrospective so long as it investigates antecedents for known outcome. Retrospective method is especially suitable for rare outcomes because the study can start after enough number of cases is assembled.

Many studies do not move from outcome to the antecedent yet are termed as retrospective in medical literature. This usage indicates the time frame and not etiological sequence. For example, Hilska et al. (2001) report 'retrospective' analysis of 150 patients with primary proximal colon cancer in Finland operated during 1981-1990. But the outcome measure was five-year survival rate. The study still is from antecedent (colon cancer) to outcome (survival). It is a prospective study under our terminology and could be called a retrospective cohort as already explained, but not a retrospective study.

Case-control Design

The dominant format of a retrospective study is **case-control** in which otherwise similar subjects with and without disease are investigated for past exposure. Those suffering from the disease or have the health condition of interest are called **cases**, and those without that particular health condition are called **controls**. All case-control studies are retrospective but all retrospective studies are not case-control. Investigating the past history of cases of Myocardial Infarction (MI) is a retrospective study but there may not be any control. Then it is not a case-control study. Control group provides a legitimate base for attributing differences in the two groups to the antecedents such as high cholesterol level and obesity in patients of MI—thus, case-control setup is considered a natural format for retrospective studies.

The term control is used generically for any reference group against which the case group is compared. In comparing patients of myocardial infarction with those of stroke for risk factors, the group with primary interest is the case group, and the other is the control group although this also is a group with disease. In a study on efficacy of diagnostic tools, if the interest is in comparing ultrasound images with tomography images, the former could be the control group and the latter the case group. Note that cases are their own controls in this situation. Since control group is not necessarily 'without disease', it is sometimes prudent to call this as a **case-referent study**.

Retrospective study is efficient for rare outcomes because it can begin with enough cases. It can simultaneously evaluate many causal hypotheses. It is efficient also in evaluation of interaction between different risk factors. As explained later in more detail, an **interaction** is the way presence or absence of two or more factors *together* modify the outcome and the extent of this modification. Case-control study allows easy control of the confounders (this also is explained later in this section). All these advantages accrue because a large number of affected cases is available in this format.

On the downside, recall lapse is common in a case-control study. Differentials such as cases easily able to recall events than controls can cause additional bias. It can be biased also because only those who already have had the required outcome can be included. Many severe cases may have already died and cannot be a part of this type of study. Case-control format is not able to establish sequence of events. The assessment of risks of adverse outcomes (or any outcome) is done in terms of Odds Ratio (OR) in this case in place of the actual Relative Risk (RR), although OR can be a good approximation of RR in most practical situations (OR and RR are explained in Chapter 11).

Nested Case-control Design

A design could combine cohort and case-control features. Consider a cohort of persons of age 40-44 years who are followed up for 15 years for development of cataract. Now the persons who develop cataract become cases for investigation of those risk factors that could not be studied in the cohort setup. This would require matched controls. They can come either from the same cohort amongst those who did not develop cataract, or from outside. Note that cohort studies start with one or two specific antecedents, but case-control format allows investigation of several antecedents. Thus, new hypotheses can be examined. The baseline data are already available from cohort study, and these data may be free of recall bias. This type of design is called **nested case-control design** since case-control setup is nested within a cohort.

EXAMPLE 5.2: A nested case-control study on inverse association between BMI and ovarian cancer

A prospective study was conducted in France to investigate any association between Body Mass Index (BMI) and ovarian cancer (Lukanova et al. 2002). Information on anthropometry, demographic characteristics, medical history, and lifestyles was obtained at the time of recruitment of subjects. (Note the advantage of availability of a lot of information in this set-up.) Women diagnosed with primary, invasive epithelial ovarian cancer (n = 122) diagnosed 12 months or later after recruitment served as cases. (Note that n was still large.) Two controls for each case matched for menopausal status, age, and date of recruitment were randomly chosen from the same cohort. This is an example of a situation where nested case-control design can be useful. Advantages of a case-control design were derived from within the cohort that was being followed any way. **Side note:** Appropriate logistic regression showed inverse association between BMI and ovarian cancer risk, i.e., for increasing quartiles of BMI, the odds ratio exhibited a decreasing trend. Such dose-response type of relationship is one of the many indicators that the relationship could be causal.

Confounders

For a valid conclusion from a case-control study, it is easy to understand that the cases and controls should be matched with respect to all those factors that do not fall into the set of hypothesised risk factors. Such extraneous factors are called confounders or concomitant variables.

Confounder or confounding factor is an antecedent characteristic that can be described as a possible explanation of the outcome in addition to the one under investigation. Thus, it is an extraneous factor that plays spoil sport. It can also be understood as the one that is related to the antecedent as well as to the outcome but is not in the causal chain. In a study on smoking and hypertension, one confounder is obesity. Smokers tend to be obese and hypertension is also related to obesity. In other words, obesity can also be at least a partial explanation for hypertension in addition to smoking and it is not in the causal chain. The effect of smoking and obesity on hypertension cannot be disaggregated unless obese and nonobese subjects are separately studied. Second confounding factor in this example is age. As age increases, the life-long burden of smoking increases for smokers, and the chance of hypertension also increases because of age-related arterial changes. Thus, again, age as a possible explanation should be ruled out. This can be done either by developing a proper design, otherwise by performing a suitable statistical analysis. This text contains plenty of information on these two methods.

One easy method of identifying confounders is to draw a list of all possible factors that might influence the outcome of interest. The list may be based on your own knowledge, wisdom of the seniors, and the review of literature. Out of this list, choose the ones that would be studied as risk factors or antecedents for their role in the outcome. The remaining in the list are confounders for that outcome and they are not in the causal pathway.

Note however that the confounders so identified would be restricted to those that are known. The knowledge could be incomplete, and the list may not be comprehensive. If so, epistemic uncertainties would remain in the results. Nothing can be done to remove this gap except to expand the horizon and look for factors that are not in the conventional domain.

Obviously, confounders should be identified before the data are collected. Previous research, clinical insight, and clarity about the disease process can help in this identification. For finding whether STD per se has a role in acquiring HIV infection, cases are HIV positives and controls are HIV negatives but they should be of same age, same gender, same sexual behaviour (such as multiple partner sex), same exposure to injectables, etc. These are the confounding factors in this study. Finding controls with so many matching characteristics is an uphill task. Thus, some may have to be adjusted at the time of analysis. If the results with and without adjustment of a factor are same, it is not a confounder. However also consider whether the cases and controls are likely to respond to the questionnaire in a similar manner, and no bias is likely to creep in due to differential pattern of responses not related to the factors under study.

Selection of Cases and Controls

The source of cases with the disease or any other outcome of interest can be hospital in-patients, or patients seen in out-door, cases identified in a survey, available in records of a health facility, etc. Control subjects should preferably come from the same setting as the cases. They can be patients of other diseases or relatives of the cases if that does not hinder the objectives. In some situations, controls can come from the population at large.

Case-control studies look simple but can produce severely biased results if not done with proper care. The case definition should be sharp so that there is no room for doubt to a third person. For example, if breast cancer cases are being studied, specify their stage. An unbiased sample survey, such as random, of the target population is preferable although that is not a prerequisite for analytical studies. The sample size must be adequate that can represent the entire spectrum of subjects and can provide reliable results. Then only the results are generalisable. Biases can appear in several other forms. These are discussed later in this chapter. For example, use of incident cases rather than prevalent cases can remove some biases such as longer survival of those with mild form of disease, or of those who are physically strong. Cases surviving for long time are more likely to have recall lapse.

Controls should be matched with cases for the confounding factors. The results are much more valid if it is one-to-one matching. That is, each case should have corresponding one **matched control**. These are also called matched pairs. The attempt should be to simulate identical twins situation so that they are exchangeable. The purpose is to be able to conclude that any difference between the cases and controls is attributable to the antecedent under study and nothing else. When the controls are available in abundance and easy to elicit, two or three controls can be taken for each case. This helps in increasing the reliability of the results without commensurate cost.

As already mentioned, it is an uphill task to match more than two or three antecedents. Generally, matching stops at age and sex that are confounders in almost every medical setup. If so, acceptable but less valid procedure is **group matching** (also called **frequency matching**). Under this scheme, controls are matched with the cases on average or with regard to pattern of presence of the confounding factors. If obesity is a confounding factor, and if 35 percent of cases are obese, then nearly the same percentage of controls should also be obese for group matching.

In addition to selection, matching should also be in ascertainment. The controls must be assessed with the same keenness and with the same methodology as the cases. Cases may be more motivated but try to extract same cooperation from the controls as well. Controls should be able to provide a correct estimate of the rate of occurrence of antecedents in subjects without the disease. Wherever possible, take help of records because they are likely to be far less biased than verbal responses. But the records should be complete.

5.2.3 CROSS-SECTIONAL STUDY

The third format for birthweight–anaemia study is that a group of deliveries is chosen irrespective of maternal anaemia and birthweight, and both are elicited. This is a cross-sectional study since both antecedent and outcome are observed at the same time. Presence or absence of either antecedent or outcome is not a consideration at the time of selection of subjects in this kind of design, but the objective still is to investigate the association. Although this kind of format is more appropriate for descriptive studies, as for estimating the prevalence of a health outcome, it is also appropriate to generate hypothesis regarding aetiology.

In some setups the distinction between antecedent and outcome is blurred. Among cleft-lip and thalassaemia in children, neither is a known cause of the other, yet dependence of one on the other can be investigated for generating a hypothesis. Such studies are analytical in this sense, and do not remain purely descriptive. A study on evaluation of concordance between two or more methods is also cross-sectional. Cross-sectional studies are more appropriate for assessing the relationship between fairly stable conditions (such as gender and hypertension) that do not change during the course of the study. Note that they provide a one-time snapshot of the status of the relationship, and not a long-term perspective.

EXAMPLE 5.3: A cross-sectional study on lifestyle and homocysteine level

Medicine is largely a science of prediction—prediction of diagnosis, prediction of outcome Lwin et al. (2002) conducted a cross-sectional study in the year 2000 on a random sample of 455 Japanese rural residents of age 40-69 years. The objective was to investigate the association of plasma total homocysteine (tHcy) concentration with 5,10–methylenetetrahydrofolate reductase (MTHFR) gene and selected lifestyle factors. After examining various associations, they concluded that higher intake of folate, vitamin B_{12}, and nonsmoking may be important to prevent mild hyperhomocysteinemia. They generated an important hypothesis for confirmation through a subsequent study.

What is an Interaction?

Interaction can work in any study but are common in cross-sectional studies. This can be explained as follows. Some factors work more effectively when other conducive factors are also present. Iron supplementation is more effective in increasing Hb level when folic acid is also given. Their combined presence is much more effective than the sum total of their individual effects. This is a positive interaction and called **synergism.** Since aspirin can reduce beneficial effect of ACE inhibiters in patients with heart failure, they possibly have negative interaction. This is called **antagonism.** Most interactions cannot be classified into any of these two categories. Osteoporosis is more severe in older women than older men [see Figure **5-2 (a)**]. Thus, age and gender interact for severity of osteoporosis. Perhaps age and gender have no interaction for Total Lung Capacity (TLC). When they are plotted, the decline in TLC with age runs almost parallel in men and women [see Figure **5-2 (b)**]. Similar pattern of response for various levels of factors, except for nearly a constant difference, indicates absence of interaction. Then they are called **additive** factors. If the responses are not parallel, interaction is said to be present. Epidemiologically, interaction is called **effect modification.**

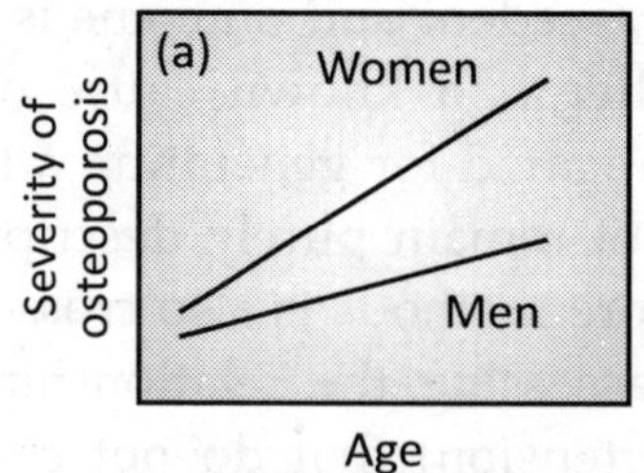

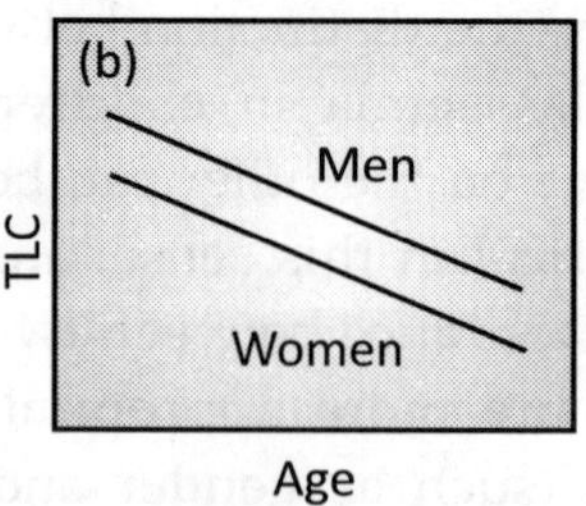

FIGURE 5-2: (a) Interaction, (b) No interaction

The term interaction is used for product of two or more antecedent factors and not for relationship between an antecedent and an outcome. Differential effect of various levels of an antecedent on outcome is not called an interaction.

Performance of a Cross-sectional Study

Cross-sectional format is rarely used for an analytical study because it fails to provide a good assessment of cause-effect type of relationship. However, it is suitable when it is not clear what is antecedent and what is outcome. In the case of peptic ulcer and milk consumption, either could be a cause of the other.

A cross-sectional study is a good tool to generate hypothesis, which can be subsequently tested by a case-control or a prospective study. Cross-sectional study is certainly good as a descriptive study. It is quick and easy to complete. It starts with a reference population, so generalisation is immediate when based on a genuine random sample. Repeated cross-sectional studies are good for detecting changes in known risk factors besides, of course, time-trend of the disease.

As explained in a subsequent chapter, it is many times helpful to obtain sensitivity-specificity or predictivities of a test procedure as indicators of its validity. The former requires a case-control study and the latter a prospective study. Sometimes a cross-sectional study is used to calculate both types of indices. When the subjects are representative of the target population, the percentage of subjects with disease and without disease would be nearly the same as in the target population. The test positives and test negatives would also be in the representative proportion. But they will be prevalent cases and not incident cases, nor 'incidence' of antecedents. With this constraint, cross-sectional data can be used to obtain both types of indices. Besides the restrictive conditions just mentioned, also note that a cross-sectional study fails to reach to severe cases that tend to be rapidly fatal.

Reporting Results of an Observational Study – STROBE Statement

Results from an observational study must be fully reported. For this purpose, a guideline on Strengthening of Reporting of Observational studies in Epidemiology (STROBE) has been framed, which is endorsed by many biomedical journals. This contains a checklist of 22 items on the contents of the article on results of observational studies. Some points are separate for prospective, retrospective and case-control studies and others are common for all observational studies.

Most of what a report on an observational study should contain is already implicit in this chapter and would be repeated in a later chapter in different context. Specifically, the STROBE statement requires that scientific background and rationale for the study should be stated. This also requires a cautious overall interpretation of results considering the objectives, limitations, multiplicity of analyses, results from similar studies, and other relevant evidence. A discussion of the existing external evidence is particularly important for studies reporting small increase in risk.

As of now, STROBE does not specifically require that new findings be put into context by conducting a *systematic review* of other similar studies. This obviously would be a positive feature as 'this could alert us about consistency of findings, allow exploration of sources of heterogeneity and would ensure, in the same way as it does for randomized trials, that research effort is not spent on rediscovering the same finding again'.

5.3 ANIMAL EXPERIMENTS AND CLINICAL TRIALS

Shift focus from natural course of events to deliberate human intervention for changing the course of events. The objective would be to find whether this intervention is effective in making the desired changes. Safety of the intervention can also be evaluated. Comparison of modalities of screening, diagnosis or other assessment also comes under this strategy. Such studies do have potential to cause harm to the subjects and the society since an unproven modality or intervention is used although the perception may be that it is beneficial.

Experiment is the most direct method to establish cause-effect relationship because the suspected causal factors can be manipulated in this strategy. Choose subjects and develop a design that suits the experimental conditions to control variations. Use methods such as randomisation to keep bias and effect of confounding under check. Temporality in the outcome can be examined by proper follow-up. Experiments are replicable if somebody wishes to verify the results. However, there are severe limitations as well. Experiments do not simulate the actual conditions where several extraneous factors also play a role. They also raise ethical issues that observational studies do not. Because of these limitations, experiments are many times carried out on nonrepresentative sample that makes generalisation even more difficult. Notwithstanding these problems, experiment is a preferred strategy where feasible. Experimental evidence for cause-effect relationship is more compelling than available from observational studies.

For reasons given later, an experiment is almost invariably carried out by including a control group that does not receive the test ingredient of intervention. However, some experiments are done without parallel controls. These are called **uncontrolled trials**. For example, one can measure oxidative stress enzyme levels in Parkinson's disease, introduce an intervention to reduce this stress, and measure again. Such an experiment can be called a **before-after study.** Not that before-after study has no control. Each subject serves as its own control in terms of its status before the intervention but there is no separate control group. The difficulty with before-after trial is that the change after intervention may be partly due to **placebo effect.** This is the psychological effect of taking some treatment – even if it is null like coloured water or saline injection. For this reason, results of before-after study are not fully believable.

Uncontrolled trial can also use earlier experience with similar patients to decide if the intervention is really effective. Pap test for cervical cancer was introduced after an uncontrolled trial.

5.3.1 LABORATORY AND ANIMAL EXPERIMENTS

The term experiment is generally restricted to laboratory experiments done on animals such as mice and rabbits, or on biological material such as cells, blood specimen, vaginal swabs, and antigen. For example, aliquots of blood sample can be given different doses of an agent to assess gene expression. Clinical trials are not counted among experiments. In the context of drug development, an experiment in a laboratory is preclinical phase and done first to obtain a formulation that has desirable biochemical properties—thus has propensity to be beneficial in either promotion of health, prevention of sickness, or treatment of a disease; and second to establish that these properties are indeed present. This exercise requires enormous inputs of theoretical knowledge about various compositions. Once such a compound is obtained, it is tried on animals to study its effect in a biological environment. A suitable animal model is chosen that can simulate human conditions. Sometimes they are genetically or physiologically altered to create suitable models. The objectives of animal experiments in the context of drug development are to study the effect of the new product on the biological system, how the product is absorbed, distributed, metabolized, and eliminated after dosing, and delineate a range of dose that could be beneficial to the human. Animal studies do raise ethical issues about which we mentioned in Chapter 1. These experiments pave the way for human experimentation in terms of clinical trials as described in a subsequent section. In fact, trying a new drug on human subjects without establishing its safety and efficacy in laboratory and animal setup is considered unethical, and is almost never allowed.

EXAMPLE 5.4: An animal experiment on HRT

To determine whether continuous or cyclic Hormone Replacement Therapy (HRT) is better, Sun et al. (2001) conducted an experiment on 142 Sprague-Dawley rats who were randomly divided into seven groups. Besides normal estrous and ovariectomised controls, the other five groups received treatments imitating clinical regimen with different combinations. The rats were sacrificed, and mitotic index and Proliferating Cell Nuclear Antigen (PCNA) were the outcome measures. Note the relevance of animal experimentation in this setup.

Side note: The results suggest that continuous regimen was better than the cyclic regimen in postmenopausal HRT rats.

Since conditions can be reasonably standardised in a laboratory, many sources of variation are automatically eliminated in this set-up. For this reason, experiments can give reliable results even when conducted on a small number of subjects. Randomisation and blinding of the experimental units, as described next for clinical trials, help to minimise bias. Some designs of experiments used in medical research are described next.

Some Designs of Laboratory Experiments and Clinical Trials

Laboratory conditions allow a lot more handle on variations and uncertainties. If the experiment is on ovariectomised mice for hormone replacement therapy (see Example 5.4) and the regimen under trial are continuous and cyclical, all this experiment needs are three groups – one with continuous therapy, one with cyclical therapy, and one control on placebo. The mice may be randomly allocated to these three groups. This is called a **one-way design**. If another factor is introduced – normal estrous – then another set of three groups is required. There will be a total of six groups – three with ovary (normal estrous) and three without ovary (i.e., with ovariectomy). Now this is a **two-way design**. Two factors under study in this case are regimen (continuous or cyclical) and presence or absence of ovary. A third factor can also be introduced that will give rise to a three-way design. And so on.

For human beings, a simple trial is on iron supplementation and folate supplementation at weekly intervals to adolescent girls to increase their Hb level. Since iron and folate interact with one-another, this trial needs four groups – one control with no supplementation (or with placebo), one with iron alone, one with folate alone, one with iron and folate both. This is called a **factorial design** since all possible combinations have been included. As an exercise, check that eight groups are needed if there is a third supplementation such as vitamin B_{12} in this example.

For conditions such as essential hypertension and diabetes, the drugs act for a limited period and they have to be administered again. Therapies with practically no carry-over effect give an opportunity to use same set of patients over and again for different therapies. For example, representative group of 90 patients of essential hypertension can be given atenolol-50 for six days, propranolol for next 6 days with a day or two in between as washout period, and acebutalol for a further period of 6 days again after the necessary washout gap for the previous drug to exit the system. The order in which various patients will receive different treatments is randomised. This is called a **cross-over design**. This can be used only when the effect of treatment can be assessed quickly. This kind of design is not suitable for cyclical diseases such as asthma and arthritis because these have natural remission periods. This design should not be used also when substantial dropout is anticipated because then the statistical analysis becomes complex.

Cases and controls can be followed-up longitudinally at predefined intervals to assess the trend of responses to the treatment. This is called a **repeated measures design**. Trials on most anaesthetic agents follow this design. This design helps to study outcomes that can emerge in short-term separately from those that emerge in long term. If the assessment is at different points of time for different subjects, it is called only longitudinal study and not repeated measures.

A useful method is to do cumulative assessment after trial on each subject or pair of subjects (test and control), and to stop the trial when a convincing result either way is obtained. This is called **sequential design**. Because of difficulty in its interpretation, this design is rarely followed.- However, **group sequential design** is becoming popular where assessment is made at pre-fixed stages of the trial, for example, after completing one-third of the trial, and then after two-thirds of the trial. This gives the opportunity to stop the trial if convincing results are available one way or the other. The trial can be stopped for futility if it is found that there is hardly any chance of the test regimen reaching to the target efficacy. It can be stopped also for adequate efficacy if sufficient evidence is available. Thus, group sequential approach can save a lot of time, efforts, and the exposure to the participants by allowing trial to stop early.

Another design gaining popularity is **adaptive design.** Under this design, interim analysis is done as in a group sequential design and at the same time, changes are made as necessary to meet the objectives. These changes could be in terms of increasing the size of the trial, changing the eligibility criteria of the participants, changing the dose, etc. Specification of what action will be taken and what stage interim analysis will be carried out is done in the protocol itself. Designing adaptive strategy is intellectually challenging and computer software is used to replace your brain cells.

A design devised long time ago but gained popularity recently is **up-and-down trial.** In this design, an anticipated median effective dose is tried on the patient such as for anaesthesia and observed if it is effective. If effective, next patient gets a lower dose. If not effective, next patient gets a higher dose. Nearly 15 to 20 patients are tried in this manner with different doses.

Features such as randomisation and blinding are also considered part of the specification of design. These are described in the next section on clinical trials.

5.3.2 CLINICAL TRIALS

Medical experiments on human beings are called **trials.** The intervention must be potentially beneficial and not harmful. This could be a drug, a surgical procedure, a medical device, behavioural change, process of care, etc. Regimen research environment is rapidly changing and safety is increasingly getting precedence over efficacy. Aspirin, with its marvellous use in cardiac problems, may not have made it to the market today with its side effects of gastric problems. The current paradigm seems to be that a new regimen should be free of toxicity while also be efficacious. Perhaps risk-benefit has taken a back seat for daily drugs. For special drugs such as against cancer, side effects are tolerated, and risk-benefit becomes more relevant.

When carefully conducted, clinical trials are the fastest and the safest way to evaluate efficacy and safety of a new regimen under controlled conditions. Although clinical trials have attained central place in product development, many breakthroughs in medicine occurred without such trials. Recent example is demonstration of bacterial origin of gastric ulcer by Marshall who infected himself with *H. pylori* and developed gastritis.

Since the subjects are humans in clinical trials, many issues crop-up ranging from ethics to profound variations. A human experimentation cannot be conducted unless sufficient reasons for doing so are present. Ethical considerations are mentioned in Chapter 1. The problems arising from variations and uncertainties are discussed in the present section. For further details of how to conduct a clinical trial, see Friedman et al. (2010).

Basics of Clinical Trials

Trials can be done on patients coming to a clinic, or on a community in the field at large. Although clinical trials are mostly for therapeutic modality, they can also be prophylactic regimen such as for amnioinfusion for meconium-stained amniotic fluid at the time of childbirth or can be for a diagnostic procedure such as comparison of prostatic specific antigen levels and ultrasound images for prostate cancer. A trial for a screening procedure can also be conducted in a clinic setup although it is generally conducted in a high risk population in a community.

The intervention in case of diagnostic trials is not an external agent but a procedure on the body that can change the diagnosis and thus, the course of treatment. Such a non-invasive procedure does not cause much anxiety except for time and cost but an invasive procedure has potential to cause harm to the health of the patient.

Therapeutic trials raise important ethical issues because they generally involve exogenous material that may have side-effects and may not be beneficial at all relative to the existing modes of therapy. For this reason, extreme care is exercised in conducting such trials. Among them, one is that the regimen must pass through rigours of preclinical phases. First of them of course is a laboratory phase to examine the biochemical properties of the test regimen, and second is an experiment on suitable animal model that can simulate human conditions. We have discussed such experiments in previous paragraphs. A clinical trial is embarked upon only after achieving success in these phases. For research on a therapeutic regimen, make sure that these phases are conducted with convincing success. This requirement is sometimes waived when the therapy or its variation is already in use for some other condition and the trial is to examine its use in a new set of conditions.

Efficacy is always related to a particular outcome. Terms such as recovery and discharge are vague outcomes. They must be specified either in terms of measurements such as glomerular filtration rate for kidney diseases, in terms of images such as x-ray of dislocation of joint, or in terms of any such objective criterion. Also, the duration after which the outcome is to be assessed should be specified—within a day, within a week, or what. This applies to death also. Everybody dies but if a death occurs three months after a surgery, should this be ascribed to the surgery? Follow-up period for different outcomes of interest must also be fully specified.

Phases of a Clinical Trial

Phase I of clinical trial is done first time on human volunteers to study the pharmacokinetic properties of the regimen, to investigate toxicity, food interactions, major side-effects, and to delineate the maximum tolerated dose. Thus, it is also sometimes called dose-escalation trial. This phase seeks to establish that the regimen is safe in human and can be pursued further.

It may not be easy to find volunteers for this kind of trial, except possibly hopeless cases who find a ray of hope in the new regimen, or courageous, many times healthy people, who agree to participate for some inducement. The inducement should be proportional to the expected discomfort and not excessive that could be frowned upon as coercive. Note that healthy subjects can be used in this phase because therapeutic efficacy is not an issue at this stage. In fact, some researchers advocate that phase I should be done on healthy volunteers only except for diseases that compromise the tolerance. Such a compromise can easily happen in cancer and many other diseases. For example, Nguyen et al. (2006) conducted phase I trial of an IV-administered vascular endothelial growth factor trap on patients with choroidal neovascularisation due to age-related muscular degeneration. Generally speaking, though, comorbidities should be ruled out so that the side-effects are not unnecessarily attributed to the drug. Symptomatic conditions in any case are part of exclusion criteria but asymptomatic conditions such as anaemia and abnormal lipid profile can also affect the outcome. These also should be excluded. This phase generally needs 20 to 40 participants.

Phase II of a trial is done on patients for which the test regimen may be eventually indicated. The objectives of this phase are to investigate potential efficacy in a clinical setup, short-term incidence of side-effects, identify a dose schedule for various kinds of cases (such as for mild, moderate, severe; or for children and adults), and to collect further pharmacologic data. Phase II trial could also compare drug induced effects in individuals with and without comorbidities or taking other drugs (in this phase there is no need to exclude such patients) that will help define exclusion criteria for phase III trial. Beware that comorbidities can skew and confound the drug effect. Do not restrict too much because generalisability would suffer.

Phase II also establishes or refutes that the new regimen is likely to meet at least the minimum level of efficacy. If this level is not met, there is no use of pursuing the regimen any further. Thus, this is also called 'proof of concept' phase. This is a crucial phase that really establishes that the regimen is going to be useful or not. The number of participants in this phase is generally 100 to 150. Sometimes it is a randomised trial with a control group on the pattern of a phase III trial. Failure of phase II helps in identifying the problems with the regimen and to go back to the basics to improve it.

Phase III is a large-scale trial to confirm the efficacy and safety that meets the regulatory standard of license. There must be a control group in this phase, and the subjects are randomly allocated to the **test arm** and **control arm**. For this reason, this is called a **Randomised Controlled Trial (RCT).** At least 300 subjects are recruited for each arm of this trial. The exact number depends on the statistical considerations described in a later chapter. The number can go upto several thousands. The follow-up must be sufficiently long in phase III for efficacy and side-effects to emerge, and to rule out that any relief to the patients is transient. It may take upto 10 years from start of phase I and finish of phase III. Phase III results are also used for preparing marketing and labelling information.

A very important research these days emanates from monitoring of side-effects of a drug after it is marketed. Patient preference due to cost, ease in ingestion, ready availability, etc., are also evaluated. This is called **postmarketing surveillance** and many times considered as **phase IV** of clinical trial. All adverse reactions or any such event attributable to long term use of regimen are monitored. This may be based on several thousands or millions of users. The effectiveness is also evaluated. Recent findings about tamoxifen carrying a risk of endometrial cancer, and arthroscopic surgery not beneficial for osteoarthritis of knee are the results partially attributable to such surveillance. Adverse drug reactions have started to gain prominence among causes of deaths in the U.S.

Randomisation

The difference in outcome can be legitimately ascribed to the intervention when the participants with and without intervention are equivalent to begin with.

Randomisation is the process by which the participants are allocated to receive one or the other treatment. It is a very potent tool to achieve equivalence and minimizes selection bias. Randomization insulates against biased allocation that can occur when the participants chose to be in a particular group. This works well for trials on a large number of participants but occasionally fails for small samples. If sample size is small, the best strategy is to identify pairs of participants **matched** for baseline characteristics, and randomly allocate one of each pair to the test arm and the other to the control arm.

Randomisation should be done with the help of random numbers so that there is no pattern. Methods such as alternation and even-odd date of birth are also applied but they can be misused. They are called **quasi-random allocations**. They may not actually bias the trial, but the intention is suspect, and is not advisable in a blinded trial as explained later. Some trials use nonrandom allocation for which the appropriate term is controlled trial because a control group is still present. Nonrandomised controlled trials are valid only when the test and control groups match for baseline characteristics.

In the wake of unaccounted variations and uncertainties, the best insurance of initial equivalence among the groups by far is randomisation, though this is not a guarantee. By giving equal opportunity to the subjects to be assigned to one group or the other, it is fair to expect that the unaccounted factors such as age, gender, and grade of disease, will be distributed nearly equally, thereby helping to achieve baseline homogeneity across groups. No group is likely to have participants of a particular type that can favour or go against the test regimen. Beware though that random allocation is not random sampling. The former is a strategy to achieve initial equivalence of the groups so that the difference emerging after the intervention can be legitimately ascribed to the intervention (internal validity). The latter is for representativeness of the target population so that the results can be generalised (external validity). The participants should closely mirror the target population.

If the number of available eligible subjects is large (say 4000) and a few (say 30, 40 and 45, in three groups) are to be randomly assigned to the three groups respectively, select 30+40+45 = 115 distinct random numbers. All these numbers should be less than or equal to 4000. The website *randomization.com* would do all this easily in a more adequate manner. In this example, the number of subjects in the groups is unequal but generally these numbers would be equal.

If the patients are consecutively attending a clinic, a systematic allocation beginning with assigning the first patient to a random group is easiest to implement. This works well when arrival of patients does not follow any specific pattern. Another method is to include all consecutive patients arriving between the pre-specified dates.

In large-scale trials, particularly in a community (see field trial later in this chapter), groups of participants such as schools or clinics are randomised instead of subjects. This is called **cluster randomisation**.

Random allocation can be open, so that concerned people know that they are randomised to which group. But the strategy of concealment of allocation is followed almost universally.

Random or nonrandom, effectiveness of allocation in achieving equivalence can be checked by post-hoc comparison of the participants in test and control groups. If there is appreciable difference, appropriate adjustments are made at the time of statistical analysis so that the net effect is obtained for valid comparison. A less realised importance of randomisation is that it provides a valid base for using statistical methods since these methods require random samples. Randomisation is not random sampling, yet it helps in providing a base to use statistical methods.

Blinding

An important method to minimise bias is blinding. When the patients do not know that they are receiving placebo or therapy then this is called **single blinding.** This eliminates the possibility of patients psychologically changing their response when they know that they are in the placebo group. They may feel discriminated against. Also, the patients who know that they are receiving a new regimen may either exhibit increased anxiety or may have favourable expectations. The objective of the trial is to assess the treatment effect and not the expectation of participants. Bias resulting from all these is called **Hawthorne effect.**

If the assessing physician also does not know that the patient belongs to the test group or the control group, this is called **double-blinding.** This removes possible bias of the physician in patient assessment — at least mitigates any subconscious influence of the assessor on the outcome such as tipping the patients as to what group they are in. Such blinding is an important criterion for validity of the results of a trial. Double-blind RCT is considered a "gold standard" to assess the efficacy of a new regimen. Sometimes the results are statistically evaluated without breaking the code for case and control group to eliminate statistician's bias. Then the trial is called **triple-blind.** The codes are broken after the analysis is over. In a broad sense, blinding is not merely concealment of allocation but also planning for similar handling of two groups so that this does not break until the results are available.

Although morality issues are attached to blinding because some information is withheld from the participants, but it has distinct scientific advantages. It not only reduces possible bias in the responses and assessments but in fact can improve compliance and retention of the subjects by clearly demonstrating that all are being treated alike. Merely stating in a protocol that blinding would be done is not enough. Give full details how the blinding is to be implemented including how the two groups would be assessed and handled similarly for medical maneuvers. The difference between the two should be only the active regimen, and nothing else that can possibly alter the outcome. If such details are not fully clarified in your report, the readers remain sceptical about bias reduction. They must be convinced that blinding was in effect until all opportunities for bias have passed.

Blinding is easily said than done. There are situations where blinding is not possible. For assessing the outcomes such as quality of life, readmissions, and falls after hip surgery, blinding is just not possible. If one maneuvre is keeping the patients in hospital for a specified number of days, and the other is early discharge and home rehabilitation, no blinding can be done. In most surgical interventions, control must be another kind of surgery, and not a 'placebo'. A sham surgery may be unethical because it exposes a patient to surgical risks. In either case, it is extremely difficult to enforce blinding in a surgical trial. The patient can be kept blind after proper consent, but the surgeon definitely knows. However, mechanism can be possibly developed that all assessments after the operations are done by another surgeon who does not know that the patient belongs to a test surgery or a control surgery.

Quasi-randomisation such as based on even and odd date of enrolment can easily break blinding if it is observed during the trial that certain effects or side-effects are occurring mostly in patients enrolled in even dates. This can happen with any systematic allocation. Thus, quasi-randomisation methods should not be used in a blinded trial.

Masking

Many times the term blinding is used to include masking but masking is apparent similarity of the regimens under trial and of the procedures followed during the trial. This is required for effective blinding. Top ingredient of masking is that the placebo or the control should have exactly same physical properties – packaging, labelling, handling, colour, size, shape, smell, and possibly taste – so that the patients or nurses are not able to distinguish, nor the physician who is assessing the outcome. The regimens must be administered in an undifferentiated fashion. If one regimen is once-a-day (OD) and the other is twice-a-day (BD), the OD group can be given placebo second dose to give an identical look. This provides an insurance against prejudiced response by the patients and prejudiced assessment by the investigators. The control subjects must pass through the same medical maneuvres in terms of physical and laboratory assessments, diet, change of wards or beds so that there is no scope: one, of deciphering the group to which the patient belongs and two, of biased response due to differential procedures. Masking is making arrangements that the identity of the groups does not break till the trial is over.

Control Group in a Clinical Trial

Controls are needed for fair comparison – like with like. Two kinds of controls can be identified. One is in the case of before-after trial or in repeated measures study where the baseline status of the subjects is used as control. In crossover trials also, the subject is its own control. The other is a separate group of subjects on control regimen. This is called **parallel control** although the term 'parallel' is many times dropped.

Controls are needed to realistically assess the difference brought about by intervention. They provide a yardstick against which the gains are measured. Parallel controls might match for baseline because of randomisation but it is also necessary that they be exposed to the same procedure and maneuvers as the cases.

In the case of a disease, ethics require that the controls be given existing proven therapy. There is always a question about using a placebo on patients who are known to have the disease because they need an active ingredient to cure their ailment. However, **placebo** can be used in the following situations.

1. No standard treatment is available, i.e., the existing treatment modality has very doubtful results—perhaps no better than placebo.
2. New evidence has emerged regarding the doubtful efficacy of the standard therapy.
3. The existing regimen is too costly or is rarely available to the population at large.
4. On patients who have already been given standard treatment and have not been benefited, and no second line of treatment is available for them.
5. The test regimen is add-on to the existing regimen. This means that all patients in the trial, including those on placebo, would receive the normally prescribed therapy any way.
6. Patients refuse to accept existing therapy and are willing to be part of a trial where they know that they can receive placebo.
7. Where for compelling, scientifically sound, methodological reasons, placebo-controlled group is necessary to determine the efficacy and safety of a regimen.
8. Where a regimen is being investigated for a minor condition and the patients who receive placebo will not be subject to any additional risk of serious or irreversible harm.
9. Where healthy controls serve the purpose such as for vaccine trials.

In situations where these conditions are not met, a group on existing therapy can serve as control. In any case, other provisions such as appropriate ethical and scientific review by a third party must be adhered to that would examine the validity of placebo in addition to the other aspects.

Sometimes randomisation is blamed for exposing some patient to an inferior or potentially hazardous substance. In fact, this is no fault of the method of randomisation but is due to wrong choice of the interventions. Including known inferior or harmful treatment itself is unethical. Placebo can be used only in restricted conditions as just enumerated, otherwise the control group receives the existing therapy. The motto "Do no harm" must be scrupulously followed in all medical research including clinical trials.

A control group studied alongwith the test group is called **concurrent control**, which could be on either existing regimen or on placebo. An apparently simple approach could be comparison of the group on new regimen with a group previously treated with an alternative regimen, called **historical control**. They must be similar subjects and on the same treatment with no alteration with the currently existing treatment. The flaw in this approach is that some factors may have changed over time such as diagnostic technology and profile of cases. Use this approach only after assuring that no such change has occurred. If a change has occurred, it should be properly accounted for in the interpretation of results.

In some situations, it is possible to give different treatment at the same time to known pairs such as two eyes or two limbs of the same persons. Twin studies also come under this category. Randomisation can be done within each pair to determine which one will receive test regimen and which control regimen. If the trial is on comparison of methods such as digital meter and mercury sphygmomanometer blood pressure readings can be taken at the same time in the two arms, and many pairs would be easily available. If the trial is for treatment regimen, it would be extremely difficult to find matched pairs such as equal severity of glaucoma in the two eyes, or both limbs with the same degree of paralysis.

EXAMPLE 5.5: A randomised controlled trial on nutritional supplementation for GIT cancer

In Italy (Gianotti et al. 2002), a total of 305 patients with preoperative weight loss <10% and cancer of the gastrointestinal tract was randomised to receive either preoperative artificial nutrition supplementation, or postoperative jejunal infusion (perioperative group), or no artificial nutrition (conventional group). There are three groups in this RCT including one control (conventional group).

Side note: The outcome variables were postoperative infections and length of hospital stay. Intention-to-treat analysis, and differences between the groups showed that preoperative supplementation was as effective as perioperative administration, and both strategies are superior to the conventional approach.

Superiority, Equivalence and Noninferiority Trials

Regular trials have objective to show that the test regimen has the minimum efficacy so that it can be adopted for larger use. In this case sampling error on either side is tolerated. The comparison could be with placebo or an existing regimen, but the objective is not to demonstrate superiority. A regimen is considered superior to the existing regimen if its performance exceeds by at least a prespecified margin. For example, if the existing regimen has 78% efficacy, you can specify that the new regimen must be at least 3% better and must have efficacy of 81% or more. If the efficacy is 80%, statistically significantly different from 78% or not, the test regimen is not considered superior.

Similarly, equivalence is different from statistically not significant difference. This also requires setting up a margin of clinical indifference within which the new regimen will be considered equivalent to the existing regimen. If the equivalence margin is ±2%, and the comparison is with a regimen with 78% efficacy, the new regimen should have efficacy confidence interval between 76% and 80%. Such equivalence is called **therapeutic equivalence** and is different from **bioequivalence** as the this is for the entire course of the disease regression from time to time. Therapeutic equivalence considers only the outcome in the end and not the course of disease.

More important these days is **noninferiority trial.** This also requires a preset margin within which noninferiority is concluded. If you set this margin as 3%, a regimen with efficacy of at least 75% would be considered noninferior to a regimen with 78% efficacy. This kind of trial is done for a regimen which otherwise is less expensive or more convenient, or more safe. If noninferiority is established, the noninferior regimen can be recommended for adoption since it is less expensive or more convenient or safe.

There are two challenges in these kinds of trials. First is setting up the margin of clinical indifference. This could be based on your expectation of random variations beyond human control, that could occur anyway, or your clinical assessment of what margin can be allowed without affecting patient management. If the features of new regimen are highly desirable, a bigger margin may be acceptable both to the physicians and to the patients.

The second challenge is the statistical. One, the analysis of such trials is in reverse gear where null hypothesis is of inequivalence instead of generally equal performance. This puts onus on the trial to show equivalence, superiority on noninferiority. Two, such trials require a larger sample because the margin of clinical indifference is generally small. Three, more care is required in conducting such trials since careless trial may unsuspectingly provide equivalence.

Also, the existing regimen under comparison must have established good efficacy. Equivalence can occur easily if both have poor performance. The same is true for superiority and noninferiority.

5.3.3 VALIDITY OF A CLINICAL TRIAL

Validity is the ability to provide correct answers to the questions under investigation. In the context of clinical trials, besides randomisation and other features of design as discussed, tools to achieve validity are proper selection of subjects, design, blinding, multiple measurements, compliance, and adequate reporting of results. Details of some of these are as follows.

Selection of Participants

Validity of results of a clinical trial depends heavily on proper selection of participants. They should really represent the target group. When an inordinately large number of eligible subjects are available that pass the inclusion and exclusion criteria, they must be randomly selected for inclusion in the trial. This allows generalisability. One method could be systematic (e.g., every fifth), and the second method is to include consecutive eligible patients arriving in a clinic/hospital within a specified period. Else random number can be used for selection.

Ethical considerations such as informed consent can preselect a biased group. Some patients or some clinicians may have strong preference for a particular therapy, and they can refuse randomisation. Some eligible patients may refuse to participate when they are told that they could be randomised for placebo or the existing therapy. Some may refuse because it is a trial and not treatment per se. Considerable efforts may be needed to keep such refusals to a minimum.

In addition, the groups should be such that there is a-priori uncertainty about the efficacy of the test therapy in them. This is called **patient equipoise** and helps to ensure that the patients are homogenous material. Another such term is **clinical equipoise** that is used for collective uncertainty among clinicians about the efficacy of the regimens under trial. (Published definitions of equipoise vary and often conflicting.) Ricotta and Piazza (2010) cites the example of carotid endarterectomy and carotid artery stenting for clinical equipoise although in their opinion these are complementary therapies. Clinical equipoise is the condition under which doctors would rationally accept randomisation for their patients. This also provides insurance against prejudiced assessment of the patients by the investigators.

Size of the Trial

The number of subjects should be reasonably large in each group so that full clinical spectrum is represented and a trend, if present, can clearly emerge. This also ensures reliability of the results. It should have adequate power (Chapter 11) to detect a minimum medically relevant difference.

Completely new treatment strategies such as Viagra are rarely discovered. Most trials are on variation of the existing modalities in the hope that some improvement in specific type of cases can be achieved. Additional benefit from such minorly different modalities is also likely to be small because the comparison is with the existing modality and not with placebo. Statistical power considerations tell that detection of small difference requires a large-sized trial. Trials involving thousands of patients are increasingly becoming norm. For comparing rtPA (altplase) and streptokinase for cardiovascular disorders, a trial on more than 40,000 patients was planned.

However, the size of the trials cannot continue to increase for ever. Large trials are expensive, difficult to manage, and run the risk of lacking uniformity. Insufficient availability of patient in one centre may force you to conduct **multicentric trial.** This is even more difficult to manage as centres may like to retain their freedom to adopt modification as per their wisdom. Thus, a balance is required. In addition, basic characteristics of cases such as food habits and nutrition level in different centres may differ that may confound the results. This can happen even when uniform eligibility criteria are followed.

For a **PG thesis,** the available time and expenses (such as for kits) limits the size of the trial. Rarely a thesis-based trial would involve more than 100 patients per arm. In many cases, only 30 cases and 30 controls are included. Less than these would not be adequate even for training purposes.

Compliance

Bias can still occur in subtle or unknown ways in an RCT despite random allocation and blinding. A major source of bias is loss to follow-up. If the follow-up requires recalling or revisiting the patients, some may not turn up or refuse to cooperate, some may be untraceable, and some could die from unrelated causes. Even if the outcome assessment is within the hospital stay, some can leave against medical advice. Another factor that could affect a clinical trial is the need to change the treatment modality mid-way if a patient develops a serious illness. Then there could be patients who did not follow the full regimen. This is called the partial compliance. Take pre-emptive steps to minimise such losses and plan to adjust the results if needed.

Realise that trials are generally done in ideal conditions that do not exist in practice. Thus, the actual performance may differ. **Efficacy** of a treatment is what is achieved in a trial that simulates ideal conditions, and **effectiveness** is what is achieved in practical conditions when the treatment is actually prescribed. For clarity, the latter is sometimes called the use-effectiveness. Effectiveness could be lower than efficacy because of lack of compliance of the regimen, inadequate care, nonavailability of drugs, etc., in practical situations. Experience suggests that nearly three-fourths of the patients do not adhere to or persist with prescriptions. Thus, the patients and maneuvers adopted during a trial do not lend the results to be generalised for patients at large. Generally, such external validity of the trials is not high. But properly conducted trials do establish the potency of a regimen to effect a change even when the participants are not representative such as due to consent, since the two groups are expected to be initially equivalent.

Effectiveness under practical conditions has brought **pragmatic trials** into focus. The patients recruited for this kind of trial are not homogeneous as in a regular clinical trial but reflect variations that occur in real clinical practice. Strategies such as randomisation and control are also not used. Because of many intervening factors in this setup, the interpretation could be difficult. Statistically, the standard deviation could be relatively large. For details of pragmatic trials, see Ford and Norrie (2016).

Another important aspect of compliance is participants intentionally flushing the drug (or placebo) in the toilet. If this is done for side effects, it certainly adds to the bias. The patient will hardly ever confess of doing so and this bias may never surface. Another instance of bias can arise if a patient occasionally takes double dose because he missed the previous one. A side effect may occur that otherwise would not if the prescription is adhered to, and the efficacy may also alter due to such aberrations. If there are few such patients, examine if these can be excluded as dropouts without affecting the validity of the trial.

Suppose two out of 500 randomized to receive placebo died of liver failure. You subsequently discover that these patients received the test drug due to an administrative error. You may have to be extra careful in a clinical trial that such errors do not occur and remain on guard while monitoring the administration process. If a lapse is found, the analysis will have to be geared to the new realities.

Another form of lack of compliance is when patients are switched from one group to the other as per their wishes.

Choosing a Design for a Trial

After describing so many types of design, it could be expedient to provide a guideline on choosing an appropriate design. The following describes the choices for experimental strategy in order of preference. Use the first type of design wherever feasible. If not, use the second. And so on.

- Whenever feasible, choose a random sample of subjects from the target population. Divide eligible subjects randomly into the test and control groups. Blind the subjects and the observers about allocation and make arrangements that this remains concealed until the results are available.
- If random selection is not possible, choose the available subjects that meet the inclusion and exclusion criteria and allocate them randomly to the test and control groups. Blinding is desirable wherever feasible.
- If random allocation is not feasible, match the cases and controls for their baseline characteristics. Use this strategy for small samples even if randomisation is feasible.
- If matching too is not feasible, use before-after strategy, i.e., assess the subjects before intervention and after intervention.
- If baseline information is difficult to assess, use existing information on baseline of another group of similar subjects.

Recommended Design to Answer Different Types of Questions

Recommended design for getting answer to different types of questions are as follows. This includes designs for observational studies as well.

Question	Recommended Design
1. What is the prevalence, or distribution of disease or a measurement, or what is the pathological, microbiological, and clinical profile of certain type of cases?	Sample survey
2. Whether two or more factors are related to one-another at a particular point of time?	Cross-sectional study
3. Whether two or more methods agree with one-another?	Cross-sectional study
4. What is the inherent goodness of a test in correctly detecting presence or absence of disease (sensitivity and specificity)?	Case-control study
5. What are the 'risk' factors for a given outcome, or what is their relative importance?	Case-control study
6. How good is a test or a procedure in predicting a disease or any other outcome?	Prospective study

Question	Recommended Design
7. What is the incidence of a disease, or what is its risk in a specified group, or the relative risk?	Prospective study
8. What are the sequalae of a pathologic condition?	Prospective study
9. Whether a particular factor is a cause or contributing to an outcome? – if the factor under study is potentially harmful animal experiment. – if the factor under study is potentially beneficial	 In rare situations, prospective study in humans Randomised controlled trial for humans, and experiment for animals or biologic material
10. Is an intervention really effective or more effective than the other?	Randomised controlled trial for humans, and experiment for animals or biologic material

Reporting Results of a Trial – CONSORT Statement

A good trial such as an RCT must also be reported in a format that could be appreciated by the readers. In view of the significance of such reporting, CONsolidated Standards Of Reporting Trials (CONSORT) have been formulated, which are revised from time to time. The basic features of these standards are the same as already stated, namely, report of the trial should indicate why the study was undertaken, should include scientific background and explanation of rationale, structured review of all pertinent literature not leaving out the opposite view, allocation of subjects and blinding, transparency regarding analytic methods including for missing data, noncompliance, etc. The revised CONSORT statement is designed to help minimize confusion and promote clarity in reporting the methods and results. This comprises 22-item checklist and a flow diagram to help ensure clear reporting of key elements of clinical trials. The objective is to achieve complete transparency. Empirical evidence suggests that not reporting complete information is associated with biased estimates. Also, such information is considered essential to judge the reliability or relevance of findings. The flow diagram depicts the passage of participants from enrolment to intervention allocation, follow-up, and analysis. Also see Chapter 13 for some more tips on how to prepare a report of an investigation. Trials that conclude that the regimen under test is not better than the existing or control are called **negative trials**. Their reporting is equally important so that other researchers do not waste resources on trying such a regimen. BioMed Central has a Journal of Negative Results in Biomedicine specifically for such trials.

Two additional points need attention. First, if interim analysis has been done, mention it explicitly including what changes, if any, were made and how the statistical results were adjusted to account for this. Second, if there is a switch over of patients from one group to the other, whether intention-to-treat analysis was done or per protocol – along with the justification.

Clinical Trials Registry

Many international medical journals now require that a trial must be registered in a freely accessible clinical trials registry. There are many such registries including one in India managed by Indian Council of Medical Research (ICMR). Registration requires certain minimum information such as the objective, details of the regimen, number of participants, process of allocation and variables under investigation. You must have all the information about the trial before proceeding to register. Among advantages of registration is that the trial can be tracked for any deviation from the protocol, whether the results published or not, etc.

5.3.4 PROPHYLACTIC AND FIELD TRIALS

Field trial is yet another form of experiment where a section of population receives some intervention. This could be for a screening procedure but generally is a prophylactic trial where population can be really involved. It could be for an agent or a procedure that promotes health or controls primordial factors. For example, a segment of population may be given iron-fortified salt and the other, equivalent segment, the usual salt. The outcome of interest could be increase in Hb level relative to the baseline. Such a trial can help to identify specific age-gender group that is most benefited, if any. Randomisation of individuals may be difficult in this setup but once equivalent *groups* are identified, they could be cluster-randomised to receive either test regimen or the placebo. Then this becomes nearly equivalent to an RCT. Such a trial may be required to evaluate efficacy of a new vaccine. For a prophylactic drug, such as aspirin to reduce cardiovascular disease, the participants must be those who are at risk for such a disease. For example, young adults may have to be excluded from such a trial.

There is a general impression that a prophylactic trial must be a field trial. This is not necessarily true. There are many procedures that are prophylactic but are tried or used in a clinic. For example, Bohner et al. (2002) report a randomised trial on prophylactic nasal continuous positive airway pressure after major vascular surgery. Another example is amnioinfusion for meconium-stained amniotic fluid in labour at the time of childbirth.

A prophylactic trial could be for a preventive strategy also such as life-style changes for coronary diseases or a vaccine as already stated or could be for vitamins—even drugs — that are stipulated to prevent occurrence or recurrence of adverse events. Giving vitamin A supplementation to infants and young children to improve their retinol level is an example of such an intervention. Although there is a fine distinction between preventive and prophylactic measures, we are including both into prophylactic category.

EXAMPLE 5.6: A field trial of vitamin A supplementation

A randomised double-blind placebo-controlled trial was conducted on children in villages of Tamil Nadu (India) by giving 100,000 IU of vitamin A to children less than one year and 200,000 IU to children one year and above (upto 3 years) three times in a year 4 months apart (Ramakrishnan et al. 1995). The other group received placebo. The outcomes of interest were diarrhoea and respiratory illness in terms of percent time ill, incidence and mean duration per episode, assessed by weekly visits. After adjustment for confounders such as age, gender, nutrition status, and economic status, they did not find any significant difference in the common morbidity in these two groups. The trial was conducted in an area where a growth monitoring research project was going on—thus the access to health care and immunisation was good. In such an area, vitamin A supplementation was not found effective in reducing common morbidities in children.

5.4 VARIETIES OF BIAS TO GUARD AGAINST

Bias occurs when something is preferred or done over the other for reasons that have nothing to do with the inherent quality of either. This can be intentional or unintentional.

Medical research results often become clouded because some bias is detected after the results are available. All biases are nasty, and you should know what to do about them. It is important that all sources of bias are considered at the time of planning, and all efforts are made to control them. Bias control is essential for achieving internal and external validity of results. Various potential sources of bias are as follows. These are not mutually exclusive sources. In fact, the overlap is substantial. Some of the biases in this list are collection of many biases of similar type. If we state all these separately, the list may become unmanageable.

1. **Bias in concepts** — Lack of clarity about the concepts that are to be used in the proposed research. This gives an opportunity to the investigators to use subjective interpretation that can vary from person to person. Sometimes the logic used can be faulty and sometimes the premise itself of the logic can be incorrect. For example, the concept of treatment of a disease is sometimes confused with the management of a patient.
2. **Definition bias** — The study subjects should be sharply defined so that there is no room for ambiguity. For example, if the cases are of tuberculosis of lung, specify that these would be sputum positive, Montoux positive, radiologically established, or some combination. Blurred definition gives room to the assessor to use subjective interpretation that can affect the validity of the study.
3. **Bias in design** — This bias occurs when the case group and control group are not properly matched, and the confounding factors are not properly accounted for at the time of analysis. Concato et al. (2001) reports another type of bias in designs for prostate cancer detection when groups were asymptomatic men who received digital rectal examination, screening by prostate specific antigen and transrectal ultrasound, but there was no 'control' group with 'no screening'. Thus, the effectiveness of screening could not be evaluated.
4. **Bias in selection of subjects** — This occurs when the subjects included in the study are not truly representative of the target population. This can happen either because the sampling was not random, or because sample size is too small to represent the entire spectrum of subjects in the target population. Studies on volunteers always have this kind of bias. Selection bias can also occur because the serious cases have already died and are not available with the same frequency as the mild cases (**survival bias**). Survival bias is common in studies based on old age patients. See also Length bias.
5. **Bias due to concomitant medication or concurrent disease** — Selected patients may suffer from other apparently unrelated condition, but their response might differ either because of this condition itself or because of medication given concurrently for that condition.
6. **Instruction bias** — When unclear or no instructions are prepared, the investigators use discretion and this can vary from person to person, and from time to time.
7. **Length bias** — A case-control study is generally based on prevalent cases rather than incident cases. Prevalence is dominated by those who survive for a longer duration. And these patients are qualitatively different from those who die early. Thus, the sample may include disproportionately more of those who are healthier and survive longer. The conclusions cannot be generalised to those

who have less survival time. Cross-sectional studies also suffer from this bias for conditions that are rapidly fatal.

8. **Bias in detection of cases** — Error in the diagnostic or screening criteria, e.g., being able to use a laboratory investigation properly in the hospital setting but not in the field setting where the study is to be actually done. In a prostate cancer detection study if prostate biopsies were not performed in men with normal test results, true sensitivity and specificity of the test cannot be determined.
9. **'Lead-time' bias** — All cases are not detected at the same stage of the disease. In cancers, some may be detected at the time of screening such as by pap smear, and some may be detected when the disease has started clinical manifestation. But the follow-up is generally from the time of detection. This difference in 'lead-time' can cause systematic error in the results.
10. **Bias due to confounder** — Failure to take proper care of the confounders so that any difference or association cannot be fully ascribed to the antecedent factors under study.
11. **Contamination in controls** — Control subjects are generally those that receive placebo or the usual therapy. If these subjects are in their homes, it is difficult to know if they have received some therapy that can affect their status as a control. In the prostate cancer detection project reported by Concato et al. (2001) and discussed in preceding paragraphs, the controls subjects are those who are under usual care. But some of these may be screened outside the study and treated. Thus, their survival rate would not be sufficiently 'pure' to be compared with the survival of those who were screened by the test procedures. In a field situation, contamination in control group occurs if it is in close proximity of the unblinded test group and learns from their experience. The neighbouring area may not be the test area of the research, but some other program may be going on there that has spill-over effect on the control area.
12. **Berkson's bias** — Hospital cases when compared to hospital controls can have bias if the exposure increases the chance of admission. Thus, cases in a hospital will have disproportionately higher number of subjects with that exposure. Cases of injury in motor vehicle accidents have this kind of bias.
13. **Bias in ascertainment or assessment** — Once the subjects are identified, it is possible that more care is exercised by the investigators for cases than for controls. This can also occur when subjects belonging to a particular social group have records, but others have to depend on recall. Sometimes this is also called **information bias**.

14. **Interviewer bias or observer bias** — Interviewer bias occurs when one can elicit better response from one kind of patients (say, those who are educated) relative to the other kind (such as illiterates). Observer bias occurs when the observer unwittingly (or even intentionally) exercises more care about one type of responses or measurements such as those supporting a particular hypothesis than those opposing this hypothesis. Observer bias can also occur if he is, for example, not fully alert in hearing Korotkoff sounds while measuring blood pressure or not being able to properly rotate endoscope to get an all-round view of, say, duodenum in a suspected case of peptic ulcer.
15. **Instrument bias** — This occurs when the measuring instrument is not properly calibrated. A scale may be biased to give a higher reading than actual, or lower than actual. The other possibility is inadequacy of an instrument to provide complete picture such as endoscope not reaching to the site of interest and giving false information from a distance.
16. **Hawthorne effect** — If a subject knows that he is being observed or being investigated, his behaviour and response can change. In fact, this is the basis of including a placebo group in a trial. Usual responses of subjects are not the same as when under a scanner.
17. **Recall bias** — There are two types of recall bias. One, arising from better recall of recent events than those occurring long time ago. Also, serious episodes are easy to recall than the mild episodes. Two, cases suffering from disease can recall events much more easily than the controls if they are currently healthy subjects.
18. **Response bias** — Cases with serious illness are likely to give more correct responses regarding history and current ailments compared to the controls. Some patients such as those of STDs may intentionally suppress sexual history and other information because of stigma attached to these diseases. Injury history may be distorted to avoid legal consequences. If the subjects can exchange notes, the response to questions might alter, in some cases might even be uniform. An unsuspecting illness, death in the family, or any such drastic event may produce an extreme response. Response bias also comes under **information bias**.
19. **Repeat testing bias** — In a pretest-posttest situation, the subjects tend to remember some of the previous questions, and they may remove previous errors in posttest—thus do better without the effect of the intervention. Observer may acquire expertise second or third time to elicit correct response. Conversely fatigue may set in repeat testing that could alter the response. It is widely believed that most biological measurements have strong tendency towards

mean. Extremely high scorers tend to perform lower in subsequent testing, and extremely low scorers tend to do better in a subsequent test.

20. **Mid-course bias** – Sometimes the subjects after enrolment have to be excluded if they develop an unrelated condition such as injury or become so serious that their continuation in the trial is no longer in the interest of the patient. If a new facility such as a health centre is started or closed for the population being observed for a study, the response may alter. An unexpected event such as an outbreak can alter the response of those who are not affected.

21. **Self-improvement effect** – Many diseases are self-limiting. Improvement over time occurs irrespective of the intervention, and it may be partially or fully unnecessarily ascribed to the intervention. Diseases such as arthritis and asthma have natural periods of remission that may look like the effect of therapy.

22. **Digit preference** – It is well known that almost all of us have special love for digits 0 and 5. Measurements are more frequently recorded ending with these digits. A person of age 69 or 71 is very likely to report his age 70 years. Another manifestation of digit preference is in forming intervals for quantitative data. Blood glucose level categories would be 70-79, 80-89, 90-99, etc., and not like 64-71, 72-79, etc. If digit zero is preferred, 88, 89, 90, 91 and 92 can be recorded as 90. Thus, intervals such as 88-92, 93-97 and 98-102, are better to ameliorate the effect of digit preference, and not the conventional 85-89, 90-94, 95-99, etc.

23. **Bias due to nonresponse** – Some subjects refuse to cooperate, injure, die, or become untraceable. In a prospective study, there might be some dropouts for various reasons. Nonrespondents make two types of effects on the responses. First, they are generally different from those who respond, and their exclusion can lead to biased result. Second, nonresponse reduces the sample size that can decrease the power of the study to detect clinically relevant differences or associations.

24. **Attrition bias** – Differential nonresponse can occur in different groups. The pattern of nonresponse can differ from one group to the other in the sense that in one group more severe cases drop out whereas in another group mostly mild cases drop out.

25. **Bias in handling outliers** – No objective rule is available to label a value as outlier except a guideline that the value must be far away from the mainstream values. If the duration from HIV infection to development of AIDS is mostly between 6 and 10 years, some researchers would call 18 years as outlier and exclude it on the suspicion of being wrong reporting, and some would include in their calculation. Some would not exclude any outlier, even if very different. Thus, the results would vary.

26. **Recording bias** — Two types of errors can occur in recording. One arising due to inability to properly decipher the writing on case sheets. Physicians are notorious for illegible writing. This can happen particularly with similar looking digits such as 1 and 7, and 3 and 5. Thus, the data entry may be in error. Second is due to carelessness of the investigator. A diastolic level of 87 can be wrongly recorded as 78, or a code 4 entered as 5 when the dependence is on memory that can fail to recall the correct code.
27. **Bias in analysis** — This again can be of two types. First, gearing the analysis to support a particular hypothesis. For example, while comparing pre- and post- values such as Hb level before and after weekly supplementation of iron, the increase may be small that will not be detected by comparison of means. But it may be detected when evaluated as proportion of subjects with level <10 mg/dl before and after supplementation. Second can arise due to differential *P*-values. When $P = 0.055$, one researcher can straight refuse to say that it is significant at 0.05 level and the other can say that it is marginally significant. Some researchers may change the level of significance from 5 percent to 10 percent if the result is to their liking.
28. **Bias due to lack of power** — Statistical tests are almost invariably used to check the significance of differences or associations. The power of these tests to detect difference or association depends to a large extent on the number of subjects included in the study—the sample size. If the study is conducted on small sample, even a big difference cannot be detected, leading to a false negative conclusion. When conducted on an appropriate number of subjects, the conclusion can change.
29. **Interpretation bias** — The tendency among some research workers is to interpret the results in favour of a particular hypothesis ignoring the opposite evidence. This can be intentional or unintentional.
30. **Reporting bias** — Researchers are human beings. Some can create a report such that it gives a premonitioned result yet based on evidence. It is easy to suppress the contradictory evidence by not talking about it.
31. **Bias in presentation of results** — Scale for a graph can be chosen to depict a small change look like a big change, or vice-versa. The second is that the researcher may merely state the inconvenient findings that contradict the main conclusion but does not highlight them in the same way as the favourable findings.
32. **Publication bias** — Many journals are much too keen to publish reports that give a positive result regarding efficacy of a new regimen, compared to the negative trials that did not find any difference. If a 'vote count' is done based

on the published reports, positive results would hugely outscore the negative results, although the fact may be just the reverse.

The purpose of describing various types of bias in so much detail is to create awareness to avoid them. Some biases are more severe than others and tend to completely invalidate the findings. They have the same role as an off-side in a hockey game where goal is not counted if an opposition player is off-side. All efforts go waste. Thus, make all efforts at least to minimize them. Some of the steps to minimise bias are listed below.

Steps for Minimising Bias

Following steps can be suggested to minimise bias in the results. All steps do not apply to all the situations. Adopt the ones that apply to your setup.

1. Develop an unbiased scientific temperament by realising that research is relentless search for truth.
2. Specify the problem to the minutest detail.
3. Assess the validity of the identified target population, and the groups to be included in the study in the context of objectives and the methodology.
4. Assess the validity of antecedents and outcomes for providing correct answer to the research questions. Beware of epistemic uncertainties arising from limitation of knowledge.
5. Evaluate the reliability and validity of the measurements required to assess the antecedents and outcomes, as also of the other tools you plan to deploy.
6. Carry out a pilot study and pretest the tools. Make changes as needed.
7. Identify all possible confounding factors and other sources of bias and develop an appropriate design that can take care of most of these biases if not all.
8. Choose a representative sample, preferably by random method.
9. Choose an adequate size of sample in each group.
10. Train yourself and coworkers in making correct assessments.
11. Use matching, blinding, masking, and random allocation as needed.
12. Monitor each stage of research, including periodic check of the data.
13. Minimise nonresponse and partial response.
14. Double check the data and cleanse it of errors in recording, entries, etc.
15. Analyse the data with proper statistical methods. Use standardised or adjusted rates where needed, do the stratified analysis, or use mathematical models such as regression to take care of biases that could not be ruled out by design.

16. Interpret the results in an objective manner based on evidence.
17. Report only the evidence based the results – enthusiastically but dispassionately.
18. Exercise extreme care in drafting the report and keep comments or opinions separate from the results.

Bias and other aspects of design can be very adequately taken care of if you could imagine presenting the results a couple of years hence to a critical but friendly audience (Elwood 2002). Consider what your colleagues could question or advise at that time, consider their reaction when you conclude that the results are significant or not significant. Can there be noncausal explanations of the results? Are there any confounding factors that have been missed? Whether chance or sampling error could be an explanation? Such consideration will help you to develop a proper design, and to conduct the study in an upright manner.

SUMMARY

Credibility of research depends, to a considerable extent, on adopting a proper design. This is the pattern, scheme, or plan to collect evidence. A design is considered good if it can give valid and reliable results quickly with least cost. Among other things, validity of results depends on proper accounting of biases including those arising from confounders. Strategies such as matching, randomisation, and blinding are helpful in enhancing the validity of results. Reliability is achieved by replication or by including a sufficiently large sample.

Basic objective of a medical study is either description such as delineation of a problem, or to analyse associations including cause-effects. The strategy used for descriptive studies is in terms of complete enumeration (census) or a sampling scheme, or a study of a case series.

The strategy used for analytical studies is either experiment or observation. The former requires introducing a deliberate intervention, and the latter is observing the natural course of events without intervention. Observational study could be prospective, retrospective, or cross-sectional, depending respectively upon that the investigation is from antecedent to outcome, outcome to antecedent, or both together. Each has its own merits and demerits. Laboratory based experiments are done either on biological material or on animals. Human experiments can be clinic based or can be conducted in a community setup. A clinic based human experiment is called a clinical trial. This requires extreme care and is done in phases. All-important is the third phase—randomised controlled trial—that provides adequate evidence for safety and efficacy of a new regimen. All studies require strict control of various biases as listed in this chapter.

REFERENCES

Bohner H, Kindgen-Milles D, Grust A, et al. Prophylactic nasal continuous positive airway pressure after major vascular surgery: results of a prospective randomized trial. Langenbecks Arch Surg 2002;387:21-26.

Concato J, Peduzzi P, Kamina A, Horwitz RI. A nested case-control study of the effectiveness of screening for prostate cancer: research design. J Clin Epidemiol 2001;54:558-564.

Elwood M. Forward projection—using critical appraisal in the design of studies. Int J Epidemiol 2002;31:1071-1073.

Ford I, Norrie J. Pragmatic trials. New Eng j Med 2016;375;454-463.

Friedman LM, Furberg CD, De Mets DL. Fudamentals of Clinical Trials, 4th ed. Springer, 2010.

Gianotti L, Braga M, Nespoli L, Radaelli G, Beneduce A, Di Carlo V. A randomized controlled trial of preoperative oral supplementation with a specialized diet in patients with gastrointestinal cancer. Gastroenterology 2002;122:1763-1770.

Green BN, Johnson CD. How to write a case report for publications. J Chiropr Med 2006;5:72-82.

Hilska M, Gronroos J, Collan Y, Laato M. Surgically treated adenocarcinomas of the right side of the colon during a ten-year period: a retrospective study. Ann Chir Gynaecol 2001;90 (Suppl215):45-49.

Korkeila J, Salminen JK, Hiekkanen H, Selokangas RK. Use of antidepressants and suicide rate in Finland: an ecological study. J Clin Psychiatry 2007;68:505-511.

Lukanova A, Toniolo P, Lundin E, et al. Body mass index in relation to ovarian cancer: a multi-centre nested case-control study. Int J Cancer 2002;99:603-608.

Lwin H, Yokoyama T, Date C, Yoshiike N, Kokubo Y, Tanaka H. Are the associations between life-style related factors and plasma total homocysteine concentration different according to polymorphism of 5, 10-methylenetetrahydrofolate reductase gene (C677T MTHFR)? A cross-section study in a Japanese rural population. J Epidemiol 2002;12:126-135.

Nguyen QD, Shah SM, Hafiz G, et al. A phase I trial of an IV-administered vascular endothelial growth factor trap for treatment in patients with choroidal neovasculari-zation due to age-related macular degeneration. Ophthamol 2006;113:1522e1-1522e14.

Ramakrishnan U, Latham MC, Abel MC, Abel R, Frongillo EA Jr. Vitamin A supplementation and morbidity among preschool children in south India. Am J Clin Nutr 1995;61:1295-1303.

Richards M, Hardy R, Kuh D, Wadsworth MEJ. Birthweight, postnatal growth and cognitive function in a national UK birth cohort. Int J Epidemiol 2002;31:342-348.

Ricotta JJ 2nd, Piazza M. Carotid endarterectomy or carotid artery stenting? Matching the patient to the intervention. Perspect Vasc Surg Endovasc Ther 2010;22:124-136.

Sun A, Wang J, Zhu P. How to use progestin in hormone replacement therapy: an animal experiment. Chin Med J (Engl) 2001;114:173-177.

CHAPTER 6

How to Take a Sample for the Study

KEY TERMS AND CONCEPTS

- ✓ Nonrandom and Random Sampling
- ✓ Sampling for Descriptive Studies
- ✓ Simple, Stratified, Systematic, Cluster and Multistage Sampling
- ✓ Sampling and Nonsampling Errors
- ✓ Determination of Sample Size

Medical decisions are almost invariably based on samples. *Sample* of blood, urine, sputum, and stool; and biopsies, are everyday occurrences. Sampling is the only feasible method in this situation since complete material of these biological entities cannot be extracted. A sample of blood from anywhere in the body gives nearly the same picture as from anywhere else because it is so thoroughly mixed inside the body. Yet repeat investigations are not uncommon. Biopsy results in many cases are not reliable, and some other form of confirmation becomes necessary. Sampling results are always interpreted with caution.

The thrust in this chapter is on sample of individuals. Whether the research is descriptive or analytical, it is conducted on a sample of subjects. *Sample is the statistical term for the group of subjects included in the study, which almost invariably would be a fraction of the target population.* Sample studies are not only cost-effective and quick but many times more reliable also because more accurate methods and better care can be exercised for a small group. Even if resources can be garnered to study all the existing cases of, say, glaucoma in the world, it would still be incomplete because the cases arising in future cannot be studied. And medical empiricism requires that the findings on existing cases be used on the future cases! Sampling is a prerequisite for this paradigm. However, if the objective is to find the prevalence of diabetes mellitus in the year 2022 among females of age 40 years and above residing in a particular city, complete enumeration is possible. If a complete registry of cancer cases in a defined population is available, perhaps sampling is not needed for assessing the *existing* situation.

Not that sampling has no disadvantage. It can create a feeling of discrimination when sample subjects get a different treatment or differential attention than the others. Sometimes explanation is necessary to dispel the feeling of discrimination. Samples can fail to provide valid results when they are not representative and can fail to provide reliable results if the size is small.

There are two dimensions of adequacy of a sample. First, it should represent the full spectrum of subjects in the target population. Various methods of sampling are adopted in different situations to meet this objective. These methods are discussed in Section 6.1 for descriptive studies and in Section 6.2 for analytical studies. A preview is given below. Some of these methods do not provide a representative sample. Second, the sample size must be reasonably large to give reliable results, without being excessively large. Size also has a role in its ability to represent a cross-section of the population for not missing an effect when present. Sample size is discussed in Section 6.4. In between in Section 6.3 is a discussion on nonsampling errors in contrast to sampling errors. Controlling nonsampling errors many times assumes importance because these also have potential to vitiate the results beyond redemption just as sampling errors have.

A Preview of the Main Sampling Methods

Purposive (Nonrandom)

- Volunteers, who agree to participate
- Snowball, where one case identifies others of his kind (e.g., intravenous drug users)
- Convenient cases such as captive medical students or other readily available groups

- Quota, with at-will selection of fixed number from each group
- Referred cases, who may be under pressure to participate
- Haphazard, with combination of above methods

Random

- Simple, that gives equal chance to all the individuals (as in lottery): consecutive cases arriving in a clinic can also be considered random when there is no bias
- Stratified, that requires separate random samples from relevant subgroups (strata) to ensure adequate representation of each subgroup such as age and gender
- Systematic, where first individual is selected at random and others follow at regular intervals
- Selection of cluster of subjects, or area sample, where blocks of cases are selected
- Multistage, wherein nested samples are successively selected within the larger units selected earlier
- Probability proportional to size, where larger units have more chance of selection—gives self-weighting scheme for statistical purposes

6.1 SAMPLING FOR DESCRIPTIVE STUDIES

The previous chapter listed sample survey, case-series, and census as the three strategies of descriptive studies. Last two do not involve any sampling. Census is complete enumeration of all individuals without leaving out anyone, and case-series is done on available subjects without recourse to sampling.

Dominant format of descriptive studies is **sample survey**. This term is generally used for a population-based study, but technically descriptive studies done on clinic subjects are also surveys. Main feature of a survey is that a selected section of the target population is investigated instead of the whole population with the objective of understanding and describing the characteristics of the population such as the prevalence rate of a health condition, its distribution in different segments of the population, and what is more common or less common and where. Study of profile of cases of a particular disease also comes under descriptive category. Cause-effect type of relationship or even association between an antecedent and outcome is not the objective of a survey. In fact, no characteristic is identified as antecedent or outcome in a survey. Sometimes surveys are done at periodic intervals in the same target population to assess trend. These are called **serial surveys**.

The term 'population' is used differently in different contexts. Statistically the term **population** is used for the whole group of units of interest to which the findings would extrapolate. More specifically, this is called the target population or target group. This could be healthy children in an area, pregnant women who register in an antenatal clinic, patients of renal disease reporting in a group of hospitals, blood units received as donation in an area, etc. This chapter is focused on individuals although other types of units such as biopsy specimens and antigens can also be studied for profiling.

Sample studies do need to make a distinction between a **unit of sampling** and a unit of enquiry. The latter is also called a **unit of study**. In a population-based study on diarrhoeas, it is possible that the ultimate unit of sampling is a family, but the unit of study could be all the children in the family, or the most recent episode of diarrhoea in the family. One unit of sampling can have two or more units of study although generally there would be only one. List of all sampling units in the target population is called **sampling frame.**

Because of profound variations mentioned in Chapter 1, it is important for validity of results of a survey that the sample of subjects included in the study is truly representative of the target population. This is especially important for descriptive studies. Representativeness depends on the method of selection as much as the size of the sample. Among the methods of selection, the following are more commonly used in medical research.

6.1.1 PURPOSIVE SAMPLING (NONRANDOM SAMPLING)

When enough of eligible subjects are not willing to cooperate in a research, **volunteers** are used. This is a purposive sample. The other possibility is to use those subjects that are easily and captively available. Many studies are done on medical students or medical professionals. This is a **convenience sample**. Another method is **snowball sampling.** This is used for obscure group of people. In this case, one eligible person such as Intravenous Drug User (IVDU) is identified, and his help is taken to identify others he knows. Then those are asked to identify others known to them. Otherwise IVDUs are so obscure that their detection and sampling is difficult. Patients **referred** to a clinic also are a nonrandom sampling. In **quota sampling,** a prespecified number of subjects is selected from various segments of population without recourse to random selection. Sometimes a mix of these procedures is followed. This is called **haphazard sampling**.

Nonrandom samples have two basic problems. First is that the larger group they represent is difficult to identify and may not match with the intended target group. This is not a limitation when generalisation of results is not required. The results would be valid for the sample itself, and they can provide useful clues for further studies that can be based on random samples. Second problem is that the statistical inference such as confidence interval and test of significance requires random sample. These methods cannot be applied on nonrandom samples. It is sometimes pretended for a clearly nonrandom sample that it is random and statistical inferences for a larger group are made. This is statistically inadmissible and can be dangerous in some situations. Yet the more important question should be whether the sample is representative of the target population or not. Randomisation is the means but representativeness is the goal (Chatfield 2002). When nonrandom samples are representative, generalisation should be possible. Practical experience suggests though that nonrandom samples are seldom representative of the target population.

6.1.2 RANDOM SAMPLING

When the sample size is adequate, basic feature that provides reasonable assurance of representativeness is random selection. This essentially means that each individual is given some chance of being included. *These chances across subjects may or may not be equal.*

What is Random and Why Random?

Random is a term that excites some and depresses others. Lottery outcome is a random event. Anything unpredictable is random. Age at death for a healthy person of age 45 years is a random event although the chance of death before age 70 years may be much less than chances of death between 70 and 95 years. *Random events can have unequal chance.* Inclusion of subjects in random sampling depends on chance and not on choice. The purpose of random sampling is to eliminate bias. This kind of sampling is expected to provide a truly representative sample, particularly if it is adequate in terms of its size. The chance that any particular group is over-represented or under-represented is minimal. Also, random samples provide a valid base for use of statistical procedures because these procedures are based on random samples.

Simple Random Sampling

When the list of sampling units (called the **sampling frame**) in the target population is available or can be prepared in a manner that each unit is assigned a number, the best statistical strategy is to use random numbers to select the sample that provides equal chance to all the units (see Example 6.1). This is called **Simple Random Sampling** (SRS), or just random sampling in short, and gives an unbiased sample. Also see Figure 6-1a. Out of 200 units in this figure, the selected 20 are shown by dots.

EXAMPLE 6.1: Simple random sampling

For illustration, consider random selection of five individuals from a total of 60 attending a Nowhere clinic. Assign them numbers from 01 to 60. The highest is 60, which is a two-digit number. Thus two-digit random numbers are required for selection. Computer can easily generate such numbers. Suppose these are as given below. Start from any random point. In this case, say number 38. Go in any predetermined direction. In the usual sequence, the first five distinct random numbers less than or equal to 60 are 38, 09, 17, 41, and 25. Individuals bearing these numbers constitute an SRS of size five out of 60. Alternatively, computer programmes (e.g., randomization.com) are available that would select five random numbers out of 60, or as many needed.

Two-digit random numbers

77	03	56	41	47	
89	60	77	74	38	← Random Start
09	17	41	78	38	
25	97	32	76	69	
28	01	35	67	90	
83	95	55	42	24	

Simple random sampling is easy when the total population is fixed and not large. In a field study, such as on hypertension in young adults in a community, the target population could be large, and it may be difficult to prepare a sampling frame. A large sample may be required and drawing a large SRS can be a tedious process. Also, in a field study, SRS may yield a sample of subjects that are located in far flung areas causing inconvenience in field work and increasing the cost and time requirements. SRS also ignores considerations such as age and gender that might be important factors influencing the parameter under study. It is possible that SRS under-represents or over-represents a particular group. For ensuring adequate representation of such groups, the best option is stratified sampling. This is described next.

Stratified Random Sampling

If factors such as age, gender and obesity are important, divide (stratify) the population by these factors where feasible and draw separate independent samples from each group using SRS method. This is called **Stratified Random Sampling** (StRS). This method of sampling ensures that all relevant groups are adequately represented. This strategy is very effective to ensure adequate representation of, for example, rare cases which otherwise would not be well-represented. The sampling frame in Figure 6-1a is divided into four strata and shown in Figure 6-1b. See Figure 6-1a carefully and note that no unit is selected from rows 8, 9, and 10 in SRS that happen to constitute second stratum in Figure 6-1b. Stratified sampling ensures that such under-representation (or over-representation) does not occur. Example 6.2 illustrates application of this method to a study of blood pressure in different groups. For a field study, stratification could be by location or areas or social groups, or any other such relevant factor.

EXAMPLE 6.2: Stratified random sampling to study BP in relation to age

Normal Blood Pressure (BP) levels are severely affected by age besides other factors. In a study to delineate normal levels in adults, it is helpful to divide them into age-groups such as 20-29, 30-39, 40-49 years, etc., and draw independent simple random samples from each age-group. Such StRS would ensure that all relevant age-groups are adequately represented in the sample.

If a central representative value such as mean is needed for all age-groups combined in a StRS, the age-specific mean is multiplied by the *population* of that age, added across age-groups and then divided by the total population.

StRS is feasible only when the sampling frame for each stratum is available or can be constructed. This requirement can be a severe constraint in many practical situations. In addition, information on the stratifying characteristic is also needed for each unit.

Strata may or may not be equal. In case of unequal strata, proportionate sample from different strata is preferable. In Figure 6-1b, the strata are unequal, and a 10 percent sample is taken across strata. If a stratum is of size 30, a sample of three units is taken and if the size is 60 a sample of six units is taken. However, proportionate sampling is not mandatory. When not proportionate, the chance of different units for being in the sample is not same although the method is still random.

Systematic Random Sampling

An easy alternative to SRS is the systematic method. If there are N subjects in the target population out of which n are to be included in the study, the **sampling fraction** is 1 in k where $k = N/n$. If this is not an integer, take the integer part of this number. If $N = 350$ subjects of liver cirrhosis are expected in a clinic in a year's time, and $n = 40$ are to be selected, then k = integer part of 350/40 = 8. Select one randomly out of first 8, and the others are automatically selected adding 8 every time. If the first randomly selected subject is 7, others are 15, 23, 31, etc., in this example. See Figure 6-1c for a schematic depiction of this method with sampling fraction 0.10.

Systematic Random Sampling (SyRS) is easy to implement in a clinic-based study where the patients come in a sequence. This method does not require a full sampling frame as needed for SRS but requires information about the total number of subjects in the target population. If the total number of subjects is not known, it is still possible to systematically select, say, five percent sample, by continuing to select one-in-twenty till the end of the frame is reached. However, in this case the sample size cannot be fixed in advance. If you want a fixed sample size, say 30, select one in five from first

150. An application of systematic sample with fixed size in a clinical set-up is in Example 6.3.

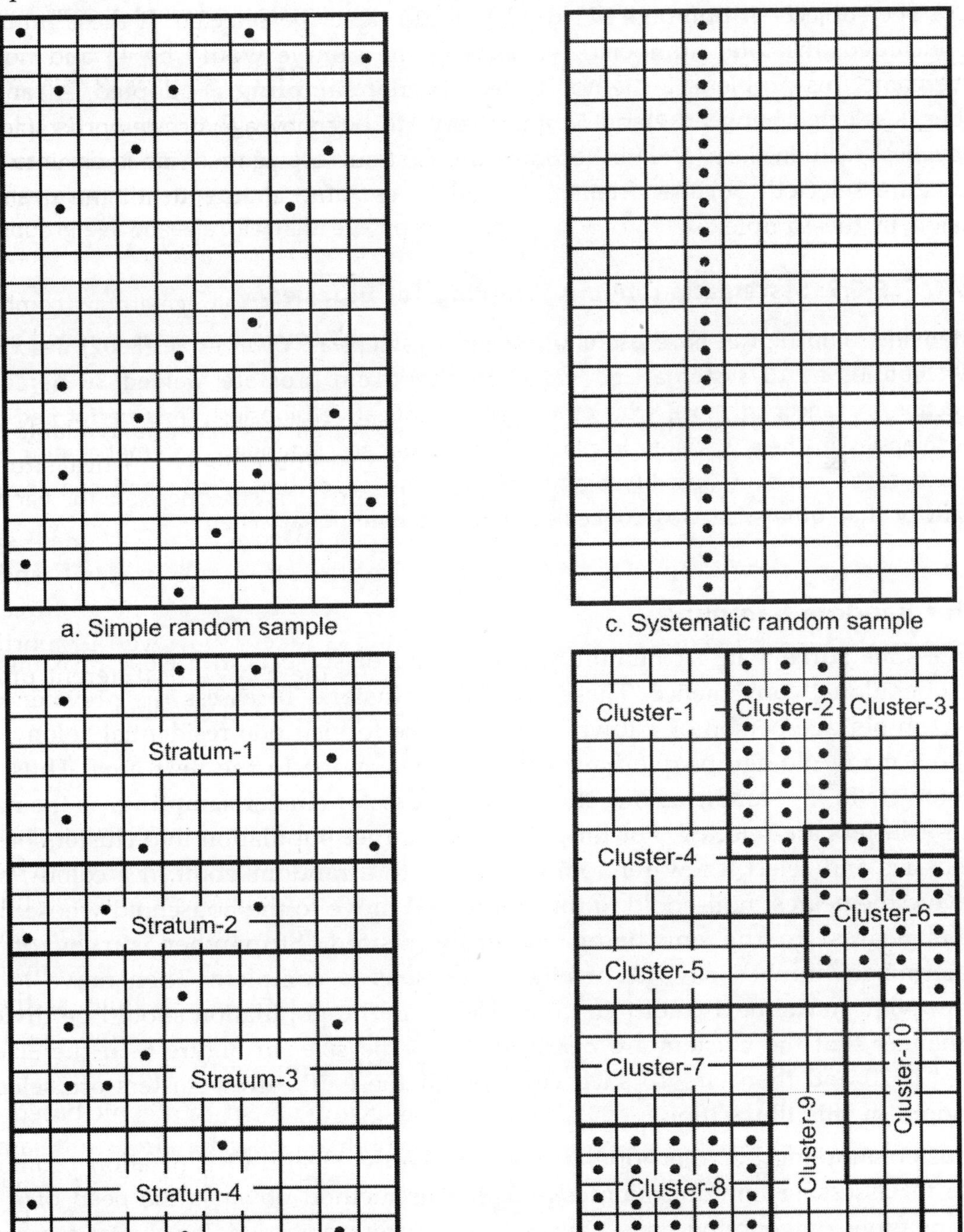

a. Simple random sample

b. Stratified random sample

c. Systematic random sample

d. Cluster random sample

FIGURE 6-1: Graphical presentation of four methods of random sampling

One difficulty with SyRS is that some subjects at the end of the list may never get selected. In the example of selecting 40 out of 350, the last number in selection would be 320. The subjects at numbers 321 to 350 would never be selected. If these numbers were included, the total number of subjects in the sample would be 43 and not 40. To overcome this problem, a method called **circular sampling** is adopted. A random number is selected between 1 and *N*, and every *k*th beginning that number is selected in a cyclical fashion, i.e., (*N*+1)th becomes the first subject again. This is done until *n* subjects are selected. Such a circular method gives same chance to all the units for inclusion in the sample.

EXAMPLE 6.3: Systematic random sampling for biopsies

Systematic sampling can have useful application in biopsies. Chon et al. (2002) describe how biopsies at 10 systematically selected sites from prostate yielded 36 percent detection of cancer in those who otherwise had negative biopsies. They performed 10 core biopsies in these patients in place of the usual six. Extended systematic sampling in such cases removes possible bias in picking the exact biopsy site and can reveal positivity that otherwise was concealed in the conventional scheme.

Cluster Random Sampling

In large-scale surveys in a community, availability of subjects in a close proximity is a big operational convenience. These are called **clusters**. To assess the prevalence of cataract in old age person of a town, you may like to visit one residential colony and find how many old-age people have cataract, then move to the next area. Thus, the full colony is in the sample as one cluster. In the case of **cluster sampling,** as the name implies, clusters are selected. For this, divide the target population into clusters of any desired size and select a few randomly. Else, go to a random point in a colony, start surveying the nearest household to this point, and move to the household whose front door is nearest to the one being currently visited. Stop when survey of the predetermined number, say 40, of eligible persons is complete. Then move to the random point in the next colony in your selection. The population should be divided in a manner that the clusters are nearly of the same size. In Figure 6-1d the size of clusters is 20 and there are 10 such clusters. Of these 10, three clusters are selected at random in this illustration.

Cluster sampling became popular after the World Health Organization promoted its use for assessing immunisation coverage. This method obviates the need of a full sampling frame of the individuals. Only a list of clusters is needed. If a cluster comprises all patients admitted in intensive care unit of a hospital on a particular day or of a particular specialty, only the list of hospitals is needed, and not of patients. This is a substantial logistic advantage in addition to convenience of getting a group of subjects together at one place.

EXAMPLE 6.4: Cluster random sampling for assessing immunisation coverage

Most prominent use of cluster sampling has been in estimation of immunisation coverage in children between one and two years of age in a population. The scheme envisages 30 clusters containing 7 children each residing in contiguous houses. This is known as **30×7 methodology.** Clusters are selected randomly, which are generally villages or enumeration blocks. In case of unequal clusters, they are selected with probability proportional to size that gives better chance to bigger clusters. This scheme provides estimate of percent of children immunized within ±10% when it is anticipated that nearly half the children are immunised.

30×7 methodology described in Example 6.4 has been used in a variety of setups, although without justification in many cases. Even for immunization coverage assessment, this methodology has lost relevance as the coverage has reached 80-90 percent in most developing countries. This methodology was based on anticipated 50 percent coverage. Nonetheless, the example illustrates the broader cluster sampling methodology that remains valid for large scale surveys.

Since persons within clusters tend to be more alike than between clusters (called **design effect**), this method requires that a larger size of sample is chosen relative to the SRS so that full spectrum of persons is represented. In Figure 6-1d, a cluster sample of size 60 is selected (three clusters of size 20 each) whereas in Figure 6-1a, a simple random sample of size 20 is selected. Three times the size may compensate for the design effect.

Multistage Random Sampling

For extremely large-scale surveys covering a full State or a full country, it is desirable that the sampling is done in stages. Select few districts randomly and then few Primary Health Centre (PHC) areas within each selected district, few villages within each selected PHC area, and few families or target individuals within each selected village. This way a relatively small sample can represent the entire population. An application is in Example 6.5. Instead of the entire sampling frame, this strategy requires only the frame of nested units that are to be selected in successive stages. Some sections of literature describe it as multistage cluster sampling, which is an erroneous label. This is another example of a method that does not give equal chance to the units but is still random.

EXAMPLE 6.5: Multistage random sampling for estimating he prevalence of obesity

Lemamsha et al. (2019) used multistage random sampling to estimate the prevalence of obesity in Libya. They selected 5 parliament constituencies randomly out 11 in Benghazi, one polling district out of each of the selected constituency and then the households by systematic sampling.

Probability Proportional to Size (PPS) Sampling

Although the details are not provided in this text, the method of estimation of a summary measure such as prevalence rate of a disease in a population depends heavily on the sampling method. Bigger strata and bigger units at different stages in multistage method must be given proportionate weight at the time of estimation. A self-weighting mechanism is to select units with probability proportional to size. Bigger units are given a better chance of selection. This is called **Probability Proportional to Size** (PPS) sampling.

EXAMPLE 6.6: PPS sampling for a study on relation of lipoprotein(a) with lipoprotein profile and anthropometric measurements

Chu et al. (2000) report that lipoprotein profile, and not anthropometric measurements, correlate with serum lipoprotein(a) values in Taipei children. They used a probability-proportional-to-size multistage sampling procedure to select 1500 students from 10 schools in Taipei city to come to this conclusion.

Other Methods of Random Sampling

The methods described in the preceding paragraphs are standard textbook methods. The situation where each is appropriate is given next. In practice, it may be convenient to include all eligible subjects that come to a clinic beginning a specific date and terminate the sampling when a predetermined size is reached. This is called **consecutive sampling**. This would provide a random sample so long as all subjects meeting the preset criteria are included and special conditions such as epidemic do not exist that can alter the basic character. This is a form of **inverse sampling** that is randomly done in sequence one by one till such time that the requisite number of subjects meeting the preset criteria is available. If you are looking for 30 males of oesophagus cancer in a cancer clinic, you go on till such time that these many are included. This method does not require knowledge of the sampling frame.

In a community study, if sampling frame is not easily available, one method is **area sampling** whereby defined areas such as colonies or blocks are randomly selected, and all eligible individuals in the selected areas form the sample. This is nearly the same as cluster sampling. The sampling frame of colonies or blocks or a map is required to execute this type of sampling. Another method, although not so popular in medicine, is **sequential sampling**. In this method, the eligible subjects from the defined target are selected one by one in a random manner and assessed. Further sampling is stopped as soon as a reliable result one way or the other is available.

For further details of the types of popular sample designs and most of the methods described in preceding paragraphs, see Indrayan and Malhotra (2018).

Where to Use Which Sampling Method?

The preferred sampling method is always SRS unless it is difficult to adopt. The estimate provided by SRS is generally the most precise. Some problems with this method are:

- non-availability of sampling frame,
- too dispersed subjects in the sample making the approach difficult,
- less representation of specific groups that are important and must be adequately represented, and
- obtaining so many distinct random numbers.

The first two problems can be handled by either cluster or multistage sampling. The answer to the third is stratified, and the remedy of the fourth is systematic sampling because it requires only one random number. Systematic method does not require the full frame also. In any case, with wide availability of computers, generating distinct random numbers is not a problem.

6.2 SAMPLING FOR ANALYTICAL STUDIES

Primary objective of an analytical study is to assess the relationship between prespecified antecedents and outcomes. This can be either an observational study (prospective; retrospective; or cross-sectional) or an experimental study (laboratory experiment or clinical trial). Sampling methods for such studies can be explained as follows.

6.2.1 SAMPLING METHODS IN OBSERVATIONAL STUDIES

Since observational studies do not involve any man-made intervention, it is relatively easy to adopt a random sampling scheme. This could be any of the six schemes discussed in the previous sections, or a new one can be generated in the context of the study.

Sampling Methods for Cross-sectional Studies

Validity of conclusions regarding association of two or more factors depends on their proper representation in the sample in proportion of their presence in the target population. Random sampling serves as a great facilitator to achieve such representation. Assessment of indicators such as sensitivity-specificity and predictivities is adversely affected if these proportions are biased in any manner. Thus, random sampling is especially important for cross-sectional studies.

The first step for sampling for a cross-sectional study is, as usual, to identify the target population to which the results would generalise. Then decide which sampling method would be appropriate. For age-gender related disease such as hypertension and diabetes, stratification by age and gender might be useful. For a community-based study in a large population, a multistage sampling involving selection of districts, villages/municipalities, and households can be adopted, or a cluster sampling might be more convenient. In a clinic setup, where subjects come in a queue one after the other, systematic sampling could be appropriate.

Sampling Methods for Prospective and Retrospective Studies

Random sampling is not so important for prospective and retrospective studies as for cross-sectional studies and descriptive surveys. At the same time, these studies too involve estimation of parameters such as incidence rate, Relative Risk (RR), and Odds Ratio (OR), finding Confidence Interval (CI) for them, and testing of hypothesis on them. These statistical procedures do require a random sample of the subjects. Whenever feasible, indeed a random sample should be taken. For example, to assess incidence and course of psychiatric disorders in a large population, a multistage cluster random sampling involving selection of states, districts, PHC areas/local body areas, villages/colonies, and cluster of families can be adopted. This would be a prospective study with follow-up, say, at 12 months and 36 months. See Example 6.7 for a nested case-control study that uses stratified sampling to assess the effect of serum selenium levels on cancer mortality.

EXAMPLE 6.7: Stratified sample for a nested case-control study

Serum selenium level is widely suspected to affect cancer mortality. But the results across studies are not coherent. Belgium has a system to follow each patient till death. A stratified (for gender – male and female) random sample of 201 cancer deaths of age 25-74 years out of a total of 343 during a 10-year period was studied for their selenium level as well as some other factors (Kornitzer et al. 2004).

Side note: Three controls were selected for each case and these were matched for age and gender. Thus, a total of 603 controls were also studied. Serum selenium level was found to be a significant predictor of cancer mortality in males but not in females.

In Example 6.7 gender-stratification of the subjects helped to come up with a conclusion that is different for males than for females. Thus, the stratification strategy paid well in this case. Also note that the investigations are from outcome (cancer death) to an antecedent (serum selenium level) and thus the study is retrospective in nature. Since controls were also investigated, it is a case-control study. It is nested because follow-up of each person is routinely done in Belgium and cases are chosen from this follow-up. Controls were easily available and choosing three controls per case helped to increase the reliability of results without corresponding cost.

On the flip side is the sample of 201 cancer deaths out of 343 and the claim that it is a random sample. Such 60 percent sample is not a norm: One can legitimately wonder why all 343 could not be included in the study. Had all these been investigated, it would still be a sample in the sense that they occurred in a specific 10-year period. Previous deaths and future deaths would still be not incorporated.

Both prospective and retrospective studies are much more useful when a comparison group is available. This group provides basis for calculating relative risk and odds ratio. In most practical situations, the comparison group is properly matched for baseline characteristics so that any difference can be safely ascribed to the factor under study. Consecutive individuals meeting the criteria can be selected. If the study is on the relationship of blood group with dengue haemorrahagic fever, other factors such as nutrition level that can affect susceptibility and Aedes density in the areas wherefrom the patients are coming that can affect quantum of infection should be the same in the cases and controls. When such baseline equivalence is assured, randomness of the sample has a limited role. Many good prospective and retrospective studies are done on nonrandom samples. At the same time, we reemphasise that random samples should be taken wherever feasible so that the external validity remains firm.

Sometimes consecutive cases attending a particular clinic within a specified period are included in the study. This procedure simulates random selection when the subjects come without preference for the study period. However, cases coming to a clinic on particular days such as on Tuesdays and Fridays may not be random because only specific type of cases may be seen in special clinics on those days, or because a particular specialist is available in those days. This causes self-selection.

6.2.2 SAMPLING METHODS IN EXPERIMENTS AND TRIALS

An essential feature of experiments and trials is human intervention. This raises ethical issues and thus random sampling may not be feasible in some situations.

Sampling Methods in Laboratory Experiments

Laboratory experiments on animals do not raise much concern about sampling methods. Generally experimental animals of one species are chosen and they can be easily considered as representative of their 'population'. However, whenever factors such as age, gender, and weight can affect findings, the animals should be either stratified for independent experiment on each stratum, or only one particular stratum of animals be investigated. For example, to study the effect of middle turbination resection on facial growth of rabbits, the animals must be of same age. For telomerase activity, which is implicated in all immortalisation and carcinogenesis, age and gender of rats are important because they affect the level of this activity. Also. in this case the strain (Sprague-Dawley, Wistar, Donru, etc.) of rats can affect the findings. Thus, separate experiments should be done in samples of rats of different strains.

Experiments on biological material such as blood specimen, vaginal swabs, and antigen are also common. If each specimen is identified and linked with a known person, the situation is back to sampling of individuals. For these the same methods as described earlier should be followed. For experiments on anonymous unlinked biological specimen, think about the possible sources of bias that can inhibit generalisation to a larger group. The specimen must represent the full spectrum of material in the target population. Whenever several specimens are available, choose a random sample of them. However, in practice, this is rarely done. Because an experiment necessarily involves an intervention, baseline equivalence of the test and control group is generally considered sufficient for validity of the results with a rider that the results are valid under laboratory conditions. Randomness of sampling in such situations has a limited role. Instead, randomness of allocation is required.

Sampling in Clinical Trials

As mentioned in a previous chapter, first phase of a clinical trial is generally done on volunteers that by nature are nonrandom. Second phase is also many times done on nonrandom sample of subjects. If it is on random sample, the following comments for third phase apply to the second phase also.

The third phase as much as possible should be done on randomly selected patients such as every fifth (SyRS) reporting in a clinic. But the requirement of consent can make it difficult to adopt such sampling. Patients agreeing to participate generally form a biased sample. If many patients with consent are available, a random sample can be taken that will minimise *further* bias. If not, a reasonably valid trial can still be carried out by random division of subjects in two or more groups and allocating them to the control and treatment groups. Though not fully, such random allocation largely takes care of the statistical requirement and helps in achieving baseline equivalence across groups. When other sources of bias as mentioned in a previous chapter are under control, the results are considered valid for those among the target group that give consent. This validity again is due to baseline equivalence of groups that allows ascribing any emerging difference to the intervention or treatment. However, the results are always interpreted with caution. They are obtained in 'ideal' clinical trial conditions and not in usual clinical practice conditions under which treatments are carried out. Thus, efficacy is correctly evaluated but effectiveness in practical conditions remains unanswered.

EXAMPLE 6.8: Random sample of control subjects but not of the cases in a trial

Abnormal mammogram can cause anxiety in some women that possibly need help. Barton et al. (2004) performed a trial in the US to evaluate the effect of an educational intervention that taught the skills to cope with anxiety. The subjects were women of age 39 years or older in seven mammography sites who came for screening. Of 8543 such women, 1439 had abnormal mammogram. These were included in the trial. A random sample of 1405 women was also taken from the remaining 7104 women with normal mammogram. Thus, these control subjects may not be matched for baseline characteristics such as age. The authors possibly expected that the age may not affect the response or expected that age structure of the controls will not be much different from that of the cases.

Side note: Subsequent investigations in subjects with abnormal mammogram showed that many of these were false positive. The authors concluded that immediate reading of mammograms was associated with less anxiety than educational intervention targeting coping skills because many were in fact false positives.

6.3 SAMPLING AND NONSAMPLING ERRORS

So-called sampling error actually is not an error. This term is used for variation across samples when repeated samples are taken. The result obtained by one sample, in all likelihood, will not be the same as on the basis of another sample from the same population. This variation is better understood as sampling fluctuation although statistically called **sampling error.** Note that this is endogenous to the investigation. On the other hand, nonsampling error is indeed an error that arises from misreporting, misjudgment, misrecording, nonresponse, etc. This is exogenous in nature. This section explains some methods to manage these two types of errors.

6.3.1 SAMPLING ERRORS

Samples by themselves are a great source of uncertainty. Yet sampling is considered a preferred strategy in most situations because of the advantages enumerated earlier. Statistical methods help in reaching to a conclusion regarding a population parameter based on just one sample. Sampling error is managed as follows.

Point Estimate

In descriptive studies, sample mean and sample proportion do provide a reasonable idea of the mean and proportion in the corresponding target population. As usual, this 'reasonability' is assessed in terms of validity and reliability. When the sample subjects represent the full spectrum of population, which is likely if one of the random methods described earlier is followed and if the sample size is reasonably large, sample mean and sample proportion are indeed valid **point estimates.** That is, they are unbiased in the sense of being able to reach to the corresponding population value when the sample size is increased, and fairly stable across samples. This statement has two underlying assumptions. First, the mean or proportion is calculated after due consideration of varying group size as can happen in the case of stratified sampling. Second, the data obtained from the sample subjects are correct, i.e., no wrong data are reported or recorded.

In analytical studies, the relative risk (RR) and odds ratio (OR) sort of summary measures based on samples are also considered a fair reflection of the true status in the population provided again that the samples are true representative. This holds for experiments and trials also.

Standard Error of an Estimate

Reliability of sample summary measures such as mean, proportion, RR and OR, is assessed by, what is called, their Standard Error (SE). SEs are also used to obtain Confidence Intervals (CIs) as discussed in Chapter 11. To understand SE, realise that samples too differ from one another—thus, mean or proportion based on one sample would be different from the ones based on another sample. This variability in summaries across samples is assessed by their SE. The size of the sample, n, is in the denominator of all SEs. The implication is that larger samples have smaller SEs. Intuition also says that large samples would not differ from one another as much as small samples would do. The other situation giving small SE for not so small sample is when the subjects themselves are homogeneous so that the variation (measured by SD) among them is small.

A large SE implies unreliable results. This could render all the efforts and time a waste. There is no way to retrieve this unfortunate situation, except by increasing the sample size. It is unethical too to expose subjects to such small-sized investigation that is not likely to produce reliable result. Thus, exercise care and conduct a study on an appropriate sample size. Determine the size by using the methods given in the next section. However, a pilot study is done on a small sample.

6.3.2 NONSAMPLING ERRORS

Samples would differ from one another no matter what you do but the nonsampling errors can be controlled—perhaps eliminated. Main sources of nonsampling errors are already stated in the previous chapters but we would like to remind them in this new context. They may arise at the time of designing, use of tools, measurement process, interviews, examinations, analysis of data, reporting of findings, etc. Most researchers do not assess or report nonsampling errors although these errors may have major influence on validity of their results. Whereas sampling errors can be directly quantified and calculated by using statistical formulae, nonsampling errors have to be only empirically guessed by using techniques such as reassessment, comparison with otherwise expected response, internal consistency checks, and replication. Ingenious method may have to be devised to measure them as illustrated in Example 6.9.

EXAMPLE 6.9: Nonsampling errors in a health interview survey in Sierra Leone

Nonsampling errors can be best illustrated by varying responses in surveys when repeat interviews are done. Evidence is provided by Fabricant and Harpham (1993), who described results of a health interview survey in Sierra Leone. Repeat interviews were conducted in 15 percent households of 1156 in the original sample. Reinterviews were done by another person after a lapse of less than one hour to overnight.

Errors in reporting of age of the ill person in the household were assessed by four indicators. (i) **Gross error rate** in the proportion of responses in reinterview that differed from the original responses. When the respondent in the two interviews was same, this error was 3.4 percent in case of adult ill-persons but 15.4 percent for ages 6-15 years. (ii) **Net bias** is the difference between proportions of answers in a particular *category*. The sum of the net biases for all response categories of each question equals zero. This was 10.8 percent for adults and –1.3 percent for children of age 1-5 years. (iii) **Relative net bias** is the net bias expressed as percentage of the proportion of the responses in the reinterview category. This was –1.1 percent for adults and -10.9 percent of children of age 1-5 years. (iv) **Mean error** in reporting of exact age (in completed years) of the ill person. This was not high because some reported higher and some lower age. All these indicators were calculated separately for those also where the respondents at two occasions were different and higher error rates were observed for them as expected.

Side note: The authors rightly comment that the interval between interviews in this study was short. Thus, a deliberate wrong reporting may have replicated and not detected. Also, the respondents may have remembered what they said earlier. In most cases, the errors seem to arise because the respondent guessed the age of the ill person and the guess differed at the reinterview.

This example is for the reporting of age of the ill person in the family. Reporting of many other variables was also assessed. Highest error rates were observed for severity of illness, reasons for choosing nonmedical treatment by those who did, and level of expenditure on treatment. This gives an idea of what kind of questions can have different responses on different occasions.

Biases

Main source of nonsampling error is bias. There is a big list of biases in the previous chapter. Any of them has potential to distort the results but the more common ones are design bias, confounding bias, ascertainment or assessment bias, response bias, and bias due to lack of power. Take care of these and other biases so that the results are not suspected.

Nonresponse

Although nonresponse is also included in our list of sources of biases in Section 5.4, this needs special mention in the context of nonsampling errors. As stated earlier, nonresponse has two types of adverse impact on the results. First is that the ultimate sample size available to draw conclusions reduces, and this adversely affects the reliability of the results. This deficiency can be remedied by increasing the sample size corresponding to the anticipated nonresponse. Second, more serious, is that the nonresponding subjects are not random component but are of specific type such as seriously ill cases who do not want to be a part of the study, or very mild cases who opt out after feeling better, or some such segment. Their exclusion can severely bias the results. A way out is to take a subsample of the nonrespondents and make intensive efforts for their full participation. Assess how these subsample subjects are different from the regular respondents and adjust the results accordingly. Provision for such extra efforts to elicit response from some nonrespondents should be made at the time of planning of the study.

Experience suggests that some researchers fail to distinguish between nonrespopnse and zero value or characteristic absent. Take care that this does not happen in your data

6.4 DETERMINATION OF SAMPLE SIZE FOR MEDICAL RESEARCH

'How large should be the sample?' is among the most asked questions in empirical research. It should be neither too small nor too large. *Conducting a study on inadequate number of subjects may be unethical because the persons are unnecessarily subjected to an investigation that is not likely to produce result either way due to limitation of its size. All the efforts and time also go waste.* A small sample is rarely able to represent the full cross-section of the population. Thus, small *n* is luxurious in most situations. The best-executed study may fail to answer the research questions if the sample size is too small. A sample of 200 for measles vaccine with 200 controls is doomed from start to have no meaning — both groups may not develop any case. At the same time, an exceedingly large sample is also wastage of resources when reliable conclusions can be drawn on the basis a smaller sample. Besides resources, it is unethical to expose unnecessarily large number of people with compromised health to an investigation when a smaller sample can provide conclusive results. If a trial on a few patients can tell you that a new chemotherapy regimen is ineffective, why try it on a large number of patients? A very big study is hard to execute and should be avoided as much as possible (Figure 6-2) unless it is multicentric. What is the right size of sample?

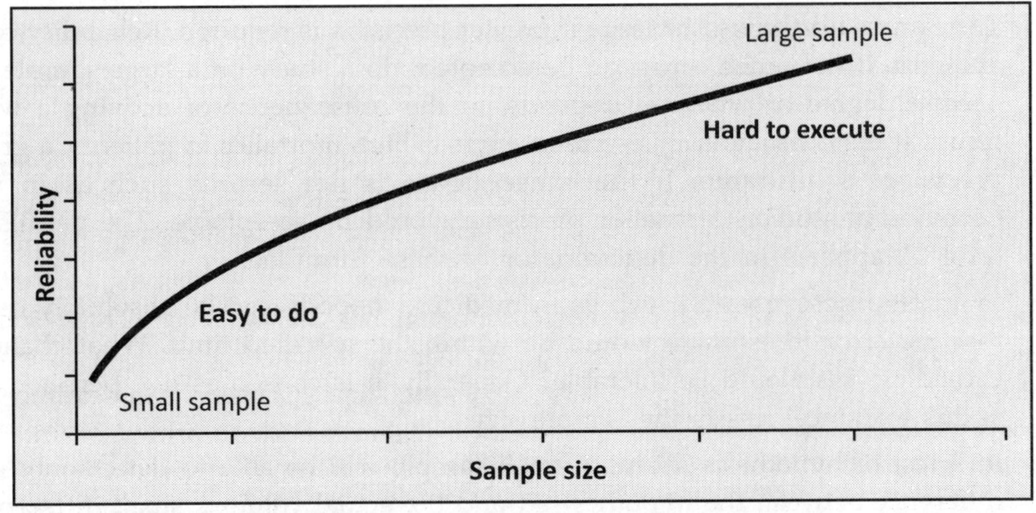

FIGURE 6-2: Sample size and reliability of results

The right number of subjects in different groups depends on a variety of considerations such as interindividual variability, chances of error in conclusions that can be tolerated, the difference aimed to be detected, confidence level desired in the results, anticipated nonresponse, etc. For example, it is easy to imagine that a small difference is difficult to detect and a big sample is required for small difference to show up. Also, if the values have high variability, detection is difficult unless a large sample is available. The general principles are given next. The formulae given later require an understanding of the concepts of level of confidence (denoted by $1 - \alpha$), level of significance (denoted by α), and power (denoted by $1 - \beta$). These concepts are explained in later chapters. We are taking liberty to use them in this chapter on sampling in the hope that the reference would be made to later chapters by those who need to understand these concepts.

General Principles of Determining Size of Sample

- The sample size should be large when the variation (SD) in the quantitative measurement of interest is large among subjects in the target population, or when the proportion (p) of subjects with the characteristic of interest is small. This sounds intuitive also.
- It is legitimate to ask as to how to know about the variation or the proportion even before the study is done. If these are known, what is the use of the study at all? This is a well-known paradox for which the most common solution is to look for a *previous study* in a similar setup. If no such study is available, the only option is to carry out a pilot study and use preliminary results to calculate the final sample size.
- The sample size would be large if greater precision is required. Reliability comes at a cost. If not much error can be accepted, do a study on a large sample. The needed degree of precision depends on the consequence of arriving a wrong result. If the consequence is serious, such as high mortality in patients, a greater precision is desirable. If the consequence is not serious such as in most behavioural studies, a smaller precision would be acceptable. The permissible error, d, appears in the denominator of these formulae.
- In an empirical research such as in medicine, nobody can be absolutely certain that the error in estimate would be within the specified limit. What chance of exceeding this would be tolerable? Generally, it is chosen as five percent. High is this tolerance, less is the sample size.
- In a test of hypothesis setup, a small sample will be able to detect only a big difference between the hypothesised and the actual value. A small difference is likely to be missed. If the comparison is between an existing treatment and a new treatment, or between an existing diagnostic modality and a new one, even a small difference could be important in this age of technology when big gains

are rare. For this set-up, a larger sample is a prerequisite. But outrageously large sample would unnecessarily find a small and medically irrelevant difference as statistically significant.

- Although ignored in most practical situations, the sample size also depends on the sampling distribution of the summary measure under study. The formulae in Annex 1 assume that this distribution is Gaussian. This would be so, or nearly so, when the sample size is large. These formulae do not apply when the anticipated sample size is small.
- The sample size also depends on the sampling scheme of the proposed descriptive study. The formulae in Annex 1 are valid for simple random sampling only. An adjustment is required for other sampling procedures. For example, if the proposed method is cluster sampling, the required sample size could be double or even more depending on how similar subjects within the clusters are. This multiplier is the same that was earlier called the design effect.
- An upward revision of sample size is generally made to incorporate possible attrition. Nonresponse is a regular phenomenon in empirical studies that can reduce the actual sample with available data to an unacceptably low level. Thus, inflate your sample size accordingly.
- Notice that the calculation of sample size is based on some prior information about the summary measure such as SD (s) and proportion (p). As already mentioned, these are the anticipated values based on previous studies or a pilot study. These priors may or may not be exactly applicable to the actual situation. Thus, inflate the sample size to some extent to incorporate this uncertainty also. Generally, inflation by a factor of 10 percent is recommended.
- Sample size requirement increases as the number of covariates under study increases.

6.4.1 SAMPLE SIZE FOR DESCRIPTIVE STUDIES (SAMPLE SURVEYS)

Primary objective of a descriptive study is to estimate a particular population parameter with a specified precision. This characteristic could be the mean of a quantitative measurement such as average homocysteine level among nonvegetarian adults, or a proportion such as the percentage of postmenopausal women who happen to have breast cancer. Sometimes a descriptive study is done to test a hypothesis that a mean or a proportion has some specified premonition value or not. General principles just enunciated demystify the process and should be intuitively appealing to those who have quantitative thinking—mainly that a larger sample implies smaller margin of error in conclusions. The statistical formulae for determining the sample size for descriptive studies in different setups are in Annex 1 at the end of this chapter.

As stated earlier, sampling is not applicable to census because that is a complete enumeration. Most case-series studies do not extrapolate results to any target population. Their results are tentative and indicative. Thus, sample size is not a relevant issue for case-series. It is always a convenience sample. This leaves only sample survey format of descriptive study for sample size consideration.

Sample size calculation for estimating a proportion requires some explanation. This could be the proportion of subjects of a particular type or a chance of occurrence of a particular event. Two kinds of formulae are available for this parameter. One uses **absolute precision** and the other **relative precision**. When absolute precision is used, the sample size is maximum for anticipated $p = 0.50$, where p is the proportion in the target population. Absolute precision is specified, for example, as ±5 percent or ±0.05, which for $p = 0.50$ implies that the sample providing estimate between 0.45 and 0.55 is acceptable. If $p = 0.06$, precision ±0.05 gives a range of 0.01 to 0.11. Relative to the small value of p, this range is too large. If prevalence of tuberculosis in a particular population is six percent and the sample estimate is anywhere between 1 and 11 percent, practically nothing is achieved. Such low precision can be a result of a small sample. Thus, precision for a proportion should be stated in terms of relative value such as 10 percent of p. Ten percent of $p = 0.50$ is 0.05 and of $p = 0.06$ is 0.006. Much larger sample size is required for such precision in anticipated small p.

EXAMPLE 6.10: Too large sample in a descriptive study on prescribing pattern of drugs for osteoarthritis and rheumatoid arthritis

Schnitzer et al. (2003) studied prescribing patterns of rofecoxib and celecoxib in 47,935 patients of osteoarthritis (OA) and 10,639 patients of rheumatoid arthritis (RA) in the US. The most frequently prescribed daily dose of rofecoxib was found to be 25 mg in both OA and RA but the most frequently prescribed dose of celecoxib was 200 mg in OA and 400 mg in RA. They did not perform any test of statistical significance because such a **big sample** would have found a medically irrelevant small difference as significant.

Despite such a big sample, the authors rightly remarked that their conclusions are limited by lack of clinical information, inability to ascertain actual use, and potential for selection bias. Note that this was not a random sample.

Side note: Although the authors called this as 'observational, retrospective cohort study' in the title, they also called it as 'primarily a descriptive study' in the text. Such confusions in the nomenclature of the study methodology are galore in medical literature.

Nomograms and Tables of Sample Size

Many researchers may find formulae in Annex 1 difficult to adopt. Two alternatives exist, although they may not be readily available. One is **nomogram.** This is a graph containing lines and curves, and needs only a ruler to read the sample size that would meet the specifications. Altman (1982) has given a nomogram for size of SRS for comparing two groups. Kumar and Indrayan (2002) have developed one such nomogram for reading off the sample size required in cluster sampling. Neter and Wasserman (1974) have given nomograms for sample size for multiple groups such as in ANOVA setup. Those weary of the formulae in Annex 1 should try to locate a nomogram for their situation. Nomogram is especially helpful to find sample sizes for several scenarios.

Second alternative is table of sample sizes. Some authors have worked out sample sizes for various situations and tabulated them. One such compilation is by Lwanga and Lemeshow (1991). Sample size required for the specified values can be directly read from such tables. An interpolation may be required when the exact specification is not in thc table.

6.4.2 SAMPLE SIZE FOR ANALYTICAL STUDIES

Analytical studies can have two purposes. One is to estimate the Relative Risk (RR) or Odds Ratio (OR) depending upon whether the study is prospective or retrospective, and the second could be to test the hypothesis that two groups have same mean or same proportion. Calculation of sample size is different in these two set-ups.

Sample Size for Estimation of Relative Risk or Odds Ratio

The basic issues in this situation are the same as already stated for descriptive studies although the formulae change. These formulae are also given in Annex 1. The formulae require specification of the relative precision. This delimits the acceptable error in the estimate. If actual odds ratio is 2.5 and the acceptable relative precision is 10 percent of OR, an estimate within 0.25, i.e., between 2.25 and 2.75 would be acceptable. Wider is this range, lesser is the requirement of sample size.

Sample Size for Testing of Hypothesis

The other problem under investigation in analytical studies is test of a hypothesis. This generally takes the form whether two or more groups have same mean or same proportion. This can also transform to examining the OR or RR. Sample size calculation for studies involving three or more groups becomes complex. For this refer to Chow et al. (2018). For comparison of two groups, the formulae are given in Annex 1. As an approximation for multiple groups, two-group formulae can be used with α-level adjusted according to the Bonferroni principle. This also is explained in a later chapter.

In place of precision of the estimate, sample size calculation in the case of testing of hypothesis requires specification of power corresponding to the least difference that would be considered medically relevant. Power is denoted by $(1 - \beta)$. This is the chance that the study is able to detect a specified medically relevant least difference. Power calculations have become important these days and have pushed sample size in research studies to at least 10-fold of what they were 40 years ago. Another consideration in case of testing is that a one-tailed test would be used or a two-tailed test. This concept is also explained in a later chapter.

Other principles regarding inflating the sample size for nonresponse and using prior values of SD and RR or OR are the same as stated for descriptive studies.

EXAMPLE 6.11: Sample size for a prospective study on disability in work-related musculoskeletal disorders

Turner et al. (2004) report a prospective study of workers in the US who file claims for work related musculoskeletal disorders. The primary outcome of interest was duration of work disability in one year after filing the claim. The purpose was to develop statistical models that could predict the duration of chronic work disability after the initial suffering from the disorder. The required sample size was calculated as 1800 workers for low-back injuries and 1200 for workers with Carpal Tunnel Syndrome (CTS). Statistical power used for these calculations were 0.96 for low-back and 0.85 for CTS, and the significance level chosen was $\alpha = 0.05$ (two-tailed) for both.

Side note: The example illustrates that the sample size could be quite large for prospective studies when statistical considerations such as power and significance level are considered. The concept of power is related to the minimum medically relevant difference, but the abstract of the article does not specify this difference. A large sample size was feasible in this case because the study is mostly based on administrative database and follow-up interviews were done by telephone.

Additional Considerations

Sample size determination procedure as discussed so far assumes that the interest is in only one variable: mean in case it is quantitative; and proportion in case it is qualitative. Note that RR and OR are ratios of the same proportion in two groups and are univariate in this sense. In practice, the interest might be in more than one variable. For example, in a case-control study on risk factors for breast cancer, the interest could be in age at menarche, age at first live birth, total duration of breast-feeding of all children put together, and the number of first order blood relatives that have positive history. Cancer prevalence would be different in various categories of different variables. If there are many variables such as in this example, which one should be used for determining the sample size? If the focus is on only one of them, say, age at menarche, and others are just concomitants to remove their confounding effect, use the cancer prevalence rate in different categories of this variable only. If there are two groups such as case and control, use OR. If two or more variables have nearly same importance, calculate sample size for each of them separately and take the largest. In any case, mean, SD, proportion, OR or RR, would have to be based on a previous study in a similar setting, and the precision in case of estimation or the medically relevant least difference in case of testing of hypothesis must be specified.

An additional consideration not accounted for in the formulae in Annex 1 is the number of concomitant variables or covariates that you want to study together. Higher this number, bigger is the requirement of sample size.

The sample size quickly multiplies and can become an enormous number if cross-classifications of several factors are under consideration. For only two factors, viz., age at menarche as <12 years and ≥12 years, and age at first live birth as <23 years and ≥23 years, the four cross-classifications are (i) menarche at <12 years and first live birth at <23 years, (ii) menarche at <12 years and first live birth at ≥23 years, (iii) menarche at ≥12 years and first live birth at <23 years, and (iv) menarche at ≥12 years and first live birth at ≥23 years. If there are four factors and all are dichotomised, the number of cross-classifications is $2^4 = 16$. Results would be reliable if each of these classifications has adequate number of subjects. No guidelines are available about the sample size that would be adequate to take care of, say, five risk factors opposed to two risk factors, but a thumb rule is that each cross-classification should have a sample of at least 30 subjects. This is applicable when the disease prevalence is large, say ≥20 percent. In our breast cancer example, the study might include only the suspected cases where the prevalence would be high. A size of at least 30 implies for four factors that there must be at least a total of 16×30 = 480 subjects, evenly distributed to the 16 categories. All these are summarized in Table 6.1.

TABLE 6.1: Requirement of larger sample

Requirement	Sample Size
Smaller Type-I error	Larger
Smaller Type-II error (Higher statistical power)	Larger
Smaller difference to be detected	Larger
Higher inter-individual variability or smaller proportion	Larger
Higher anticipated nonresponse	Larger
Higher number of subgroups	Larger
Higher number of variables to be considered together	Larger

The sample size many times depends on the resources and time available for a project. For a **Master's thesis,** less than 2 years are generally available with practically no funding. Thus, the sample size would be small regardless of what the formulae say. Our advice in such situations is to choose a topic for which adequate number of subjects are available within one year and restrict to the investigations that are feasible. Perhaps Master's thesis should not be done on rare diseases. Else, be clear that it would be a pilot study in nature whose results would not have much reliability but can provide important clues to plan a major study.

Even for big studies, resources and time constraints sometime dictate the sample size. Vickers (2008) gives this interesting example: A colleague points out that the drug under trial is safe and inexpensive and could be advocated if it is able to reduce average pain score by even half a point. A recent paper shows a SD = 2 for the change. For these values, the formula gives n = 774. Fund limitation does not allow to do such a big trial. What if SD = 1.5? The sample size reduces to 380 but it is still high. Lower the bar and aim at detecting pain score reduction by 0.75 instead of half a point. Now n = 170. This is doable. If this is chosen, the size of the study is dictating the research objective whereas actually the research objective should dictate the sample size. In practice, this happens and accepted.

Thumb Rules

Thumb-rules lack scientific basis, and many scientists dislike them. When no baseline information for computation of sample size is available and the constraints do not permit pilot study either, the following thumb rules can be used.

A large-sized medical trial should include nearly 300 subjects in *each group,* a mid-sized trial nearly 100 in each group, and a small-sized trial at least 30 in each group. The last can be used for postgraduate theses where the time and resources are limited. Bigger study is multicentric with these numbers in each centre. Same norms can be used for retrospective or case-control study. However, in the case of a prospective study, the number to be followed up should be such that at least 30 persons are finally available with the outcome of interest in *each group.* This applies to field trials also. In this case, extremely large group may be needed to yield an outcome such as HIV infection in at least 30 subjects after administration of a protective vaccine. To calculate exact numbers, use the formulae given in Annex 1.

For running a quantitative regression, a thumb rule is that values on a minimum of 10 subjects must be available per independent (regressor) variable. If there are 5 regressors, the sample size must be at least 50. For logistic regression, the least likely category in cross-classification with minimum number must have at least 5 subjects. This can transform into an enormous number. If there are 6 dichotomous regressors, the number of categories is $2^6 = 64$. Each of these categories will have subjects with and without disease that you are studying as outcome. If the disease is rare, say with prevalence 10% in your target population, there must be at least 5 subjects with disease (total 50 subjects if prevalence is 10%) in each of these 64 categories. The total number of subjects then becomes at least 64×50 = 3200 when uniformly distributed. Most likely the subjects will not be uniformly distributed, and the required number will be higher.

For a descriptive study that seeks to find normal levels in healthy subjects, the thumb-rule is to include at least 120 subjects in each group for which norms are required, although in this case also exact number can be calculated using an appropriate formula. For pathological levels in patients, the group-size could be smaller. Depending upon the targeted reliability of the results, exact sample size requirement can be calculated. However, all these may have to be modified because of feasibility considerations when the resources and time are limited. Such limitations obviously compromise the reliability.

Sample Size for Laboratory Experiments

Experiments on animals such as mice are done on small numbers per group yet provide reliable results. One might wonder why the statistical formulae do not apply to this setup. There are two reasons. One, experimental animals are much more homogenous such as of same strain – thus, inter-individual variability is small. Second, laboratory conditions are fairly well standardised, and the factors are under good control. Thus, any difference found between groups can be legitimately ascribed to the treatment. For this reason, experiments on 5-6 mice per group are norm than exception. This cannot be said about clinical trials or observational studies. When data from experiments on small samples per group are analysed, exact or nonparametric methods may have to be used.

Smaller–than–Desired Samples

Situations exist where a large sample is not feasible. A small-scale study is better than no study at all. But two precautions are required. First, as already mentioned, realise that a study based on smaller-than-desired sample is pilot in nature that may not give conclusive results. Second, a separate class of statistical procedures is used to analyse data based on small samples. One set of methods is nonparametric that we discuss in a later chapter. The other is the set of exact methods. These require extensive calculations – much more than the usual methods. Separate statistical software such as StatXact and LogXact should be used to draw inferences from small samples. These methods help to find, for example, that the difference between the test and the control group is large enough to be statistically significant or not. Generally, only very large difference would turn out to be statistically significant in case of small samples. This may not be so for experiments on animals for reasons stated in the preceding paragraph.

SUMMARY

Although nonrandom methods of sampling can be used in early phases of a study but the final results should be based on a random sample, particularly if the objective is to describe the features of disease in one or more segments of population. Popular methods are simple random sampling, stratified random sampling, systematic random sampling, cluster random sampling, multistage random sampling, and probability proportional to size sampling. The choice of the method would depend on the size and spread of the target population, and the distribution of the characteristic under study across different segments of the population.

Among analytical studies, cross-sectional study should also be based on a random sample of the target population. For prospective and retrospective studies too, a random sample is preferable. But valid conclusion regarding effect of a factor on an outcome can be drawn based a nonrandom sample also, provided the case group and the control group are adequately matched for baseline characteristics.

For laboratory experiments on animals, it is generally believed that the animals are randomly chosen even when a limited number is available with no opportunity for sampling. Experiments on biological material can be carried out on nonrandom samples if the material with and without intervention are similar. This largely applies to the human subjects in third phase of a clinical trial as well. First phase in any case is carried out on a nonrandom sample, and in second phase too randomisation is not a prerequisite.

Number of subjects to be included in the study (sample size) depends on a host of considerations such as inter-individual variability, precision required, statistical power and the level of significance. Formulae are available to calculate the sample size for different situations.

REFERENCES

Altman DG. Practical Statistics for Medical Research, 2nd ed. Chapman and Hall, 2006.

Barton MB, Morley DS, Moore S, et al. Decreasing women's anxieties after abnormal mammograms: a controlled trial. J Natl Cancer Inst 2004;96:529-538.

Chatfield C. Confession of a pragmatic statistician. The Statistician 2002;51(Part-1):1-20.

Chon CH, Lai FC, McNeal JE, Presti JC Jr. Use of extended systematic sampling in patients with a prior negative prostate needle biopsy. J Urol 2002;167:2457-2460.

Chow SC, Shao J, Wang H, Lokhnygina Y. Sample Size Calculation in Clinical Research, 3rd ed. Chapman & Hall/CRC Press, 2018.

Chu NF, Makowski L, Chang JB, Wang DJ, Liou SH, Shieh SM. Lipoprotein profiles, not anthropometric measures, correlate with serum lipoprotein(a) values in children: Taipei children heart study. Eur J Epidemiol 2000;16:5-12.

Fabricant SJ, Harpham T. Assessing response reliability of health interview surveys using reinternews. Bull World Health Org 1993;7:341-348.

Indrayan A, Malhotra R. Medical Biostatistics, 4th ed. CRC Press, 2018.

Kumar R, Indrayan A. A nomogram for single-stage cluster sample surveys in a community for estimation of a prevalence rate. Int J Epidemiol 2002;31:463-467.

Kornitzer M, Valente F, de Bacquer D, Neve J, de Backer G. Serum selenium and cancer mortality: a nested case-control study within an age- and sex-stratified sample of Belgian adult population. Eur J Clin Nutr 2004;58:98-104.

Lemamsha H, Randhawa G, Papadopoulos C. Prevalence of overweight and obesity among Libyan men and women. Biomed Res Int. 2019 Jul 15;2019:8531360.

Lwanga SK, Lemeshow S. Sample Size Determination in Health Studies: A Practical Manual. World Health Organization, 1991.

Neter J, Wasserman W. Applied Linear Statistical Models: Regression, Analysis of Variance and Experimental Designs. Richard D. Irwin, 1974:pp 827-828.

Schnitzer TJ, Kong SX, Mitchell JH, et al. An observational, retrospective cohort study of dosing patterns for rofecoxib and celecoxib in the treatment of arthritis. Clin Ther 2003;25:3162-3172.

Turner JA, Franklin G, Fulton-Kehoe D, et al. Prediction of chronic disability in work-related musculoskeletal disorders: a prospective population-based study. BMC Musculoskelet Disord 2004;5:14.

Vickers AJ. Let's dance! The sample size samba. www.medscape.com/viewarticle/584026. (Posted 2008 - Last accessed 3rd January 2021).

ANNEX 1

1. SAMPLE SIZE FORMULAS FOR DESCRIPTIVE STUDIES (SAMPLE SURVEYS)

Estimation

1. Estimation of mean with specified precision:

   $n = z^2_{1-\alpha/2}\sigma^2/d^2$, where d is the specified precision on either side of mean

2. Estimation of proportion with specified absolute precision:

   $n = z^2_{1-\alpha/2}\pi(1-\pi)/d^2$, where d is the specified absolute precision on either side of the proportion

3. Estimation of proportion with specified relative precision:

   $n = z^2_{1-\alpha/2}\pi(1-\pi)/(\varepsilon\pi)^2$, where ε is the specified relative precision in terms of fraction of π

Test of Hypothesis

4. Test of hypothesis for a mean:

$$n = \frac{\sigma^2(z_{1-\alpha/2} + z_{1-\beta})^2}{(\mu_0 - \mu_a)^2},$$ where μ_0 is the value under the null hypothesis and μ_a is under the alternative such that the medically relevant difference to be detected is at least $\mu_0 - \mu_a$

5. Test of hypothesis for a proportion:

$$n = \frac{[z_{1-\alpha/2}\sqrt{\pi_0(1-\pi_0)} + z_{1-\beta}\sqrt{\pi_a(1-\pi_a)}]^2}{(\pi_0 - \pi_a)^2},$$ where π_0 is the value under null hypothesis and π_a under the alternative hypothesis such that the medically relevant least difference to be detected is $\pi_0 - \pi_a$.

Note: For one-sided estimations and one-sided tests replace $z_{1-\alpha/2}$ by $z_{1-\alpha}$. This is the value from Gaussian table corresponding to the 100(1–α)% level of confidence or 100α% level of significance. Similarly $z_{1-\beta}$ is the Gaussian value corresponding to the power 100(1–β)%.

Source: Adapted from Lwanga and Lemeshow (1991), and Indrayan and Malhotra (2018)

2. SAMPLE SIZE FORMULAS FOR ANALYTICAL STUDIES

The following formulae are applicable when there are only two groups and both have same sample size. Thus, the situation with multiple controls is excluded.

Prospective Study – Estimation of RR

1. Estimation of an incidence rate with specified relative precision:

   $n = (z_{1-\alpha/2}/\varepsilon)^2$, where ε is the specified relative precision as fraction of the anticipated incidence rate on either side

2. Estimation of RR with specified relative precision:

$$n = \frac{[z^2_{1-\alpha/2}[(1-\pi_1)/\pi_1 + (1-\pi_0)/\pi_0]}{[\ln(1-\varepsilon)]^2},$$ where ε is the relative precision in terms of fraction of RR (RR = π_1/π_0, and π_1, π_0 are the anticipated incidence rates in the exposed and unexposed groups, respectively)

Prospective Study – Test of Hypothesis

3. Test of hypothesis for an incidence rate:

$$n = \frac{(z_{1-\alpha/2}\lambda_0 + z_{1-\beta}\lambda_a)^2}{(\lambda_0 - \lambda_a)^2},$$ where λ_0 and λ_a are the incidence rates under the null and the alternative hypothesis respectively, i.e., the least difference considered medically relevant for detection is $\lambda_0 - \lambda_a$

4. Test of hypothesis for difference in incidence rates per year (attributable risk):

$$n = \frac{[z_{1-\alpha/2}\sqrt{2f(\lambda)} + z_{1-\beta}\sqrt{f(\lambda_1)+f(\lambda_2)}]^2}{(\lambda_1-\lambda_2)^2}$$, where $f(\lambda) = \lambda^3 T/(\lambda T - 1 + e^{-\lambda T})$ if the duration of study (in years) is fixed as T (censored observations), and $2f(\lambda)$ is to be calculated at $\lambda = (\lambda_1 + \lambda_2)/2$. (When T is not fixed, replace $f(\lambda)$ by λ^2, $f(\lambda_1)$ by λ_1^2 and $f(\lambda_2)$ by λ_2^2; λ_1 and λ_2 are the anticipated incidence rates in the two groups.)

5. Test of hypothesis for RR:

$$n = \frac{[z_{1-\alpha/2}\sqrt{2\pi(1-\pi)} + z_{1-\beta}\sqrt{\pi_1(1-\pi_1)+\pi_0(1-\pi_0)}]^2}{(\pi_1-\pi_0)^2}$$, where $\pi = (\pi_1 + \pi_0)/2$, and medically relevant least RR is π_1/π_0

Retrospective Study – Estimation of OR – Unmatched

6. Estimation of OR with specified relative precision (for small disease prevalence):

$$n = \frac{[z^2_{1-\alpha/2}[1/\{\pi_1(1-\pi_1)\}+1/\{\pi_0(1-\pi_0)\}]}{[\ln(1-\varepsilon)]^2}$$, where ε is the relative precision in terms of fraction of OR. ($\text{OR} = \frac{\pi_1/(1-\pi_1)}{\pi_0/(1-\pi_0)}$, and π_1, π_0 are the anticipated exposure rates in the case and control groups, respectively.)

Retrospective Study – Test of Hypothesis – Unmatched

7. Test of hypothesis for OR:

(a) 1 control per case:

$$n = \frac{[z_{1-\alpha/2}\sqrt{2\pi_0(1-\pi_0)} + z_{1-\beta}\sqrt{\pi_1(1-\pi_1)+\pi_0(1-\pi_0)}]^2}{(\pi_1-\pi_0)^2}$$, where the medically relevant least OR is π_1/π_0 (When exposure rate among the controls, π_0, is known with high precision, else replace $2\pi_0(1-\pi_0)$ by $2\pi(1-\pi)$ where $\pi = (\pi_1 + \pi_0)/2$)

(b) C controls per case:

$$n_1 = \frac{[z_{1-\alpha/2}\sqrt{(C+1)\pi_0(1-\pi_0)} + z_{1-\beta}\sqrt{C\pi_1(1-\pi_1)+\pi_0(1-\pi_0)}]^2}{C(\pi_1-\pi_0)^2}$$

and $n_0 = Cn_1$ (number of controls)
with condition as stated in 7(a).

Any Type of Study – Estimation

8. Estimation of difference in two means with specified precision:

   $n = z^2_{1-\alpha/2}(\sigma_1^2 + \sigma_2^2)/d^2$, where d is specified precision on either side of the mean difference

9. Estimation of difference in two proportions with specified absolute precision:

   $n = z^2_{1-\alpha/2}[\pi_1(1-\pi_1) + \pi_2(1-\pi_2)]/d^2$, where d is the specified absolute precision on either side of the difference

Any Type of Study – Test of Hypothesis

10. Test of hypothesis on difference in two means:

    $(\sigma_1^2 + \sigma_2^2)(z_{1-\alpha/2} + z_{1-\beta})^2/d^2$, where d is the least difference considered medically relevant for detection

11. Test of hypothesis on difference in two proportions

    $$n = \frac{[z_{1-\alpha/2}\sqrt{2\pi(1-\pi)} + z_{1-\beta}\sqrt{\pi_1(1-\pi_1) + \pi_0(1-\pi_0)}]^2}{(\pi_1 - \pi_0)^2},$$ where $\pi = (\pi_1 + \pi_0)/2$, and the least difference considered medically relevant for detection is $\pi_1 - \pi_0$
    (This formula is the same as for test of hypothesis on RR)

Note: For one-sided estimations and one-sided tests replace $z_{1-\alpha/2}$ by z_α. This is the value from Gaussian table corresponding to the 100(1–α)% level of confidence or 100α% level of significance. Similarly $z_{1-\beta}$ is the Gaussian value corresponding to the power 100 (1–β)%.

Source: Adapted from Lwanga and Lemeshow (1991), and Indrayan and Malhotra (2018)

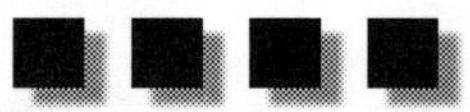

CHAPTER

7

What Data to Collect and How to Manage

KEY TERMS AND CONCEPTS

- ✓ Primary and Secondary Sources of Data
- ✓ Record Linkage
- ✓ Interview, Examination, and Investigation
- ✓ Questionnaire, Schedule, and Proforma
- ✓ Structured and Precoded Forms
- ✓ Quality of Data
- ✓ Data Accuracy and Data Editing
- ✓ Pilot Study and Pretesting
- ✓ Training and Supervision
- ✓ Quantitative and Qualitative Measurements
- ✓ Metric, Ordinal, and Nominal Scales
- ✓ Dichotomous and Polytomous Variables
- ✓ Indicators, Indexes, and Scores
- ✓ Standardisation of Values

The word data is a plural for datum and stands for a collection of measurements. The measurements are not necessarily quantitative: They could be qualitative also. Signs and symptoms are qualities yet are 'measurements' in statistical sense. Blood pressure, creatinine level, peak expiratory flow rate, etc., are measurements any way. Qualitative data too convert to numeric when summarised for a group. For example, if the measurement is presence or absence of ascites for a group of 50 patients with complaints of pain in abdomen, one can say that ascites was present in 18 of them. Thus, qualitative data also become quantitative when related to a group. This would invariably happen in a primary medical research set-up.

All measurements are easily understood as **variables** since they do vary from person to person. Thus, there are qualitative variables and there are quantitative variables. This distinction is important since the method of inference is different. Merits and demerits of various types of measurements will help to decide which ones to use for different kinds of assessment in research. We discuss these in detail later in this chapter. First is the choice of sources that can provide quality data. Various secondary and primary sources of medical data are listed in Section 7.1. Methods for maintaining data quality are in Section 7.2. Types of measurements such as qualitative-quantitative and discrete-continuous are discussed in Section 7.3. Before the data are put to analysis, many times they are converted to indexes and scores, and need standardization and adjustment to make them comparable across groups. The methods for these also are in Section 7.3.

7.1 SOURCES OF MEDICAL DATA

Empirical research requires data. Where from to get these data? Obviously, the most important source is the person or the patient himself. This information can be obtained either by asking (interview) or by examination. But medicine is not such a straight science. Laboratory and imaging investigations are important sources. Then there are records either with the person or with the doctor, clinic, or hospital. Each source has its own strengths and weaknesses.

7.1.1 SECONDARY AND PRIMARY SOURCES OF DATA

Data sources are of two types. **Primary sources** are those that provide data through direct interface with the person. Interview, examination, and laboratory investigations are the methods to obtain primary data. The other type is **secondary,** in which there is no interface with the person concerned. Data in records are secondary. Original source of these data also is primary but primary today becomes secondary tomorrow for someone else.

Secondary Data

Secondary source of data is the most inexpensive and readily available source when access is available. Among easily accessible secondary sources are the following. For details, see Indrayan and Satyanarayana (2019).

1. Medical records of patients in clinic, nursing home, or hospital.
2. Disease registries such as of cancer and thalassaemia.
3. Internet-based databases such as on COVID maintained by several organisations.
4. Reports of the surveys conducted by the government agencies such as various fertility and mortality indicators for various segments of population available in annual report of the Sample Registration System in India or surveillance data giving prevalence of HIV in different segments of population as brought out by the National AIDS Control Organisation of India.
5. Periodic reports of the government and nongovernmental organisations such as National Health Profile of India published by the Indian Ministry of Health & Family Welfare every year, and periodic reports of Cancer Society of India.

Some of these can enormously help in research. For example, hospital records of cases of hernia over 10 years can provide invaluable information on their age distribution, duration of hospital stay, factors responsible for quick recovery, effectiveness of different surgeries, time trend, etc. At the same time, they can be highly biased also as they represent only those cases that come to that hospital. Case-histories may be very incomplete, and some may be missing. There might be errors in classification. They may not be adequate to meet a particular research objective such as of finding aetiological factors. Researcher has almost no control or influence over the content of secondary data. Diagnostic and surgical criteria may change from surgeon to surgeon and over time depending upon new knowledge and improvement in diagnostic, radiological and surgical facilities. Treatment modality may also vary from physician to physician and over time. Thus, it may be necessary to filter secondary data properly, or make appropriate adjustment before they are used for research.

Many useful studies have been done on secondary data. Historical cohort, about which we mentioned in an earlier chapter, is almost invariably done on secondary data. Case-control studies are also many times done by using past records. In many cases, secondary data can be effectively used as a supplementary to the primary data to augment or confirm findings.

Primary Data

Primary source provides authentic data that can be tailored to the research needs. In case some information looks unusual, reinvestigation or reprobing can be done while collecting such data. Thus, more reliable information can be obtained. But this source is expensive, particularly if the information is required on many subjects. It may require expensive investigation and may need substantial time and efforts. Quality is difficult to sustain when the information flow is slow. But when the past information is not available, as would commonly happen in medical research, primary is the only source of data.

The easiest source of primary data are the patients who are interviewed and investigated during the normal course of interactions. Once you decide what cases to be included, you can be more careful about obtaining the correct and full information from them that otherwise in a routine set-up many not be so accurate. Many PG thesis are done on such data.

Record Linkage

Patients do have a tendency to take advice from more than one physician in different institutions, particularly for long-term illness. A record is generated at each point of contact. *Linkage is the process of pooling of disparate data to make a comprehensive single record for each person.* This process is routinely followed for admitted patients in a hospital when results of laboratory and imaging investigations are sent to the main folder of the patient. But linkage of records in different hospitals pertaining to the same patient, or with private practitioners, is a difficult process.

Disparate data are generated on patients under research if they get some treatment outside the protocol. This treatment can influence the results. Thus, linkage to that extent is necessary.

7.1.2 INTERVIEW, EXAMINATION, AND INVESTIGATION

Primary data on subjects of your choice can be obtained by interview, examination, and investigation. In most situations, all three methods are deployed that supplement each other. But the data obtained by different methods are not equally reliable.

Interview

History taking by personal interview is an integral part of medical maneuver. This is the most direct method of obtaining the data. But the interviewer must go down or come up to the level of the respondent to elicit correct response. Make sure that the person is not casual or evasive, and not giving misleading information as on commercial sex in the case of Sexually Transmitted Disease (STD), or on knife injury that may have legal implication. Guard against recall lapse. Elderly people may not report about cataract or cough perceiving them as a natural consequence of old age. For such reasons, assess if the interviewer requires some training to be able to elicit full and correct response.

In a community-based research, interviews can be done by mailed questionnaire, telephonic conversation, or personal interface. The response of mailed questionnaire could be low, and highly selective. It is applicable only to the educated segment of the population who can read and understand the questions. Telephonic interviews can be done only of those who have telephones, and thus, could make the sample highly biased. Also, the refusal rate can be high. Face-to-face interviews are the commonest and most valid form of eliciting the information. The kinds of information that can be obtained by interview are:

(i) facts such as age and sex,

(ii) complaints or symptoms,

(iii) behaviour such as smoking, feeding practices, and hygienic practices,

(iv) knowledge about health practices, and services, and

(v) opinion such as on contraception, or preference for system of treatment.

Resist the temptation to collect too much of information from a person lest the focus is lost, and the person loses interest: He may evade the questions and start giving casual answers. Only necessary information as required under the protocol should be collected.

Examination

Examination is the most reliable source of getting the medical data on a subject. Besides signs and symptoms, this includes measurements such as weight, body temperature, and blood pressure. There could be some hiccups, though. You may find spleen palpable in a case that the other physician cannot. You may like to observe and note pallor in a suspected case of leukaemia whereas another physician may consider it inconsequential. In a research set-up, take steps to achieve standardisation. Perhaps the same physician should examine all the patients, and with uniform dexterity. Same examination should be carried out for all the subjects.

Investigation

Radiological and laboratory investigations are gradually gaining centrality in establishing a diagnosis, and in monitoring the progress of a patient. Although there are many physicians who believe that nothing can replace clinical acumen, their number is dwindling. Because of relatively higher objectivity, investigation results get much more weightage in research than clinical observations. Ensure though that the laboratory is reliable, and the investigation results are believable.

Decide before hand what specific information is to be obtained by the respective methods. They should corroborate or supplement each other. If a male patient of age 55 years or more complains of increased frequency of micturition, poor stream, large prostate on rectal examination, but normal prostate specific antigen on laboratory examination, then they provide corroborative evidence of enlarged prostate, namely, the Benign Prostatic Hyperplasia (BPH). If corroboration is lacking, the patient may not be of enlarged prostate, and possibly not suitable for inclusion among cases for research if that is on BPH.

7.1.3 QUESTIONNAIRE, SCHEDULE, AND PROFORMA

It is always desirable in a research to follow a pre-defined pattern for collecting data and record them in a standardised format. A form is a big help in retaining the focus on the objectives and in ensuring uniformity and also serves as a repository of information for later reference. In view of such important functions, ample time and thought should be invested in designing forms. The format could be a questionnaire or a schedule or a proforma for master chart. There is a considerable confusion among medical fraternity about these terms. The contents however of all three formats are basically the same as outlined below. These include information on variables that characterise the subjects, the interventions, and the outcomes.

Broad Contents of a Form of Data Collection for Medical Research

- Identification data (name, address, ward, patient ID, date, name of the observer, etc.)
- Demographic characteristics (age, gender, area, ethnicity, education, income, etc.)
- Basic measurements (height, weight, addictions, sexual practices, blood pressure, pulse rate, etc.)
- Disease measurements (signs-symptoms, duration, severity, biochemical measurements, pathological assessments, etc.)
- Intervention received (treatment facility, prescriptions, actual intake, surgery, etc.)
- Health outcome (mortality, residual disability, quality of life, duration of survival, side-effects, duration of hospitalisation, etc.)

Questionnaire

As the name implies, **questionnaire** contains a series of questions that are required to be put to a subject in verbatim at the time of interview. Thus, the phrasing of questions and their sequence are important. Such features have potential to change the response. For side-effects, for example, asking generally about any problems caused by the treatment may elicit much less response than asking separately for each possible side-effect. But in the latter case all possible side-effects should be known at the time of framing of questionnaire. Also, the last asked side-effect is likely to be reported much less than the first asked. Sensitive questions such as on sexual behaviour should be asked as late as possible because that can change the course of the interview. Suppose the interest is in finding whether a couple had undergone sex determination of a foetus in relation to their knowledge of legal provisions in this respect. If knowledge about legality is asked first and the respondent says 'yes, he knows that it is illegal', he would be bound to say 'no' to the question regarding sex determination actually practiced by him. The right sequence is to first ask about any sex determination undertaken and related questions, and then ask about his knowledge regarding legal provisions in this respect.

Avoid questions such as "Don't you use pain killers for acute pain?" They suggest answer and are called **leading questions**. Such questions are not recommended. Also avoid double negative question such as 'you believe that not smoking does not cause lung cancer'. Also do not seek two pieces of information in one question. The wordings must not be ambiguous. Minimise hypothetical questions on future or regarding attitude because the response to such questions depends on mental frame at the time of the interview. The response may change when asked second time. It is sensible to concentrate on questions on facts rather than opinion. In place of asking what he would do in a particular situation, ask what he did last time in that situation. For regularity of condom use, for example, do not elicit response as never, sometimes, regular, and always, but ask how many times condom was used in the last, say, four sex encounters.

The language used in framing the questions should be focused on the research question. Avoid long questions and the questions that can have dual answers. Initial questions should be such that the respondents feel that answering them is in his interest and the sequence should be such that can sustain the interest. Questions based on long memory and requiring deep intelligence should be avoided. Each item of enquiry must have separate question.

A questionnaire could be self-administered also where the subject fills responses without interface with an interviewer. For this to be successful the respondent must be fully literate to understand and interpret the questions properly and the questionnaire must contain all the explanations and instructions for its completion. Use simple language for the respondent to understand with correct perspective. If the language of the questionnaire is different from the language of the respondent, the translation should be appropriate. Despite all these precautions, portions of a self-administered questionnaire are likely to be left blank. But more accurate information can be obtained by this method on sensitive issues such as sexual behaviour. Face to face interview may not yield the same quality of response on such sensitive issues.

In postal questionnaires, increase the chance of response by offering incentives, advance contact, personalized letter, stamped return envelope, follow-up contact, etc.

In case you are using translation of a standard questionnaire such as on quality of life, back translate to the original language and see if you get the same expression.

Schedule and Proforma

Schedule contains only the items on which the information is to be collected. Framing question to get that information is left to the interviewer in this case. Schedule will have an item – Age. Questionnaire will have 'What is your age?' A bed-head ticket or a case-sheet is a schedule since it contains only the items of information.

Proforma is the prototype or a sample providing the items of information on which the information is to be collected. It is neither a questionnaire nor a schedule. Perhaps this can be used to prepare columns in a register where information for each patient can be recorded in one line as done in a database or master chart.

Features of a Form

Whether a questionnaire, a schedule, or a proforma, the following should be kept in mind.

1. It should be properly formatted with headings and subheadings, and spaces as required. Use capitals, bold, italics and different fonts to emphasize the thrust of the information you are seeking. The layout of the form should be aesthetically pleasant.
2. Printed form with logo and immaculate appearance instils confidence in the interviewer and the respondent alike. Photostat or cyclostyled forms do not do that.
3. The unit of recording for each piece of information should be specified, e.g., whether duration of symptoms is to be recorded in days or weeks or months. Age of a neonate of 4 hours is recorded as 1/6 day if this information is to be used for analysis along with such information on other neonates whose age is recorded in days.
4. Specify how the measurement is it to be rounded off. If age is 13 years and 8 months, is it to be recorded as 14 years, which is the nearest integer, or in completed years 13 as is generally done all around the world in a medical record? Do not make categories such as 15-19, 20-24, etc., in the data collection form. Such categories can be made later at the time of analysis or presentation.

5. The questions or the items should be framed in a manner that the chance of bias in the responses is minimum.
6. Questions or items that need to be skipped for being not applicable in certain cases should be specified. If there is an item on cause of death that is to be asked only if there is a death in the family, the item should have a remark that this is to be skipped in other conditions.
7. Nonstructured questionnaire is used for informal surveys. For medical research, **structured questionnaires** are used. For this, follow the guidelines provided in a short while.
8. If multiple response is admissible, this should be clear to the investigator. **Multiple response** means that one question or one item can have more than one answer. Complaints could be many in one person. Thus 'complaints' is a multiple response question.
9. The forms can be **precoded** that will make computer entry simple. In any case, text responses such as signs and symptoms are be coded either at the time of recording or later at the time of computer entry. But remember that codes are not grades nor scores, and they cannot be added, subtracted, etc.
10. The form should be comprehensive so that all information on one subject or one patient could be recorded together. Investigation results may have to be obtained separately but they should be transferred to the main form. Post-operative details should be recorded together with pre-operative findings. Each page of the form should have the same identification number, which would be unique for each subject.
11. The information should be elicited only on the items that are really required to meet the study objectives. Unnecessary information can dilute the quality. Overly detailed form can be tedious and boring, and wasteful of the time of the interviewer and the respondent. It is difficult to sustain interest of a respondent for more than one-half of an hour unless there is some inducement. Nonetheless, obtain all the information committed in the protocol.
12. As far as possible, restrict to the collection of objective information. Opinions and attitudes should be separately identified.
13. Standardise the form after **pretesting** on a small number of subjects from the same target population for which this is going to be finally used. Pretesting helps to identify ambiguities or potential biases in the responses. Investigators can be trained accordingly. It also helps to assess the time and resources required to administer this kind of instrument to various types of respondents. For a large-scale study, two or more rounds of pretesting may be required.

A short schedule is in Example 7.1 that can give leads on how to prepare such a form.

EXAMPLE 7.1: Suggested design of a structured precoded close-ended schedule

(Note: This is part of the form for illustration purpose only)

College of Medical Sciences

LOGO

DEPARTMENT OF INTERNAL MEDICINE

Oxidative Stress in Type II Diabetes Patients

Name ______________________ Group (1/2/3) [ ]

Age last birthday [ ] years Case no. [ ][ ][ ]

Sex (M/F) [ ] Date ___/___/___

Address ____

I. DIABETES

Age at detection of diabetes (in completed years) [ ] years

Duration (calculate later: age last birthday – age at detection) [ ] years

II. PERSONAL HABITS

(Write zero if not taken during last one year;
if taken during last one year, write **average since the beginning**)

Cigarettes smoked: average [ ] per day, since (duration) [ ] years

Alcohol intake: average [ ] per day, since (duration) [ ] years

Tobacco chewing: average [ ] per day, since (duration) [ ] years

III. COMPLAINTS (tick that are present)

Increased frequency of urination [ ] since (duration) [ ] months

Tremors [ ] since (duration) [ ] months

Constipation [ ] since (duration) [ ] months

Nausea/Vomiting [ ] since (duration) [ ] months

Acidity [ ] since (duration) [ ] months

IV. VITAL SIGNS

Body temperature [ ] °C

Pulse rate [ ] per minute

Respiration rate [ ] per minute

Systolic BP: sitting [ ] mmHg Diastolic BP: sitting [ ] mmHg

Structured Questionnaire

A questionnaire is called structured when the language and the order of the questions are fixed. When the list of possible answers is also given and the respondent is required to just tick one or more as applicable, this becomes **close-ended.** One possible answer can be 'Any other (specify)' to cover the possibility of the list not being exhaustive. A question can be framed close-ended only when enough is known about the type of responses so that the responses under 'other' category are minimum, say, not exceeding 10 percent. If they are more, this reflects that the questionnaire was not prepared with sufficient thought. If responses cannot be anticipated, do a pilot study to find out what responses are common that need to be separately listed in a close-ended fashion. If substantial responses occur under 'other' category despite best efforts, invoke the 'specify' component and identify which responses are common that can be separated. Remember that a large number of responses for 'other' without identifying what, can throw your research out of gear. Also, at the time of statistical analysis and conclusions, this other category can cause problems because it contains the assorted leftovers that defy interpretation.

Probing is allowed provided no suggestion is made regarding the reply, and the interviewer is trained. The objective of close-ended questions is to make it friendlier to the respondent, and for easy data processing and analysis. However, care must be exercised in providing the list of possible answers. The choices for 'How often do you get bouts of depression?' can be never, sometimes, often, and frequent. These are subjective terms. Instead try 'less than once a year', 'more than once a year but less than once a month', 'more than once a month but less than once a week', etc. In addition, for a close-ended question the instruction should be clear about how to correct mistakes in a filled-up form without making it ambiguous.

Online Forms

Online forms can be used for short surveys where the number of questions or items does not exceed, say, 10. Facilities are now available to drag and drop to reorder questions when needed. The possible answers in a structured questionnaire can be customised as per the need. The response to such forms is automatically stored in a format (such as Excel) you specify. Thus, the efforts needed to prepare a master chart are saved. Descriptive analysis for the number of subjects with different responses, averages, percentages, etc., can be easily done.

7.2 QUALITY OF DATA

'Garbage-in garbage-out' is a very appropriate phrase for medical practice. If correct information is not elicited about the patient, do not hope that prescriptions or surgery would still bear fruit. If sufficient care is not adopted about the information collected during research, the results would be equally sloppy. Much of the medical research in some countries fails to attract attention because of a general feeling that some research workers in those countries are not sufficiently careful. Such 'researchers' also tend to undermine the work of others in the same country who use immaculate care. It is not so much about using expensive instruments or procedures, but about being careful about whatever is being done. If blood pressure is being measured, the subject in comfortable position without any stress, resting arm, and three readings if required – all this makes up the quality of measurement. Whatever tools are used, be it glucometer or Magnetic Resonance Imaging (MRI), must be valid and reliable. A large part of modern medical research is devoted to searching methods and instruments that are inexpensive and fast, yet valid and reliable. Accuracy, completeness, relevance, etc., are the other dimensions of quality of data.

Remember that anecdotal evidence lack scientific basis and plural of anecdote is not data. Secondly, as Tukey once remarked, the availability of data and the aching desire for an answer do not ensure that a reasonable answer can be extracted.

7.2.1 RELIABILITY, VALIDITY AND ACCURACY OF DATA

The concept of reliability and validity are discussed at length in a previous chapter in the context of a study as a whole. These are the two most important components of quality of data also. Reliability is also called consistency, reproducibility, repeatability, and precision. Question to sex workers about the number of sex partners in one week has no reliable answer; first because it may have large variation from week to week, and second because of failure to recall correctly. Memory based questions are always less reliable. Reliability of measurements is assessed by coefficient of variation and of an instrument by test-retest, split-half, and Cronbach's alpha methods.

Validity has several dimensions – face, content, concurrent, construct, criterion, and internal and external validities as discussed in an earlier chapter. The statistical indicators of validity are sensitivity, specificity, and predictivities.

A telling example illustrating the difference between reliability and validity of data is assessment of age by asking how old the subject is, asking what his date of birth is, and by inspecting birth record that may be the ultimate truth. Agreement between the first two is reliability, and agreement with the third is validity. Thus, an assessment could be reliable without being valid and *vice-versa.*

Various biases discussed in a previous chapter are threats to validity. Assuring confidentiality helps in some cases to get correct information. Implement it faithfully by deleting all the items of information that could identify the respondent. Also take precaution if presence of other people at the time of interview can affect the response.

Accuracy of Measurements and Recording

Accuracy is confused with validity and reliability, but it is neither. It is the correctness of the measurement. The measurement should be devoid of error and recorded to the last digit for it to be accurate. But the term has other ramifications as well.

The data, whether obtained in terms of quantities or in terms of verbatim text, should be clearly and correctly recorded. Before grinding it through computer for statistical analysis, scrutinize the data for their internal consistency. For example, make sure that sysBP = 126 is not written as 162 mmHg, or presence of a disease is not recorded with its contradictory features. Scrutiny of the forms should be done immediately after they are filled up when memory is fresh. Incomplete forms, unclear information, and illegible writing can be easily corrected at that time without revisiting the subject. If any information is suspicious, repeat contact should be made for verification. The information should look about right. All forms must be signed and dated so that the responsibility can be fixed.

There might be errors in keying the data to the computer. It is not unlikely that an adjacent key is pressed such as 8 for 9. Also guard against misreading visually similar digits such as 1 for 7, and 5 for 3 in a hand-written form. A decimal might be missed. Check also for internal consistencies. A systolic level 152 mmHg can rarely go upto 180 mmHg after taking an antihypertensive therapy. Similarly, a woman of 22 years can rarely have a child of age 10 years. Double check such records for accuracy. The investigator who has been a part of the data collection or data recording process may not be able to detect own errors. Whenever feasible, all checking should be done by an independent person.

Errors occur in reversing the codes for males and females, and in calculating severity score of patients, for example, based on columns 10, 11, 12, 25, and 26 where 10, 11, 12, 24, and 25 should have been used. The score incidentally turned out as expected and did not arouse suspicion and detected on second scrutiny. In another instance, one set of values was unwittingly exchanged with another set of values and one row was copied to another at the time of data entry. In another case, while computing change from pre- to post-, minus sign was missed. Such errors may be inadvertent but substantially compromise the credibility of research.

Coding errors can occur by itself as human do make mistakes but also because the responses in forms are not standardized. For example, lymphoma may be wrongly stated in the form as lipoma. Second, one form may say hyperplasic and the other hypertrophic, and getting separate codes. They do have subtle difference, but both are generally used for enlargement.

7.2.2 OTHER ASPECTS OF DATA QUALITY

Quality of data is adhering to the defined standards. This innocuous looking concept is difficult to implement. It encompasses validity and reliability for sure as already explained but also includes completeness, timeliness, relevance, etc.

Completeness

Completeness of data can hardly be overemphasized. Incomplete data can lead to erroneous conclusions. Simple rules for completing a form are given below.

To ensure completeness, check all the filled-up forms for errors, omissions, and discrepancies. These lapses can easily occur with self-administered questionnaires and will not be uncommon in interviewer filled questionnaires. Call back to the respondents is in any case needed for those who were not available at the first contact, but it may also be needed for whom the information was incomplete or inconsistent.

Rules for Completing a Form

- Give enough time to the respondent in an interview for him to think or recall and to give correct answers.
- Write the responses faithfully without imputing your own views or interpretation.
- Ensure that the responses are consistent across various items. If a patient says he is diabetic, his plasma glucose level without drug can rarely be 100 mg/dl.
- Do not leave blank for any item. Write 'Not Applicable', 'Not Available', 'Refuse to Cooperate', 'Died', etc., as applicable. All missing data should have sufficient reason, and none should be due to carelessness or casual attitude.
- All writing must be legible. Remember that scrutiny of the form may be done by a third person and data entry in computer by yet another. They should be able to read the writing properly.

While framing the items for collecting the information—either as questionnaire or as schedule, it is necessary to assess that those items adequately answer each objective of the research. Also, it should be clear as to how various medical parameters are going to be measured. If the outcome of interest is recovery of the patient, whether this would be in terms of physiological parameters, or ability to do certain activities, or based on imaging evaluations. The endpoints should be clear and relevant for the research in hand. Whether these would be assessed every day, or once in two or three days, etc., should also be specified. Who would assess them, with the help exactly what tools, if any, should be a part of the protocol. In this context pilot study and pretesting are valuable steps. The details are as follows.

Pilot Study and Pretesting

Protocol writing can be a frustrating experience when baseline information regarding the subjects or the disease is missing. In such a case, it is advisable to carry out a small-scale preliminary investigation on the same type of subjects that are proposed to be studied. Such a forerunner, which is done to get a feeling of the subjects and of the conditions, is called a **pilot study.** Specifically, such a study helps in the following.

- Assess feasibility of the study as a whole and of various measurements proposed to be taken.
- Confirm that the collected information fulfils the objectives.
- Standardise the tools.
- Evaluate the reliability and validity of tools.
- Get an idea of expected variation among subjects that helps to determine the size of sample.
- Anticipate the problems that might come up during the implementation.
- Assess the time frame within which various phases of the study would be complete.
- Get a feedback that the instructions are not confusing or incomplete.
- Assess the requirement of staff and discover the training and supervision needs, including for data management.
- Assess the adequacy of logistical support.

Pilot studies have extremely important functions yet get little attention in research methodology training. They help refine the data collection procedures and tools, and also in preparing a better protocol. For a large-scale study, pilot study is considered an essential step. For a small-scale investigation such as for Master's thesis, this may not be needed although in this case also a preliminary investigation may be needed to finalise the protocol. Although it is possible to conduct pilot study on a subsample of the subjects of the main study, but it is many times difficult to include these observations in final analysis since they could be incomplete or inconsistent with the main phase of the study.

Another forerunner that helps in increasing the quality of the study is **pretesting.** When tools of investigation and of data collection such as scoring system and schedule are developed, they are tested under actual conditions for their performance. In the case of questionnaire, for example, pretesting would indicate whether the sequence of questions is logical, the wordings are clear, list of possible answers is exhaustive, respondents are able to answer correctly, space for open-ended questions is adequate, etc. In the case of measurement tools such as pulse oximeter, testing may have to be done at regular intervals to check its validity. Standardisation of laboratory procedures can also be tested. Modifications as needed are made after pretesting. Some features of this exercise such as standardisation of tools may overlap with those of pilot study.

Despite pilot study and pretesting, it will not be uncommon that the data collection form or the procedure requires further changes while the study is in progress. If this change is done, ensure that the corresponding changes are also made in the data already collected.

Missing Values and Outliers

Some genuine missing values can be nonserious. If a patient missed taking a drug one or two days in a 4-week trial this is not serious. If required for statistical purposes, perhaps such missing values can be imputed using the trend on other days. Such **imputation** helps to retain the data for that patient in the analysis that otherwise will have to be excluded. If many patients are dropped like this, the final available sample could be substantially reduced. Thus, imputation does help in certain situations (see, e.g., Little and Rubin 2002 for imputation methods). Imputation is advisable when the missing data are neither too few nor too many.

A patient absenting for two weeks in a 4-week trial is a serious breach of protocol. Taking prohibited concomitant drug for a considerable period is also a serious violation. Such patients may have to be excluded from analysis. If the pattern of such exclusion is similar in the two groups under comparison, this may not affect the tenor of results except reducing the sample size.

Treatment related dropout should be counted as not cured by the treatment. An unrelated dropout such as due to accidental death can be excluded or impute their values for the unobserved follow-up period by following one of the standard procedures.

Outliers are difficult to identify and manage. Although statistical methods are available to identify outliers, it is advisable to depend on common sense. If in doubt, give benefit and leave it in the dataset. If you are confirmed that a particular value is an outlier, first step is to assess if it is due to an error in recording, coding, or data entry. If so, restore the correct value. Outliers have potential to distort all the results. The usual practice therefore is to exclude such values. A genuine outlier will have a biological explanation. Retain the one that can be reasonably explained. It is safe to analyse the data with and without the outliers and see what difference they make.

Training and Supervision

Correct implementation of a protocol in a big research may require a full manual of instructions on how to approach the subjects, the strategies needed to elicit correct data, when to substitute the subject if at all by another subject, how to get cooperation of various agencies, an explanation of the terms and concepts, where to go for help if needed, etc. But the best bet for quality assurance is training and supervision. The data collectors and health assessors should be trained to follow uniform procedures in an as identical fashion as possible. Erroneous data can never lead to right conclusions, no matter how meticulously analysed. Obtaining correct information cannot be overemphasized. In a long-term study, periodic refresher training may be needed after feedback is received. The staff may behave in a responsible manner, yet supervision is needed from time to time. This is needed to ensure that no digression occurs from the predefined protocol. Supervisors should be equipped to tackle any problems that interviewers or assessors might face. Adequate training and periodic supervision go a long way in improving the quality of data.

The other aspects of training are improved techniques of questioning and quality interviews that help to elicit correct information with minimal nonresponse. These aspects are sometimes overlooked in medical research, but they can have bearing on the conclusions where history and other enquiries are important components. The interviewer should reassure the respondent about the confidentiality of the information and should scrupulously maintain this assurance. He should have perseverance and patience.

7.3 TYPES OF MEASUREMENTS

Loading this text with statistical terminology will defeat the purpose of keeping it intelligible to medical research workers. At the same time, it is necessary to be conscious of the type of measurements and their consequences. We try to explain all this in simple terms.

Blood group is a quality and blood glucose level is a quantity. The former is assessed in terms of words or attributes whereas the latter in terms of numerics. As already mentioned, both are 'measurements' in technical sense. Various types of measurements are as follows.

Types of Measurements

Categorisation I — Quantitative/Qualitative Types

Quantitative — Measured for each individual in numerics such as body temperature, haemoglobin level, and creatinine level. The other name for the same is metric.

Qualitative ordinal — Assessed for each individual as a quality that can be graded such as disease severity into mild, moderate, serious, and critical categories. The number of categories must be three or more—thus it is always polytomous.

Qualitative nominal – Assessed for each individual as a quality that cannot be ordered such as site of injury as head, chest, limbs, etc. This can be of two types—dichotomous when the number of categories is two, and polytomous when the number of categories is more than two.

Intensity of pain when measured by visual analogue scale as 7 out 10 is quantitative; when measured by verbal rating scale is mild, moderate, or intense is ordinal; when measured as present or absent is nominal as well as dichotomous. Most scientists prefer quantitative measurements to qualitative measurements.

Categorisation II — Continuous/Discrete Types

Continuous – A measurement that can take innumerable number of values within a given range, such as age that can be 45.126 years or 42.78 years (although there is hardly any need to measure it to that accuracy). BP also is continuous but measured in terms of integer values only, mostly even integers.

Discrete – A measurement that can take only finite—generally small—number of 'values'. All qualitative variables are discrete. Family size is discrete although it is quantitative. The details of both these categorisations are given in the following sections.

7.3.1 QUANTITATIVE MEASUREMENTS

A large number of variables in health and medicine are quantitative. Age, blood pressure, body temperature, creatinine level, and time to recover, are all quantitative. When an appropriate instrument is available, they can be measured exactly.

Metric Scale

Quantitative measurements are said to be measured on **metric scale.** Such measurements are mostly summarised in terms of average to get an idea of the central value and in terms of Standard Deviation (SD) to get an idea of their dispersion. As a corollary, OPD number, though numeric, is not quantitative. Statistically, quantitative is the most appropriate form of measurement. Use such measurements wherever feasible—even at some extra cost in terms of time and resources. Kelvin dictum says that when you can quantitatively measure a phenomenon, you know something about it, and when you cannot your knowledge is meagre and unsatisfactory. Some medical professionals follow this dictum literally and have developed scoring systems (also called rating scales) for differential diagnosis and to assess severity of a condition. Such scoring systems are discussed in a previous chapter. We mention them again later in this section. The point here however is that such scoring systems are relatively 'soft' options. Very rarely widely acceptable rating scales are available, and they are considered subjective. Prefer hard measurements, e.g., blood pressure instead of hypertension. If they do not exactly measure the characteristic of interest such as quality of life, use scoring. Scores might be better than qualitative information. If the efforts required for hard measurements are enormous such as in measuring size of brain, or when no quantitative scale or scoring is available, use qualitative measurement as described in the next section.

Metric scale can be interval or ratio. In the case of body temperature, differences are valid, but ratios are invalid. It would be naïve to say that 103°F is just 3 percent higher than 100°F. Thus, ratios are not applicable. Such measurements are said to be on interval scale. Many medical measurements do not have absolute zero, and thus have interval scale. Calendar dates, size of kidney, and birth weight are on interval scale. A measurement such as duration of stay in a hospital is on ratio scale. The duration of eight days is twice of four days. Age, parity, and gain in weight are other examples of measurements on ratio scale.

Continuous and Discrete Measurements

It is important in research to distinguish between two types of quantitative measurements. First are those that can take, at least theoretically, any value in a specified range. They can be measured arbitrarily to many decimal places. Albumin level can be 3.4 g/dl or even 3.432 g/dl although it does not help to measure it that accurately. Such measurements are called **continuous**. Second type of quantity is parity that cannot be 2.7 or 3.2. Such measurements are called **discrete**. The method of analysis of discrete data is different from the method of analysis of continuous data.

Any count is always discrete but if the number of persons has a large range such as the number of hypertensives in various cities, it is treated as continuous for the purpose of statistical analysis. It is seen that treating them as discrete gives nearly the same results as treating them continuous, and the methods for continuous data are generally simpler and well-known.

This distinction is important if you plan to analyse the data yourself. Otherwise, the statistician would take care.

7.3.2 QUALITATIVE MEASUREMENTS

Sign-symptoms are qualities, and so is severity of an injury. However, the latter has grades that generally is not the case with the former. Thus, there are various scales of measurement. We have already mentioned about metric scale. Others are as follows.

Scales of Qualitative Measurements

How do you measure severity of injury in a patient? Perhaps by the sites affected and the extent of damage to the vital organs. It is difficult, although not impossible, to measure severity of injury in terms of numerics. It is far too easy to categorize an injury as mild, moderate, serious, and critical. Histopathologically, grades of acute cholecystitis can be (i) only mucosa inflamed, (ii) mucosa and submucosa involved, and (iii) whole gall bladder wall affected. These are text-words and thus are qualitative, but they also have an order. Such measurement is called to be on **ordinal scale**. Stage in cancer is ordinal. Note that these variables are in fact quantitative but measured ordinally because no satisfactory or generally acceptable metric scale is available. There is a danger though. What is mild for one physician may be moderate for another. Very rarely these terms are tightly defined and there is a great likelihood that subjectivity will creep in. Thus, be cautious while using ordinal scale. Further caution is required if scores are 0 for none, 1 for mild, 2 for moderate, 3 for serious, and 4 for critical. Such scores assume that the difference between mild and moderate is the same as between none and mild, and serious is three times of mild, etc. This obviously is not true.

Analysis of ordinal data is difficult and there could be pressure to reduce ordinal scale to only two categories for easy analysis. This expediency can be counterproductive. Do not succumb to this pressure except when the number of subjects in one or more categories is too small to allow use of standard statistical methods. Ordinal categories provide much more useful information in most situations than two categories when sample size is adequate. These could be used to investigate a trend.

Medicine is a science governed mostly by qualities than quantities. In place of saying that Hb level is 8 g/dl, it is many times convenient to say that the patient is anaemic. Diseases such as hypertension, diabetes and glaucoma are quality expressions for quantitative measurements. Such expressions are very commonly used, and you may also like to use them in your research. But use acceptable cut-offs for such labelling. Identifying such cut-offs may not be easy. Despite extensive deliberations, physicians still do not agree that hypertension cut-off for starting drug therapy in old age should be 140/90 or 160/95 mmHg. Also, it is not clear what to do if BP is 138/92. If cut-off 140/90 is acceptable, it should also be clear in a research setup that a person with exact level 140/90 would be called hypertensive or not. The definition of anaemia can vary from place to place, and perhaps it is different for females than for males. This problem is not so acute for diseases such as diabetes mellitus because the definition is fairly well established. The real problem arises when these conditions are graded as mild, moderate, and serious. Then a consensus is required regarding the criteria for such grading because, otherwise, one grading may not match with the other, and one would wonder how the results are at variance.

At the bottom end are the variables such as gender. It has only two 'values' — male and female. Such variables are called **dichotomous** or binary. All attributes when assessed as 'present' or 'absent' are dichotomous. Death is either yes or no. There is no grading. Visual acuity can have grading but wearing glasses is dichotomous. Diagnoses such as hepatitis, cirrhosis and malignancy are also of this type. In addition, there are many characteristics that can have grading but are generally assessed as either present or absent. Splenomegaly in malaria, myocardial infarction, and renal failure come in this group.

In contrast to dichotomous, there are variables that are **polytomous**, i.e., those with more than two categories. Blood group is a polytomous variable with O, A, B, and AB categories. These categories are names, and such a variable is called **nominal**. Categories such as normotensive, probably hypertensive, and definitely hypertensive are also polytomous, and simultaneously they are ordinal also. They are not nominal in that sense. Age is a quantitative variable but becomes qualitative ordinal when divided as child, adult, and old. For this, again, acceptable age range should be used. That is, the decision that a person of age 16 years would be called a child or not should be based on some rationality in the context of the research. There should be sufficient justification of the chosen categorisation such as to call adults with BP <120/80 mmHg as definitely normotensive, between 120/80 and 129/84 as probably normotensive, between 130/85 and 139/89 as border line, between 140/90 and 159/94 as probably hypertensive, and 160/95 or more as definitely hypertensive. One can question what is so wonderful about digits 0 and 5 in such categories, and a convincing answer must be available.

All qualitative data are necessarily **categorical**. Quantitative data also becomes categorical at least for the purpose of presentation, such as diastolic level (mmHg) divided into 70-74, 75-79, 80-84, etc, categories. Quantitative data in such categories are called **grouped data**.

Care in the Count Data

All qualitative variables, whether nominal or ordinal, are assessed in terms of counts. Sometimes episodes are counted instead of persons. One child can have several episodes of diarrhoea, and a person can have many attacks of asthma. Angina, epileptic seizures, adverse reactions, hospitalization, and sometimes even fractures and myocardial infarctions can occur repeatedly in the same person. Sometimes organs such as eyes and kidneys are counted instead of persons. This goes on all the time for counting units of blood transfused even when the same person has received multiple transfusions. Thus, exercise care that the persons are being counted or the episodes are being counted.

EXAMPLE 7.2: Various types of measurements used in research on abortion-miscarriage relationship

Sun et al. (2003) reports a study on perinatal epidemiology in Shanghai in which two cohorts were recruited – an abortion cohort who had induced abortion in the first trimester, and a reference cohort of primigravidae. They concluded that induced abortion by vacuum aspiration is associated with an increased risk of first-trimester miscarriage in the subsequent pregnancy.

Among various types of measurements, they used for this research are as follows:

Maternal age at conception (years) – Metric and continuous but categorised as – 25, 25-29, 30+

Maternal education – Polytomous ordinal and discrete, categorised as – Middle, High, College

Maternal occupation – Nominal and discrete as white collar, blue collar

Family income (Yuan/month) – Metric and continuous but categorised as – 500, 500-1499, 1500+

Habit of smoking/alcohol – Dichotomous as no, yes

Body mass index (kg/m^2) – Metric and continuous but categorised as – 19.1, 19.8-25.9, 26.0+ (no value between 19.1 and 19.8)

Disease during pregnancy – Dichotomous as no, yes

Gestational age at recruitment (days) – Metric and continuous but categorised as – 49, 50-56, 57-63

Conception season – Polytomous nominal as spring, summer, autumn, winter

As an exercise, check that the name of each type of measurement mentioned in this example is the same as described in this text.

7.3.3 INDICATORS, INDEXES, AND SCORES

Factor is a characteristic and indicator is its measurement. Lipid profile is a characteristic and levels of various lipids are the indicators. There might be many indicators for the same factor. Sometimes one indicator is not enough by itself and it has to be seen in combination with one or more of the others. A combination of two or more indicators is called an **index**. Simplest of these is the body mass index, which considers weight and height together. Smoking index may incorporate indicators such as number of cigarettes smoked per day, duration of smoking, age at initiation, duration elapsed since quitting, etc. A further problem in measurement is converting qualities such as signs and symptoms into quantities. This is done by scoring systems. All these are explained in this section.

Choice of Indicators

An attribute like obesity can be measured by body mass index, waist-hip ratio, or skin-fold thickness. Results could differ depending upon what criterion is used. All three are quantitative but measure different aspects of obesity. There is a debate among research workers that waist-hip ratio is a better marker of obesity in the context of coronary heart disease or body mass index. This can happen with any characteristic for which multiple indicators are available. If resources permit, use all such indicators, and examine which one is a better correlate of the disease under investigation, and possibly look for reasons why others are not equally good.

Pain can be assessed by visual analogue scale, verbal rating scale, or McGill Pain Score. These methods do not necessarily agree with one another. The choice should depend on validity considerations for the research in hand. Sometimes feasibility is an over-riding consideration. McGill Pain Score may look better for a particular research but that could be too complex for the patients if they are not educated, or it may be too time consuming.

Despite all the advances that medical science has made, there still are factors that defy any kind of measurement. Psychological feelings such as compassion, love, and affection come under this category. They can be important variables in a psychiatric research. The same is true for anxiety and depression. They also affect recovery rate of some somatic disorders. Such characteristics may have to be measured approximately in a tentative manner till such time that an acceptable scale is developed.

Scoring System

Quantities are often preferred over qualities in research because they introduce exactitude. When adequate in describing underlying qualities, quantities do tend to increase the objectivity. How to convert qualities such as signs and symptoms into quantities? Through scoring system. APACHE score and Apgar score are everyday examples. A large number of such scoring systems are used in different contexts, and the use is increasing, as the new ones are devised everyday.

We discussed some scoring systems for diagnosis and for gradation of severity in an earlier chapter. The purpose there was to highlight their role in reducing epistemic uncertainties. That indeed is the dominant reason for developing and using scoring systems. The reason for mentioning them here in this section is that scoring is one of the several methods of measurement of various medical factors, and that this method could be useful in some research. While using a scoring system, ensure that this is a tested system and has been found valid for your type of setup.

7.3.4 STANDARDISATION OF VALUES FOR DATA COMPARABILITY

Sometimes the measurements make more sense when they are standardised. The term "standardised" here is not for the methodology but is for individual measurements. Weight of children are commonly standardised by z-score where $z = (x - \text{mean})/SD$. These standardised scores are used to categorise child as undernourished if $z < -2$ for him or her or obese if $z > +2$. For comparison of one measurement of a person with another measurement in the same person, such as pulse rate and diastolic level, both can be standardised and checked for their correspondence in the sense that both give nearly the same z-score.

Another form of standardisation is called normalisation. This is obtained as $(x - \text{minimum})/(\text{maximum} - \text{minimum})$, and converts a value on 0 to 1 scale. If albumin level in a kidney patient is 5.0 g/dl where the maximum seen is 22.0 and the minimum is 2.0, the normalised albumin level of this patient is $(5.0 - 2.0)/(22.0-2.0) = 0.15$. This is the relative value on 0 to 1 scale.

This standardisation is for individual measurements. We will discuss standardisation of group-based rates in one of the next chapters.

SUMMARY

Medical measurements can be done in a variety of ways. Hypertension can be measured as present or absent, or as none, mild, moderate, serious depending upon the BP level, or in terms of systolic and diastolic levels themselves. The statistical processing of various types of measurements is different and the conclusions too are dependent on this type. Thus, choose your measurements carefully that adequately meet the objectives of your research.

Two basic categorisations of measurements are qualitative and quantitative. Qualitative can be nominal or ordinal (both can be dichotomous or polytomous), and quantitative is always on metric scale. Measurements with limited number of possible values such as gender and parity are called discrete variables, and measurements with unlimited possible values such as age and body mass index are called continuous variables. Parity is an example of a variable that is metric yet discrete. Statistical analysis of discrete variables is different than of continuous variables.

Some measurements become more meaningful and easier to interpret when juxtaposed with one or more of the other measurements. For example, for liver function, various proteins and enzymes are studied together. For some measurements, an index such as BMI is calculated. Qualitative and quantitative measurements are pooled by scoring systems.

Measurements sometimes cannot be used straightaway because of underlying aberration due to intervening factors and are standardised so that they become valid for comparison.

REFERENCES

Indrayan A, Satyanarayana LS. Simple Biostatistics, 5th ed. Delhi: Brillion Publishing, 2019.

Little RJA, Rubin DB. Statistical Analysis with Missing Data (Second edition). New York: John Wiley & Sons, Inc., 2002

Sun Y, Che Y, Gao E, Olsen J, Zhou W. Induced abortion and risk of subsequent miscarriage. Int J Epidemiol 2003;32:449-454.

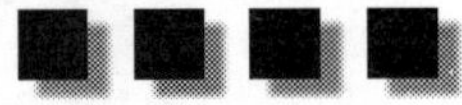

CHAPTER

8

How to Assess Health and Disease

KEY TERMS AND CONCEPTS

- ✓ Univariate and Multivariate Assessments
- ✓ Types of Medical Factors
- ✓ Distal and Proximal Factors
- ✓ Morbidity and Disease Spectrum
- ✓ Mortality and Duration of Survival
- ✓ Statistical Summaries – Mean, Median, Mode, SD, and Percentiles
- ✓ Normal and Abnormal Levels

Health and disease may be a matter of perception for individuals but for the society at large it has some objective meaning. Medical fraternity is required to strike a balance—give due recognition to their own and the patient's perception while dealing with individuals and also be consistent with the societal expectations. This text does not dabble with clinical assessment that has to be geared to individual needs; instead concentrate on conclusions from the groups that work for individuals in the long run but can fail in specific cases. Individuals are extremely important for medical maneuvers but assessments in research are mostly epidemiological as they are based on study of groups. Knowledge of the methods for assessing health and disease is needed before the protocol is framed.

8.1 ASSESSMENT OF MEDICAL FACTORS

To clarify semantics, 'factor' in our terminology is a characteristic, and 'indicator' is its measurement. Obesity is a factor and Body Mass Index (BMI), Waist-Hip Ratio (WHR), and skin-fold thickness its indicators. Condom use is a factor, and its regularity can be measured, for example, as always/regular/irregular/never, or more specifically as number of times used in last four sexual intercourses. These are the indicators. Nutrition status is a factor and serum albumin level, retinol level, and haemoglobin level its indicators. Indicator converts a factor into its operational definition. This distinction is important for implementation of research. Enough thought must be given at the time of protocol writing for identifying relevant indicators. For example, depending upon what aspect of obesity is most relevant for research, decide that BMI is more appropriate indicator or WHR or skinfold thickness or any other.

8.1.1 INTRICACIES OF ASSESSMENT

Besides identification of indicators for various factors of interest, empirical research requires that the factors be correctly assessed. Some aspects of data quality that include correct assessment were discussed in an earlier chapter. In addition, the timing and circumstances of all assessments should be standardised to minimise the variation. For example, decide for Blood Pressure (BP) measurement that the patient would be supine or sitting, how much time is to be given for rest before BP reading, what would be the gap between two measurements, what instrument would be used, what time of day will it be measured, whether rounding off would be to even number or nearest integer, etc.

Decide also that the research interest is in the average of a quantity or in occurrence of an 'event'. Iron deficiency in a group can be measured either by mean haemoglobin level or by finding how many have level <11 g/dl. The two indicators may give different results. Incidence of a disease may give different results from prevalence, and efficacy is different from effectiveness. Similarly, decide that the appropriate indicator to meet the objective is relative risk, attributable risk, or relative risk reduction. The interest may be in duration of disease in some situations and in survival in others. Sensitivity-specificity have different implications than positive and negative predictivities. The choice is dictated by the objectives of the study and by the specific hypotheses formulated at the time of protocol writing.

While using two or more indicators for the same factor, beware of the threats posed by possibly different results. For example, finding for cholesterol levels may disagree with those on triglyceride level—which one would you believe? The advantage is that the correspondence between two or more such indicators increase the level of confidence in findings, and the difference prompts us to look for the reasons for such differences.

Risk perception can be different: if a celebrity is affected, the risk is highlighted many folds even if it is one in a million. Secondly, stating it as 0.001 is perceived differently than one in a thousand although both are same.

Univariate and Multivariate Assessments

Occurrence of hypertension depends on heredity, diet, exercise, obesity, stress, etc. Generally, presence of several factors together is required to trigger the disease. Thus, hypertension has multifactorial aetiology. Compare this with malaria. Its occurrence solely depends on mosquito bite. Thus, malaria is a univariate disease with single factor aetiology. When parasite is not detected, malaria diagnosis is multivariate since then it depends on presence of fever with rigors, splenomegaly, etc. Hypertension is a univariate disease since diagnosis is based only on blood pressure level alone but has multifactorial aetiology. Thus, exercise caution while using terms such as univariate and multifactorial disease.

Further implication of univariate and multifactorial terms is in risk assessment. Lung cancer can occur from certain diet constituents, smoking, exposure to radiation, asbestos dust, etc. Any one of these factors can cause cancer. Also, one risk factor such as smoking can cause many diseases (lung cancer, asthma, coronary disease, etc.). Assessment of medical factors in a research should give due consideration to such distinctions. In the case of noninfectious diseases, the latent period from exposure to onset can be long and the presence of other factors during this period can complicate the assessment.

8.1.2 TYPES OF MEDICAL FACTORS

It is important in research to make distinction between factors that can be modified and factors that cannot be modified. Age and gender may be important risk factors for many chronic diseases, but nothing can be done to change them: Only precaution can be advised. Most genetic factors too are unmodifiable although counselling and perhaps engineering can handle some. The primary target of research should be factors such as diet, life-style, biochemical, and pathological parameters that can be modified either through advice such as for diet and exercise, or by physical intervention such as drug and surgery.

A convenient division of medical factors is distal, proximal, physiological, pathophysiological, pathological, morbidity, mortality (Figure 8-1). Some examples of these factors are given below. Note that distal factors can seldom be outcome and mortality can never be antecedent for the same person. All others could be antecedent in one situation and outcome in the other. Lipid profile is an outcome for dietary changes but antecedent for coronary diseases.

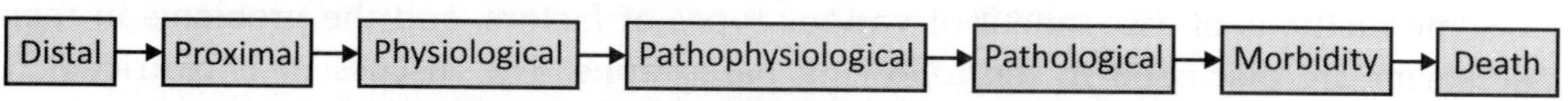

FIGURE 8-1: Types of medical factors and their flow

Some Examples of Medical Factors

It is difficult to list all the factors. The following is a partial list that illustrates the factors of different types that can be considered in a research. Further details will be presented in a short while.

Distal factors — Socioeconomic status (literacy, income, and occupation); culture and behaviour; living conditions and quality of life; genetic predisposition; climate and pollution; age structure, population density and sex ratio; health infrastructure including health care and water-sanitation; inequities; legislations and policies; etc.

Proximal factors — Diet and nutrition; obesity, exercise, and physical activity; quality of life, stress and strain; smoking and other addictions; health and hygiene practices; personality traits, attitudes, etc.; family history; etc.

Physiological and pathophysiological factors — Levels of blood pressure, heart rate, etc.; blood and urine chemistry; liver, kidney, and lung functions; cognitive and psychomotor functions; electromagnetic status; gestation, childbirth, growth; menarche, reproductive history, and menopause; anthropometry; immunity level and tolerance; etc.

Pathological factors — Blood constituents; urine, blood tests for pathogens; histology and cytology of cells and tissues; images; serology; etc.

Morbidity — Type of disease, infirmity, injury, etc.; signs and symptoms; onset and remissions; previous history; prevalence, duration, and severity; parts affected; medical treatment and surgery; side-effects and complications; etc.

Mortality — Population–based death rates (crude, standardized, age and cause-specific); standardised mortality ratio; livebirths-based mortality (still-births, perinatal, neonatal, and infant mortality, under-five mortality, maternal mortality); proportional deaths; case-fatality.

Duration of survival – Expectation of life; survival with residual disability and quality of life; healthy life expectancy; years of life lost; etc.

The above list may help in identifying factors that are relevant for research and also possibly not to miss out any, or to demarcate factors for future research. A categorisation and flow (see Figure 8-1) may help in assessing the role of various factors and in assessing their modifiability that may have deep implications in arriving at implementable conclusions. All this is done for writing a good protocol before the actual study is conducted.

Some methods of assessment of various types of factors, and the problems in their assessment are discussed in the following paragraphs. The discussion is restricted to commonly studied factors: perhaps a representative of their category. Mortality and survival require special methods that are discussed separately in the next section.

Distal Factors

Distal factors work from behind and give opportunity to proximal factors to emerge when other favourable conditions are present. Most prominent distal factors are socio-economic status and inequities, cultural practices, and environment. Socioeconomic status is measured as social class I (highest) to class V (lowest) depending upon the level of education, income, and occupation. Indrayan and Malhotra (2018) have devised one such classification that can be internationally used.

Cultural practices include vegetarianism that affects nutrition, gender preference that could mean foeticides and neglect of girl child, belief in supernatural powers (such as *tantrik*) that could affect utilisation of health facilities, and family bonds that provide social security including at the time of serious illnesses. No widely acceptable scoring system is available to convert these factors into measurable indicators. The only way to assess them is present/absent, or in some situations in full/partial/nil type of categories. Because of difficulty in their assessment, cultural factors tend to be ignored in most medical research. Do not ignore these factors if the disease under investigation is significantly affected by varying cultural practices in your target population.

Environment can be studied by climate and the resulting flora and fauna such as thriving pathogens and vectors, by pollution inside and outside home and workplace, by the kind of housing, traffic and roads, and such other factors. Many of these cannot be appropriately defined at individual level. They are societal or community-based factors.

Demographic structure of the population indirectly affects health in a variety of ways. Age-sex structure determines the per capita availability of specialised health facilities such as of paediatric and geriatric care, and rural-urban distribution that sometimes highlights the disparities. Age-sex structure can be assessed directly or by indicators such as dependency ratio and sex ratio.

Health infrastructure comprising hospitals, doctors, health centres, system of treatment, and particularly water and sanitation facilities, is an important distal factor. Iodine and fluoride level in potable water are glaring examples. Indicators such as doctor-population ratio and percent population receiving potable water are used to measure health infrastructure. The COVID pandemic has highlighted the availability of PPE kits, ventilators, testing facilities, and some drugs.

Distal factors do affect individual diseases, but their application is more common in public health research. Nevertheless, some of these may be important for clinical research as well.

Proximal Factors

Factors directly affecting health are called **proximal.** They are also called risk factors in classical sense. Prominent among them are nutrition, obesity, addictions, health practices including hygiene, stress and occupational hazards, and sexual practices.

Problems in assessing proximal factors can be very aptly described by using smoking as an illustration. Many times, it is assessed only as never smoker, past smoker, and current smoker. But smoking has many dimensions. One is the type of smoking: cigarette, bidi, hukka, cigar, pipe, etc. Further dimensions of cigarette smoking are number smoked per day that can vary from year to year, years of smoking, filter or nonfilter cigarette, age at start, and time elapsed since quitting by ex-smokers. In addition are finer aspects such as depth of inhalation, early morning smoking, and the size of the butt left. Most commonly used indicator of smoking is the person-years smoked. This obviously ignores other dimensions of smoking. It also assumes that the 'burden' on health of smoking 10 cigarettes for 20 years is the same as smoking 40 cigarettes for 5 years. Do you agree with this equivalence? No correction is available for this discrepancy. However, Indrayan and Malhotra (2018) have developed a comprehensive index on the premise that the burden of smoking on health is rapid in the beginning but increases slowly later as the cigarette-years accumulate. It also considers age at start, filter/nonfilter cigarette, variation in smoking from year to year, and time elapsed since cessation.

Indicators for assessing a factor such as **health practices** are neither available nor easy to develop. Health practices include personal hygiene; awareness and adoption of good health practices such as balanced diet, exercise, and good sleep; utilisation of health care facilities such as when a doctor is consulted, and where; and child feeding such as mother's milk and supplements. Separate information on each relevant item may have to be obtained.

Height and weight are used as indicators of nutrition as well as for assessing obesity. Several indicators are available for different age-group such as ponderal index and birth-weight ratio for neonates; weight-for-age, weight as percent of median, z-score for children; and BMI, waist-hip ratio, waist-height ratio, Broca index and conicity index for adults. Such complexity can arise for many factors. Judicious choice is not always easy. Some guidelines for this choice are as follows.

- Indicator should have documented validity and reliability for the specific objective of the research.
- It must be precise, unambiguous, and measurable.
- It must also have biological relevance and appropriate for the topic of research.
- It should be sensitive so that it reflects changes over time or across groups and specific in the sense that it reflects changes only in the situation concerned.
- It should be simple, feasible, inexpensive, and should require less effort and time. Thus univariate indicator is preferable over multivariate index.
- It should not require repeat measurements at the same time.
- It should be least inconvenient to the subject and easy to implement for the assessor.

For an outcome indicator, convention is to talk about Clarity, Relevance, Economic, Adequacy, and Monitorability, acronymed as **CREAM.** All other features are the same as mentioned above but additional requirement for an outcome indicator is that it should be amenable to independent validation.

Physiological and Pathophysiological Factors

Blood pressure and pulse rate; blood and urine chemistry; evoked potential; lung, kidney, and liver functions; are examples of physiological factors. All these are directly measurable. However, cut-offs for normal, marginally abnormal, and abnormal levels are many times not clear. A level of 50 mg/dl of serum urea may be considered normal by one physician and abnormal by another. Peak expiratory flow rate of 4 l/sec and intra-ocular pressure of 22 mmHg are also borderline values. Thus, there is always a risk of misdiagnosis and missed diagnosis. Normality or otherwise of a measurement should be assessed after considering the values seen in healthy and sick subjects with sufficient precaution for overlapping values.

Pathophysiology refers to functional changes that accompany a disease. For example, kidney and liver functions change in diseases affecting these organs. These are generally measured in terms of indicators such as urinary creatinine and blood urea nitrogen levels for kidney function, and albumin and serum bilirubin level for liver function.

Similar indicators are used for other diseases. Problems in their assessment are the same as mentioned in the preceding paragraph.

Pathological Factors and Disease

Problems in assessing pathological factors are similar to physiological factors. For example, pain assessment can be done in several ways: Visual Analogue Scale (VAS), Verbal Rating Scale (VRS), McGill score, and Global Perceived Effect (GPE). Some make a distinction between intensity of pain and quality of pain. Prefer a scale for which reliability and validity is documented for your target population. Once a choice is made, implement it as faithfully as possible. For example, for assessing pain by VAS, ensure that the patient has understood the scoring and that he is providing a correct response.

Precautions are required not only for subjective assessments such as pain and other symptoms but also for relatively objective signs also. Judging size of prostate per rectum could be difficult, particularly if the enlargement is marginal. Spleen may be palpable for one physician and not for the other. Rashes can be interpreted differently. Even Electrocardiogram (ECG) is sometimes interpreted differently by different physicians.

Whereas objective criteria are generally available for laboratory based quantitative investigations such as platelet count, Erythrocyte Sedimentation Rate (ESR), and serum ferritin, but this is not so for histology, cytology, and images. Different physicians can interpret same x-ray differently. All such assessments should be based on a standard set of criteria and followed uniformly throughout the research, preferably by one observer who is fully trained for this purpose.

Medical tests can be false positive or false negative. Urine culture may show exotic pathogens because of contamination or may not be able to grow the microbe. Fine Needle Aspiration Cytology (FNAC) may not agree with mammogram for lump in breast. Plan in advance to take care of such anomalies.

Disease assessment also has several dimensions. It can be based exclusively on clinical picture, on laboratory investigations, on images, on scoring system, response to therapy, etc. Generally, a combination is used but acceptable criteria can be difficult to devise. Assessment of severity of a disease on which prognosis depends is even more difficult. If the interest in research is to find whether a particular intervention can inhibit a severe sequalae, or the interest is in delaying the onset of disease or its consequence, take care that the assessment is appropriate for these objectives.

Duration of follow-up of cases depends on the kind of disease and the type of response of interest. For research on an anaesthetic block, a few minutes follow-up may be enough in some situations. To assess response of a drug, cardiovascular system may reveal changes within a week, respiratory system may take a month, and central nervous system would need perhaps six months. Parameters such as Creatine Phosphokinase (CPK) level, coagulation time, and immune functions may take even longer.

For a serious disease such as cancer, the concern may be the duration of survival and quality of life. For less serious diseases, the focus may be on progression of disease such as blood count. In the latter case, the pre-existing level is important.

EXAMPLE 8.1: Various types of medical factors in research on antidepressant medication use and breast cancer risk

Steingart et al. (2003) report a case-control study on Antidepressant (AD) medication use and breast cancer risk among women in Ontario, Canada. Cases were 3077 women with primary breast cancer, and controls were randomly sampled from female population of Ontario. Various medical factors studied by them can be grouped as follcws:

- **Distal:** Education, income, and marital status
- **Proximal:** Smoking, alcohol, physical activity, breast cancer in first degree relatives, and oral contraceptive use
- **Physiological:** Age at menarche, age at first live birth, parity, history of breast feeding, age at menopause, height, and weight
- **Pathophysiological:** None
- **Morbidity:** Ever diagnosed with depression, traumatic stress, anorexia, history of benign breast cysts, hormone treatment, use of antidepressants (regularity, duration, time since last use, time since first use, class of depressant)

Note the classification of factors.

Side note: The study found a modest association between ever use of AD and breast cancer, which evaporated when known factors for breast cancer risk were adjusted.

8.1.3 DISEASE SPECTRUM

The term spectrum of disease is used in at least three senses. This can be illustrated by considering pain. First, one can think of pain characteristics such as throbbing, intermittent, local, etc. Second is the magnitude of pain—mild, moderate, severe, etc., or 7 on a 10-point scale. Third is the progression. The last is very aptly described for infections from susceptibility to pathogenicity and virulence. The first is the exclusive domain of clinicians. The second is quantitation of disease that we have been concerned all through this text. The third is illustrated in Figure 8-2.

In the context of research, disease spectrum has two applications. First is proper use of the terms such as pathogenicity and virulence. Second is their correct assessment when required for research. These are aptly illustrated by the COVID pandemic where various shades of disease have appeared.

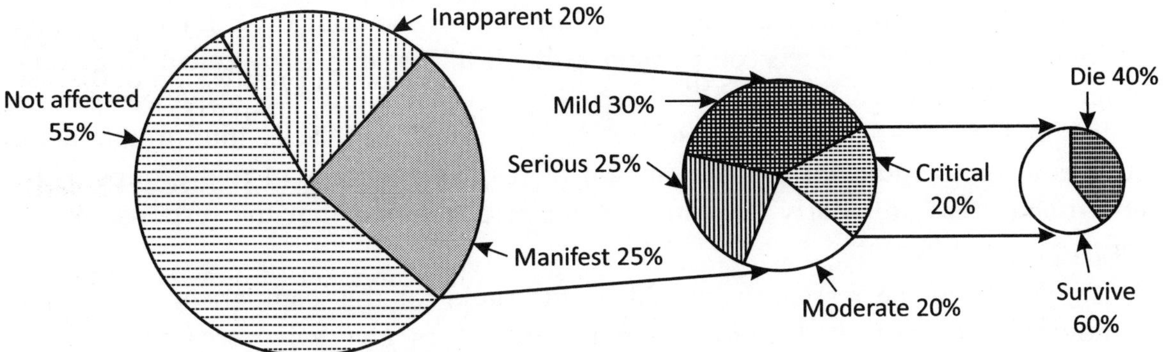

FIGURE 8-2: Disease spectrum

Severity of Disease

It is customary in medicine to categorise a patient into mild, moderate, serious, and critical phase of disease. Such categorisation helps to focus the research according to severity and helps in assessing the outcomes in right perspective. Such ordinal classification may be different for different diseases. For example, malignancies are classified as stage I, stage II, etc., hypertension as borderline, probable, and definite, and proteinuria on dipstick testing as –, ±, +, ++, and +++.

The trend now is to give exactitude to severity by quantifying it. For this, various scoring systems are used as discussed in earlier chapters. In research, scoring is preferable because it reduces subjective elements. But scoring should be used only if it is properly validated for the kind of subjects under research.

EXAMPLE 8.2: Scoring systems for predicting outcome after multiple trauma

The most widely used scoring systems for predicting outcome after trauma are Injury Severity Score (ISS) and TRauma and Injury Severity Score (TRISS). In a review, Chawla et al. (2004) found that no ideal scoring system is available for trauma injuries. In their opinion, the task of incorporating factors such as pre-existing morbidity, immunological differences and different genetic predispositions in these scores is extremely arduous. They advise caution while using any of the existing scoring systems.

Area Under the Curve

Another aspect of disease spectrum is the pattern of response or how a disease progresses or regresses over a period of time. When the pattern of response across subjects is nearly the same, average pattern for a group can be obtained. Such time trends for two groups such as cases and controls can be compared for equivalence. One popular method of such comparison in medical research is by calculating **Aarea Under the Curve** (AUC). This is the area between x-axis and the response curve as shaded in Figure 8-3a. This by itself is rarely useful and lacks interpretation but becomes a useful indicator for comparison of response pattern in two groups. If the pattern and areas are nearly the same, it can be concluded that the response in two groups is not different.

The *pattern* in the responses should be the same for this comparison to be valid as shown in Figure 8-3b. Widely different pattern can give same area as shown in Figure 8-3c. In this figure, one response curve is the inverse of the other. In such a situation, comparison of AUC can give fallacious results.

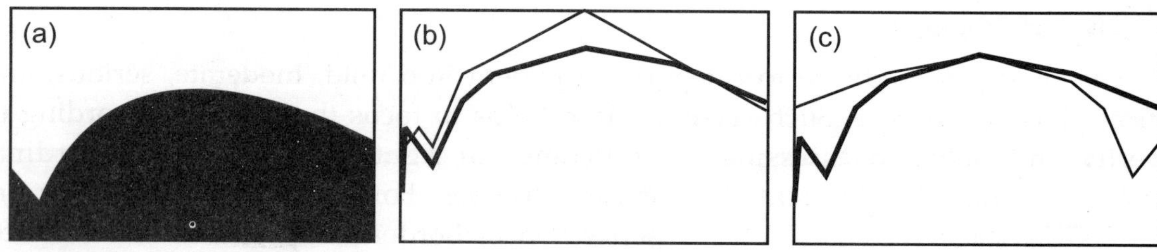

FIGURE 8-3: (a) Area under the curve, (b) and (c) two different curves with the same area

8.2 ASSESSMENT OF MORTALITY AND DURATION OF SURVIVAL

Death is inevitable yet it agitates. One of the basic aims of medical science is to reduce the levels of mortality. Realise however that death cannot be avoided: it can only be postponed. The level of mortality is reduced through postponement. We will discuss duration of survival and quality of life later in this section, but the initial concern is with the level of mortality — either in general population or in specific groups such as among infants and in the cases of cardiovascular disease.

8.2.1 ASSESSMENT OF MORTALITY

Mortality is assessed either in conjunction with the population, with live births, or with the cases of a particular type. Different denominators may give different results.

Population-based Death Rates

Crude Death Rate (CDR) is the number of deaths per 1000 population in an area at mid-year. This rate disregards the age composition of the population. Since death is closely linked to age, a higher death rate in people of old age may not be as bad as in a young population. Thus, quite often, **Age-Specific Death Rates** (ASDRs) are calculated. For public health research, such as to evaluate impact of an educational campaign for utilization of medical care facilities, death rates before and after can be compared. These rates can be calculated separately for different areas or for different age-gender groups to find which segment of population has been the prime beneficiary or has not benefited much.

CDR and ASDRs can also be calculated for cases of specific types. One such illustration is in Example 8.3 for cases of peritonitis.

EXAMPLE 8.3: Crude and age-specific death rates (ASDRs) in cases of peritonitis in a hospital over a 10-year period

Consider the following hypothetical data from imaginary Anamika Hospital.

Age (years)	Number of Cases	Number of Deaths	ASDR (%)
0-9	43	19	44
10-19	15	5	33
20-39	16	2	12
40-59	20	4	20
60-69	36	12	33
70-79	21	8	38
80+	5	3	60
Total	156	53	34=CDR

The CDR in the bottom row of the table indicates that nearly one-third cases of peritonitis in this hospital died. However, ASDRs vary from 12 percent to 60 percent. ASDR is higher in children and cases of old age, and lower in age 20 to 59 years. If this rate is plotted against age, the shape will be U-like. The example illustrates how CDR by itself in some situations fails to convey the entire story.

Note that the death rates in Example 8.3 are the same as the **case-fatality.** A death for a condition such as peritonitis is counted in case-fatality only if it occurs in the hospital. If a patient dies next day after discharge, that death is not counted. Case-fatality for any condition is calculated on the basis of deaths within a reasonable period after onset or detection so that they can be attributed to the disease. For uniformity, death in a subsequent period, even if associated with the disease, is not counted in case-fatality.

Livebirths Based Mortality

What happens if the mortality in a group is assessed in relation to the corresponding births? Many measures such as infant mortality rate, maternal mortality ratio, and probability of death before reaching age five years has number of live births as the denominator. A full list of such indicators is given below, including population-based indicators. For their definition and formulae, see any elementary biostatistics book such as by Indrayan and Labani (2019).

Livebirths based measures of mortality are extremely important for public health research such as for assessing the impact of vitamin A supplementation to a child population in an area, or impact of providing adequate immunisation coverage. Early neonatal mortality, which is the number of deaths within seven days of life per 1000 live births, can be used to assess the quality of natal services in a hospital.

The probability of death within a specified period transforms to the question of duration of survival that will be discussed in a short while. This duration can be assessed either from the time of birth or from any other onset such as the time of detection of leukaemia and the time of getting HIV infection.

Population-based death rates — Crude death rate, age-specific death rate, standardised death rate (direct and indirect), standardised mortality ratio, cause-specific death rate.

Live-births based mortality rates — Still birth ratio, perinatal mortality, neonatal mortality (early and late), infant mortality, child mortality, maternal mortality ratio.

Proportional mortality — Percentage deaths in specific age-group, percentage deaths due to specific cause or groups of causes.

Disease specific — Case-fatality.

Duration of survival — Probability of survival (or death) for a specific period, median survival time, expectation of life at birth and at other ages, healthy life expectancy, years of life lost.

Global measures — Equivalent years of life lost due to disability, i.e., disability adjusted life years (DALYs) lost.

Quality of life — Physical quality of life index for communities, activities of daily living index, quality of life score based on various questionnaires, duration of disability, severity of disability (disability weights).

Death Spectrum—Are there Desirable and Undesirable Causes of Death?

Since the probability of death is one, various causes of death tend to compete with one another. Depending upon the biologic, environmental and demographic factors, the causes only change hands. One cause replaces the other or others. If I do not die of tuberculosis, I may die of cancer. If I had not died in infancy, I may die at the age of 90 years. Over a period, the spectrum of causes of death and age at death has undergone dramatic transition. Due to various health promoting steps in many developing countries, infant deaths have substantially reduced and corresponding deaths due to chronic diseases such as cancers, diabetes and coronary artery diseases have increased. This **epidemiologic transition** is a direct result of increase in longevity.

This raises the question whether some causes of death are more desirable than others. Medical science seems to have completely ignored this issue. The thrust all around is to control all the causes. That simply is not possible. Time has come to debate which causes should in fact be promoted for death in *old age* and which should be controlled. Indrayan (2001) has emphasized this aspect. In his opinion, more people prefer sudden death in old age instead of protracted slow death, which necessarily will be painful. There is no condition yet that would bring slow death but would still be not painful. A disease such as Alzheimer's may not cause physical pain but is an intense psychological trauma. In his opinion, myocardial infarction (MI) could be the most desirable cause of death in old age since it causes sudden death in many cases. But sudden death has negative features also. The person does not get time to meet the near and dear ones, to pass on the messages, or to settle the accounts. Since the concern here, is with death in *old age*, one can counter-argue that the person should do all this at the time of reaching old age, say at 80 years or earlier, and not when death approaches.

If the contention that MI is the most desirable cause of death in old age is accepted, the whole research around the world will have to be reoriented. The risk factors for such deaths in old age have to be identified not for control but to cultivate so that the chances of death by this 'desirable' cause increase and correspondingly for other painful causes such as cancer decrease.

Perhaps a choice should be available to decide to die suddenly or slowly. The choice will be exercised not at the time of death but during the lifetime by controlling risk factors of one type and promoting the other types that increase the chance of death by the promoted factors.

All this is for deaths in old age only. Deaths in young age by any cause including MI, have to be averted as much possible. Thus, there is a need to differentiate between risk factors of death in old age and risk factors of death in young age—the former to be promoted and the latter to be controlled. This kind of orientation is currently missing from medical research.

8.2.2 DURATION OF SURVIVAL

As mentioned earlier, the crux of medical research is prolonging life and to make it liveable. Levels of various mortalities have a role but more important probably is the duration of survival and quality of life. We first discuss assessment of duration of survival and other medical durations, and then move to the issues related to quality of life.

Any period between a beginning and an endpoint is the duration. It is the time-to-event. Of special interest in medical research are duration of disease, duration between two episodes (such as of asthma), incubation period, time to reach peak concentration of a drug, duration of stay in the hospital, and duration of treatment. All these can be assessed similarly to the duration of survival. The following discussion is focused on survival but apply to the other durations also.

Special Methods for Assessment of Duration

Special methods are required to study durations because of three reasons. (i) In some cases, the information on full duration is not available. Quite often the follow-up is terminated before the endpoint is reached in some cases. Some subjects are lost to follow-up. These are called incomplete segments or **censored observations**. It is usually not appropriate to consider censored observations as missing values because they do provide at least some information. Summary measures, such as mean and SD, cannot be calculated when such incomplete segments are present. ii) The duration of survival and most other durations generally do not follow a Gaussian pattern. The distribution is right skewed. Lack of Gaussianity inhibits use of conventional statistical methods based on mean and SD such as *t*-test and ANOVA. (iii) The main interest for duration is rarely in mean or median but in finding the percentage of cases with different durations such as five-year survival rate. For these three reasons, a special method called **survival analysis** is used. When no censored observation is present, usual methods of analysis can be used, possibly after transformation to correct for skewness.

The duration of survival can be assessed either from birth, from any age, from the time of onset of a particular disease, etc. If a patient lives through the normal course of life after an intervention such as organ transplantation, it can be claimed that the intervention has been totally successful. The basic summary measure used in survival analysis is the chance of survival for a specific duration, or of attaining a particular duration for reaching to any other outcome of interest. Median or average is also used in situations where censored observations are none or negligible.

Survival Analysis

Life table method of survival analysis is slightly different from the classical life tables used in calculation of expectation of life. Survival analysis keeps a provision for censored observations that a classical life table does not.

The duration of survival or age can be grouped into intervåls such as 0-1, 1-4, and 5-9 years. Because of such grouping, it is not necessary to be continuously observing the subjects. For example, in an experiment on a carcinogenic agent that kills mice, a visit can be made each morning to note down the number still surviving. The survival duration would be available as 0-1 day, 1-2 days, 2-3 days, etc., and not as 30 hours, 58 hours, etc. However, wherever feasible, exact duration should be recorded.

The plot of probability of survival at different points of time is called the **survival curve** (Figure 8-4). Because of incomplete segments, this probability is not the same as percentage of survivors. Also, this probability is serially calculated on the basis of the probability in the previous interval.

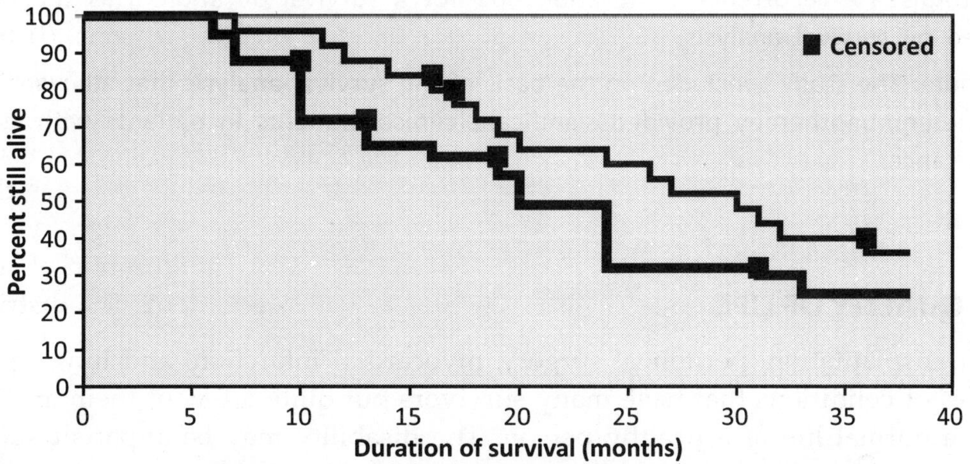

FIGURE 8-4: An example of a survival curve for patients of lymphocytic leukaemia and mylogeneous leukaemia

Dropouts and those not followed-up for full period till reaching the defined end point (such as death) are considered to have been lost at the mid-point of the next interval. If a patient was known to be alive at five years but was not traceable at six years, he is considered to have been lost at 5½ years. In this case it is not known that the subject is alive or dead at six years. No assumption is made regarding their time of death. The probability of survival is calculated with this assumption.

When survival duration is noted exactly instead of intervals, use **Kaplan-Meir method** of survival analysis. In this method, the censored values are counted only upto the time the subjects are seen alive. After that they are ignored. The probability of survival is serially calculated at each time point based on the known deaths out of known survivors. For details see Indrayan and Malhotra (2018).

As was mentioned earlier, the method of survival analysis can be used to assess any duration, and not just duration of survival. Also, survival can take many forms. Example 8.4 illustrates one such application.

EXAMPLE 8.4: Use of the method of survival analysis in assessing various kinds of durations

Hanna et al. (2001) performed three multi-institutional randomised controlled trials for assessing the therapeutic effect of post-resection adjuvant active specific immunotherapy in patients with stage II and stage III colon cancer. All outcomes of interest were durations: time-to-disease recurrence, overall survival interval, disease-free survival interval, and recurrence-free survival interval. Last three illustrate various types of survival duration. All these durations were studied by Kaplan-Meir method. Note that time-to-disease recurrence is duration but not a survival duration. This too can be studied by survival analysis.

Side note: The study concluded on the basis of the **survival analysis** that adjuvant active specific immunotherapy provided significant clinical benefits in patients with stage II colon cancer.

8.2.3 QUALITY OF LIFE

Organ transplantation, peritoneal surgery, myocardial infarction, and lung cancer are examples of conditions that have many survivors but quite a few of them are not able to lead a normal life of a healthy person. The disability may be apparent such as in walking and talking, or more subtle as in doing hard work for long hours. Quality of life assessment is gaining importance as more and more can live longer due to medical intervention but have disability of one kind or the other.

Health-related Quality of Life

In severe conditions, particularly in old age, quality of life is assessed in terms of Activities of Daily Living (ADL) index that incorporates scores on the level of independence in walking, bathing, use of toilet, and dressing. In the case of chronic patients, this may contain information on sleep, appetite, sexual functions, social participation, work performance, etc. Conventionally, a quality of life questionnaire has domains such as physical health, psychological well-being, level of independence, social relationships, and environment.

Quality of life has intimate local context. But development of a quality-of-life questionnaire to suit local conditions is a long-drawn process involving pretesting, testing, and retesting. If quality of life is an issue in your research, try to locate an already available questionnaire that has been validated for your kind of setup. For example, there is a well-tested World Health Organization Quality of Life (WHO-QOL) questionnaire with 100 items of information. Its brief version contains 26 items. There is another short form with 36 items called SF-36. These can be used on healthy persons as well. For specific conditions such as visual impairments and cardiac diseases, separate questionnaires are available. All these may require some modification, particularly regarding the language, to adapt them to the local conditions.

Quality of life assessments should be interpreted with abundant caution. These mostly reflect perception that can quickly change. A patient in an advanced stage of malignancy may still report a good quality of life.

At the community level, quality of life index takes an entirely different format. It is customary to measure physical quality of life in a community by a combination of literacy rate, expectation of life at one year, and infant mortality rate. Each is rescaled zero to 100 from minimum seen to the maximum plausible, and an average is taken. By its very nature, it excludes psychological aspects such as happiness and satisfaction in life.

8.3 DATA SUMMARIES

Data summaries such as mean, median, mode, standard deviation, percentiles, and inter-quartile range have tremendous role in assessing health and disease in the groups of cases under study. At least an elementary knowledge of these summaries is essential for conducting a successful research. These concepts are used in the protocol at the time of describing the proposed methods of analysis and interpretation.

8.3.1 REPRESENTATIVE SUMMARY MEASURES FOR QUANTITATIVE DATA

Primarily two types of summary measures are used in medical research. One that represents location of the distribution such as the central value and the value is seen in, say, more than 75 percent subjects, and the other that describes how different are values from one-another.

Mean, Median, and Mode

Levels in a group can be represented either by a single value, or by a range of values. The representative single value is called the central value. It is computed in terms of either mean, or median or mode. Mean is the usual average that need not be explained any further. Statistically inclined researchers understand that the usual mean is **arithmetic mean**. The other types of mean are geometric and harmonic. Geometric mean has application in multiplicative measurements such as antibody titre and gamma radiation count (where log values are used), and harmonic mean is sometimes used for averaging rates. Such special applications are avoided in this text because the emphasis is on the basics.

Median is the most middle value obtained after arranging the data in ascending (or descending) order. It is an intermediary value that divides a group in to two equal halves. Median is a good representative of central values when extremely high or extremely low values (outliers) are present. If the duration of admission after a surgery is mostly 3 to 5 days but one or two patients have to be in the ward for 30 or 40 days because of complications, the mean will be highly vitiated. Use median in this situation because such outliers do not affect median. Use median also for highly skewed distribution also such as of IL-6 values.

Mode is the most commonly occurring value. If the most seen incubation period from exposure to appearance of rash for measles is 10 days, this is the mode. Mode can be used for ordinal data also. For example, one can say that the most common response to the occurrence of nosocomial infection in a hospital is 'slight' when this possibility is graded as none, slight, moderate, or strong. Similarly, mode can be used for nominal variables also. Mean and median do not have this flexibility. Also, for quantitative measurements, more than one mode can exist. This would happen when the distribution has two or more peaks although one peak can be smaller than the other. Age distribution of Hodgkin's disease and leukaemia is bimodal with one (smaller) peak around 20 years and the other (bigger) peak at age around 60 years.

EXAMPLE 8.5: Mean, median and mode

Imagine survival duration (in years) after detection of cervical cancer in a group of 12 patients with radical hysterectomy:

7 4 7 5 2 29 8 6 24 3 5 2

The **mean** survival duration is 92/12 = 7.6 years. This obviously is not representative of these values since 9 out of 12 patients have survival less than this average. Mean is vitiated in this example due to extreme values 29 and 24 years for patients who probably lived their normal life. In such situations, the appropriate measure is **median**. For n = 12, this is the average of sixth and seventh values after arranged in increasing order. These values are 5 and 6 years. Thus, the median is 5.5 years. This looks like a good representative value in this example. Apparently there are three modes in this example—2 years, 5 years, and 7 years—each occurring 2 times. Multiple **modes** are rarely acceptable. No mode can be obtained in this example until the data are available for more patients.

Calculating mean, median, and mode is simple, but their usage requires caution. Saying that *a person with head in oven and feet in freezer is comfortable* epitomizes the caution required. It must always be accompanied by a measure of dispersion such as Standard Deviation (SD) that we describe in a short while. The number of observations should also be mentioned. Mean of values in three subjects has little meaning. The mean value in 300 subjects may be the same but has very different reliability. Outliers have tremendous impact on mean. Can a person drown in a channel with an *average* depth of 12 inches? Yes, if there is a 8 feet deep pit somewhere!

Conclusion based on mean alone without considering other correlates could be misleading. If an antihypertensive drug is able to reduce diastolic BP by 10 mmHg on average after one week of use by hypertensives, the other considerations such as side-effects, cost, and convenience of intake cannot be ignored altogether while evaluating the usefulness of the drug. Mean, median, and mode are much more meaningful when they are based on homogenous group. For example, mean survival period of assorted patients admitted in a hospital could be an inappropriate measure of efficiency since there would be cases of hernia with minimal risk of death and cases of advanced malignancy with grave prognosis: The survival periods could be widely different.

Percentiles

Sometimes the interest is not in the central value but is in a threshold seen in certain percent of the subjects. These are called **percentiles.** In child growth, it is common to say, for example, that 14 kg is the 90th percentile of weight for 2-year old girls. This implies that 90 percent girls of age 2 years have weight 14 kg or less. The method to obtain *k*th percentiles is to pick up ($k \times n/100$)th value after arranging the data in ascending order. For survival duration in Example 8.5, 70th percentile is the $70 \times 12/100 = 8$th value in ascending order, which is approximately 6 years.

EXAMPLE 8.6: A good use of percentiles for assessing the risk of heart disease

Evidence is growing that children with low birthweight but with rapid gain in weight and increase in body mass index after the age of one year are at greater risk of coronary heart disease later in life, particularly males (Eriksson et al. 2001). Rapid gain implies that a child who was at lower percentile for birthweight reaches to a higher percentile at, say, age 8 years. A boy with birthweight in the bottom 10 percent (10th percentile) who rapidly gains weight to reach in top 25 percent (beyond 75th percentile) at age 5 or 10 years is at much greater risk of coronary heart disease. This is called **crossing the centiles** and illustrates a very apt application of the concept of percentiles.

Quartiles, tertiles, and deciles are special percentiles. Twenty-fifth, fiftieth, and seventy-fifth percentiles are called first, second and third **quartiles,** respectively, because they divide total subjects into four groups of equal size. Tenth, twentieth, etc., percentiles are called **deciles** since they divide the subjects in ten equal groups. If a man's height is 188 cms, he may be in top decile. Less than 10 percent men will have that much height or more. **Tertiles** are the cut points that divide the group in three equal parts.

Standard Deviation and Variance

Some measurements such as body temperature in healthy subjects do not vary much across healthy individuals whereas others such as cholesterol level are highly variable. Thus dispersion (scatter) is important. A universally accepted measure of dispersion is Standard Deviation (SD).

Dispersion is the difference one value has with the other. Instead of calculating so many differences, it is convenient to find the difference each value has with group mean. Some of these differences would be negative and some positive, and the sum will be zero. To get rid of negative values, a standard statistical practice is to square them. All differences are squared. The average of these squared differences is called **variance.** To retrieve the original units (*i.e.*, μg in place of μg^2 for square), square-root is taken. The value so obtained is the SD. Thus, SD actually is the root-mean-square-deviation and measures dispersion around the mean. If SD of systolic blood pressure (BP) in males of age 40-49 years is 8 mmHg and in females 10 mmHg, it shows that the systolic level varies more in females of age 40-49 years than in males of this age.

An important property of SD in a Gaussian distribution is that the range from (mean – 2SD) to (mean + 2SD) covers nearly 95 percent values. This is called mean ±2SD range. If mean of fasting blood glucose level among healthy subjects is 90 mg/dl and SD is 7.5 mg/dl, then this range will be from (90 – 2×7.5 =) 75 to (90 + 2×7.5 =) 105 mg/dl. Nearly 95 percent of such subjects would have levels between 75 and 105 mg/dl. This property is extensively used in medicine to delineate normal levels of various measurements.

Standard deviation must be interpreted with caution when comparing variability of one measurement with the other. A small looking SD such as 0.2 mEq/l for serum magnesium is in fact high compared to SD = 10 mg/dl for cholesterol since the mean is only 2.0 mEq/l for serum magnesium while it is 150 mg/dl for cholesterol. A unit-free measure of variability for comparison of dispersion in different measurements is **Coefficient of Variation** (CV). This is calculated as

$$CV = SD \times 100 \div mean.$$

In the above example, CV is 0.2×100÷2.0 = 10 percent for serum magnesium and 10×100/150 = 6.67 percent for cholesterol level. Thus, variability in magnesium is relatively higher. A higher CV indicates that the measurement is less reliable, and its research utility is less. The CV cannot be calculated when mean is zero and should not be calculated when mean could be very small. This can happen when negative values are also present. For example, average gain after a treatment over the baseline level could be very small in some situations.

Variance, although in square units, is a more popular term particularly in the context of attributing part of variation to certain set of risk factors. For example, 60 percent of the variance in P3 amplitude (a measure of cognitive functioning) explained by genetic factors implies that 60 percent of the differences among individuals in P3 amplitudes are attributable to the differences in their genetic factors.

EXAMPLE 8.7: Differentials in SDs

While reporting results of a case-control study on heavy vs. nonheavy drinking as a risk of intracerebral hemorrahage in Australia, Thrift et al. (1999) state the mean and SD of body mass index also while studying its confounding effect. Among males (n = 200 each), the mean Body Mass Index (BMI) in cases was 26.2 and in controls 25.8. There is not much difference in the means. But the SD of BMI was 4.5 among cases and only 3.6 among controls. Authors have not commented on this aspect but different SDs show that the cases could be quite different for BMI from one another relative to the controls. This can influence the final results.

8.3.3 SUMMARY MEASURES FOR QUALITATIVE DATA

Not many options are available to summarise qualitative data. Either the count itself or the percentage of subjects possessing a particular characteristic or meeting a set criterion is used as a summary measure. Statistical equivalent of percentage is **proportion** that is stated in terms of fraction considering the whole group as one. If 27 patients of peritonitis survive out of 48 admitted in a hospital in one-year period, the percentage survival is 56.25, and the proportion is 0.5625. This proportion is denoted by p.

What is a Binomial Distribution?

As stated earlier, a variable is called **dichotomous (or binary)** when it has only two possible outcomes. They must be mutually exclusive. Birthweight is a quantitative measurement but becomes dichotomous when categorized as <2.5 kg and ≥2.5 kg: sometimes labelled as low birthweight and not low birthweight. Probabilities relating to such variables are obtained by a binomial distribution.

In a Sexually Transmitted Disease (STD) clinic, the attendees are identified either with STD or without STD (cases with psychosexual problems or nonSTD genital diseases). If it is known from experience that 82 percent (p = 0.82) of the clinic attendees have at least one STD, what is the probability that in a randomly selected group of four attendees, all turn out to have STD? This is a simple problem for those who are familiar with probability concepts. Use of multiplication rule tells that this probability is $(0.82)^4 = 0.45$—not really high. There is a 55% chance that at least one of these four will be a nonSTD patient.

Such probabilities are immensely useful for dichotomous variables when the group size n is small. When n is large and the proportion p not too small so that np is not small (say, ≥8), the binomial probabilities can be reasonably approximated by Gaussian form. In such cases, there is no need to worry about specially using binomial method.-

Power of Descriptive Statistics

All summary measures described in this section are descriptive statistics in the sense that they describe the state of health for a group. Strength of descriptive statistics is generally underestimated. In fact, they are the ones that drive many medical conclusions. Policies regarding diagnosis and treatment or for provision of services at macro level are based on descriptive summaries. Finding that 65 percent of diabetic retinopathy cases are proliferative has a different implication than the finding that only 12 percent have such severe form.

SUMMARY

Before embarking on actual data collection, a researcher must be aware how to use the proposed data to assess various medical factors. Assessment is relatively easy, and the research is focused when medical factors are divided into antecedent and outcome, modifiable and unmodifiable, and distal, proximal, physiological, pathophysiological, and pathological. All factors must be converted to measurable indicators. When many indicators are available to measure the same factor, a judicious choice is required.

Several indicators are available to assess levels of mortality. Choose the one that focuses on your objective. Duration of survival, or any other duration (such as duration of disease) is assessed by the method survival analysis, including Kaplan-Meier method.

Mean, median, mode, percentiles, standard deviation, and proportion are commonly used parameters for assessing the state of health. These are the summary measures and called descriptive statistics when calculated for the sample values.

REFERENCES

Chawla MN, Hildebrand F, Pape HC, Giannoudis PV. Predicting outcome after multiple trauma: which scoring system? Injury 2004;35:347-358.

Eriksson JG, Forsen T, Tuomilehto J, Osmond C, Barker DJ. Early growth and coronary hearth disease in later life: longitudinal study. BMJ 2001;322(7292):949-953.

Hanna MG Jr, Hoover HC Jr, Vermorken JB, Haris JE, Pinedo HM. Adjuvant active specific immunotherapy of stage II and stage III colon cancer with an autologous tumour cell vaccine: first randomized phase III trial show promise. Vaccine 2001;19:2576-2582.

Indrayan A., Malhotra RK, Medical Biostatistics, 4th ed. CRC Press, 2018.

Indrayan A, Labani S. Simple Biostatistics for Medical, Nursing and Pharmacy Students, Fifth Edition. Delhi: Brillion Publishers, 2019.

Indrayan A. Can I choose the cause of my death? BMJ 2001;322:1003.

Steingart A, Cotterchio M, Kreiger N, Sloan M. Antidepressant medication use and breast cancer risk: a case-control study. Int J Epidemiol 2003;32:961-966.

Thrift AG, Donnan GA, McNeil JJ. Heavy drinking, but not moderate or intermediate drinking, increases the risk of intracerebral hemorrhage. Epidemiology 1999; 10:307-312.

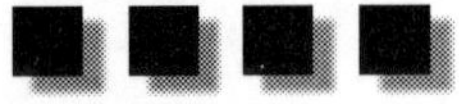

CHAPTER 9

How to Prepare the Research Protocol

KEY TERMS AND CONCEPTS

- ✓ Choosing a Research Topic
- ✓ Objectives and Hypothesis
- ✓ Contents and Structure of Protocol
- ✓ Timeline
- ✓ Inclusion and Exclusion Criteria

The information provided in the previous chapters is required for preparing the protocol. This is the document that describes the proposed research in its entirety, comprising the elements such as title, statement of the problem, objectives and hypotheses, the design and the sample size, the variables of interest, the method of collection of the data, the method of the analysis strategies, and the timeline. Protocol is the backbone that supports research in all steps of its execution. Thus, sufficient thought must be given to its preparation. Many times, it gradually evolves as more information becomes available and progressively examined for its adequacy. Most important aspect of protocol is the statement of the problem, objectives, and hypotheses. This deserves a separate discussion.

9.1 THE PROBLEM, OBJECTIVES, AND HYPOTHESES

A full section in one of the previous chapters is devoted to the selection of the problem for research and how to state it. In brief, the title should be precise to include what is proposed to be investigated and how. For example, if it is a Randomised Controlled Trial (RCT), state that in the title. If it is an observational study, mention that it is prospective, case-control, or cross-sectional. For stating the problem, follow the guidelines stated earlier, including a reference to the lacuna in the existing knowledge. Extensive literature search and a search of all the related databases may be required to make a convincing case that the proposed problem indeed requires a study and will help develop the medical science. Guidelines for setting and stating the objectives and hypotheses are as follows.

9.1.1 OBJECTIVES

Even the focused area of the problem may have several smaller components. Formulating objectives is breaking down the problem into a parsimonious set of questions to which answers would be sought. These questions are reworded as objectives in a measurable format. Statement of the objectives in this manner also helps to assess the feasibility and the limitations of the study. Actual relevance of the study also becomes clear when the broad and specific objectives are framed.

Broad and Specific Objectives

Broad objective is generally the one that specifies the area of research, and specific objectives delineate the specific aspects of the problem. As mentioned earlier in a different context, a primary medical research can have two types of broad objectives. One is to describe features of a condition such as clinical profile of a disease, prevalence in various segments of population, and the levels of medical parameters seen in different types of cases. The second type of objective is to study associations and cause-effect type of relationships. This is called analytical and involves comparison of two or more groups. The broad objective would determine the methodology to be followed.

A broad objective would generally encompass several dimensions of the problem. These dimensions are spelt out in specific objectives. For example, the broad objective may be to assess whether a new diagnostic modality is better than the existing one. The specific objectives in this case could be separately stated, on its (i) positive and negative predictivity, (ii) safety in case it is an invasive procedure, or side effects, (iii) feasibility under a variety of settings such as field, clinic, and hospital, (iv) acceptability by the medical community and the patients, and (v) cost-effectiveness. Another specific objective could be to evaluate its efficacy in different age-gender or disease-severity groups so that the kinds of cases where it works well are identified. Specific objectives relate to the specific activities and they identify the key indicators of interest. Do not use umbrella type of terms such as 'To study the role of …' Instead say direct, for example, 'To estimate the relative risk of …'

Keep the specific objectives as few and focused as possible. Do not try to answer too many questions by a single study especially if its size is small. Too many objectives can render the study difficult to manage. Whatever objectives are set, stick to them all through the study as much as possible. Changing them mid-way or at the time of report writing signals that enough thinking was not done at the time of protocol development.

In the case of clinical trials, the objective could be to establish superiority of one regimen over the other, or equivalence or non-inferiority. This objective is different from establishing efficacy such as that it is at least 70% or safety that says, for example, that no more than 5% experience significant side effects. Superiority, equivalence, and non-inferiority require that a margin is pre-fixed that will be inconsequential in managing the cases. Some details of this are given later in this chapter.

Operationalise the objectives into variables you plan to study. If the outcome is recovery, specify that it is in terms of relief in pain, ability to walk, improvement in lung function, etc. If you can also specify the exact quantity of improvement, the research quality will improve. If the objective is to estimate safety, specify that this will be in terms of which side effects, complications, duration of adverse reactions, or whatever is applicable.

In short, the objectives should follow the **SMART** format – **S**pecific, **M**easurable, **A**chievable, **R**elevant, and **T**imely.

9.1.2 HYPOTHESES

A **hypothesis** is a precise expression of the expected results regarding state of a phenomenon in the target population. Research is about replacing the existing 'hypotheses' by the new ones that are more plausible. In medical research, hypotheses could purport to explain the etiology of diseases, prevention strategies, screening and diagnostic modalities, distribution of occurrence in different segments of population, the strategies to treat or to manage a disease, to prevent the recurrence or adverse sequelae, etc. Consider which of these types of hypotheses can be investigated by the proposed research.

Hypotheses are not guesses, they reflect the depth of knowledge of the topic of research. They must be stated in a manner that can be tested by collecting evidence.

The hypothesis that dietary pattern affects the occurrence of cancer is not testable unless the specifics of diet and the type of cancer are specified. Antecedents and outcome variables, or other relevant variables, should be exactly specified in a hypothesis. Generate a separate hypothesis for each major expected relationship.

The hypotheses must correspond to the general and specific objectives of the study. Thus, carefully examine each objective and assess which of these generate a new hypothesis. Whereas objectives define the key variables of interest, hypotheses are guide to the strategies to analyse the data.

Beware that objectives and hypotheses are governed by the current knowledge. For example, nobody wants to know how music aptitude affects cancer risk, although future endeavour may reveal an association between these.

9.2 PROTOCOL CONTENT

Protocol is the focal document for any medical research. It is a comprehensive yet concise statement regarding the proposal. Protocol is generally prepared on a structured format with headings such as introduction containing background that exposes the gaps needing research, review of literature with details of various views and findings of others on the issue including those that are in conflict, a clear-worded set of objectives and the hypotheses under test, the methodology for collection of valid and reliable observations, a statement about methods of data analysis, and the process of drawing conclusions. These components are listed more systematically next. Further details are given later in this section.

Administrative aspects such as sharing of responsibilities should also be mentioned. In any case a protocol would contain the name of the investigator, his qualification, institutional affiliation, and the hierarchy such as guides in the case of Master's and Doctoral work. The place of the study such as the department and institution should also be mentioned. The year the proposal was framed is also required. Appendix at the end includes the form of data collection, the consent form, etc. The main body of a protocol must address the following questions with convincing justification.

9.2.1 BROAD AND SPECIFIC CONTENTS OF THE PROTOCOL

Protocol is a precise document with no frills. We first describe the broad contents and then come to the specifics. These are further explained in the next section.

Broad Contents

Title

1. What is actually intended to be studied—whether the title of the study is sufficiently specific?

Introduction

2. How the problem arose? In what context?
3. What is the need of the study—what new is expected that is not known so far? Is it worth investigating? Is the study exploratory in nature, or definitive conclusions are expected?
4. To what segment of population or to what type of cases the problem is addressed?

Review of literature

5. What is the status of the present knowledge? What are the lacunae? Are there any conflicting reports? How the problem has been approached so far? With what results? What are the lacunae in knowledge and how your work relates to this lacuna?

Objectives and hypotheses

6. What is the broad objective and what are the specific questions or hypotheses to be addressed by the study—are these clearly defined, realistic, and evaluable?

Methodology

7. What are the subjects, what is the target population, what is the source of subjects, how are they going to be selected, how many in each group, and what is the justification? What will be the statistical power of your study to detect a clinically relevant difference? What are the inclusion and exclusion criteria? Is there any possibility of selection bias, and how is this to be handled?
8. What exactly is the intervention, if any—its duration, dosage, frequency, etc.? In what way, if any, this intervention is different from the routinely prescribed. What instructions and material are to be given to the subjects at any time?
9. Is there any comparison group? Why is it needed and how will it be chosen? How will it provide valid comparison?
10. What is the exact design of the study? Is it descriptive or analytical? If analytical, is it observational (prospective, retrospective, or cross-sectional), experimental or a human trial? If trial, is it without parallel control (before-after, cross-over, repeated measures, etc.) or with a parallel control group? Whether it is a superiority trial, equivalence trial, or a noninferiority trial? Experimental design is one-way, two-way, or what?

11. What are the possible confounders? How these and other possible sources of bias are to be handled? What is the method of allocation of subjects to different groups? If any blinding, how will it be implemented? Is there any matching?
12. On what characteristics would the subjects be assessed—what are the antecedents and outcomes of interest? When these assessments would be made? Who will assess them? Whether these assessments are necessary and sufficient to answer the proposed questions?
13. What is the operational definition of various assessments? What methods of assessment are to be used—are they sufficiently valid and reliable? What information will be obtained by inspecting records, what by interview, what by laboratory and radiological investigations, and what by physical examination? Is there any system of continuous monitoring in place? What is the schedule? What mechanism is to be adopted for quality control of measurements?
14. What form is to be used for eliciting and recording the data? (Attach it as Appendix) Who will record? Whether or not it will contain the instructions?
15. What system is to be followed to obtain and record data, or to ensure their accuracy? What mechanism would be in place to check for internal consistency and for errors in recording?
16. What is to be done in case of contingencies such as dropout of subjects or nonavailability of the kit or the regimen, or development of complications in some subjects? Or, when protocol violations occur? What safeguards are provided to protect the health of the participants? Also, when to stop the study if a conclusion emerges before the full course of the sample? Under what conditions a subject will be withdrawn from the study?
17. What is the period of the study and the timeline? (See Figure 9-1)

Data analysis

18. How do you plan to check the correctness of entries in your worksheet for mistyping, unintentional copying, errors in calculating scores based on entered data, etc.?
19. What estimations, comparisons and trend assessments are to be done at the time of data analysis? Whether the quality and quantity of available data would be adequate for these estimations, comparisons, and trend assessments?
20. What statistical indices are to be used to summarise the data? Where would you use percentages, where mean, where odds ratio, etc.? Are these indices sufficiently valid and reliable under the condition of the study?
21. How the data analysis is to be done—what statistical methods would be used and whether these methods are really appropriate for the type of data, and to provide correct answer to the questions? What level of significance or the level of

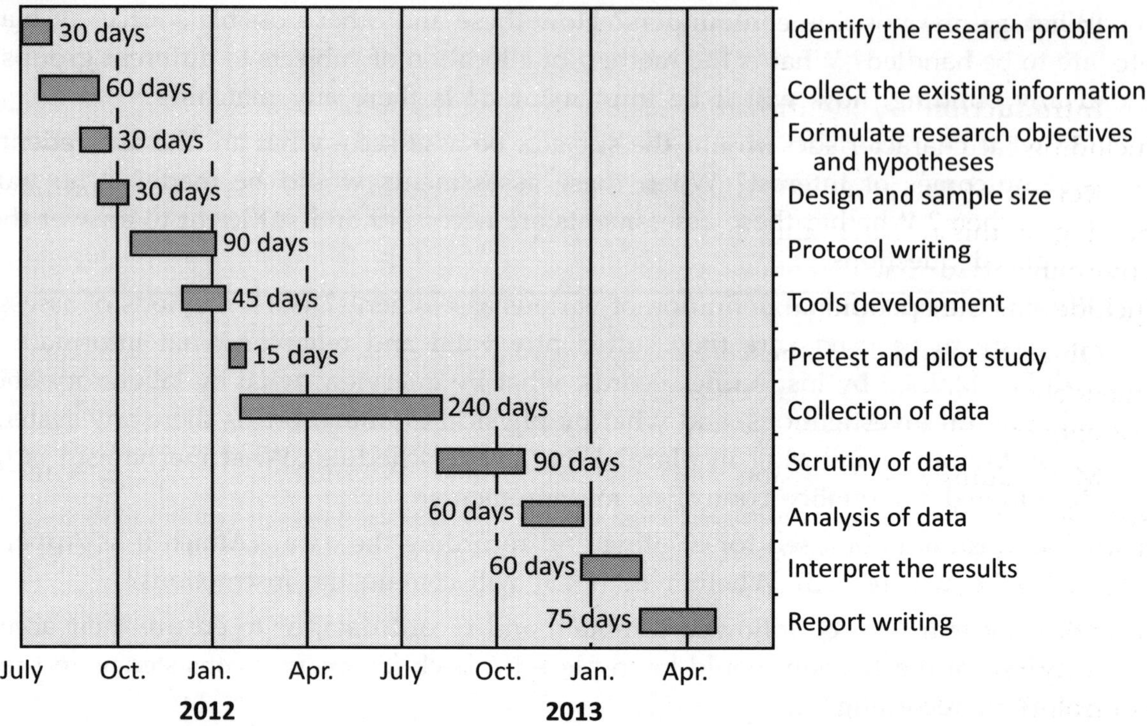

FIGURE 9-1: An example of a timeline (Gantt chart) for a medical research project

confidence is to be used? How the missing data, noncompliance, and nonresponse are to be handled?

22. What is the expected reliability of the conclusions? What are the limitations of the study, if any, for generalisability or applicability?

Logistics

23. What resources are required, and how are they to be arranged?
24. How the responsibilities are to be shared between investigators, supporting units (e.g., pathology, radiology, biostatistics), hospital administration, funding agency, etc.?
25. What are training needs, if any, and who would conduct this training?

Specific Elements of a Medical Research Protocol

At the risk of some duplication, we give the specific elements next so that nothing is missed.

Title — Clearly worded but concise title that aptly describes the gist of the study.

Investigator(s) — Name, qualification, affiliation, supervisor/advisor, degree, year, etc.

Introduction — Identification of the problem area, background information including lacunae and gap in knowledge, and why is it important to fill this gap.

Review of literature — Critical appraisal of the findings of others that could have bearing on this research; this may have global overtones but must be focused on local environment so that the relevance is clearly established; confine it to the topic and include latest developments.

Objectives and hypotheses — Clear-worded short statement of what exactly is intended to be achieved by this research, and for what segments of population or patients would it apply; statement of what hypotheses are under test.

Methodology — Inclusion and exclusion criteria for subjects as described next, specification of various groups, number of subjects to be included in each group with justification, method of selection of subjects, method of allocation of subjects to different groups, blinding and other strategies to reduce bias, matching criteria with justification, specification of intervention if any and the treatment schedule, definition of variables to be assessed, assessment of compliance, identification of confounders and their control, method of eliciting information, validity and reliability of devices, and time-sequence of collecting data and their frequency.

Ethics — List of ethical problems and how are they proposed to be resolved, including protocol deviations, and safeguards for the participants.

Statistical evaluation — Methods to be used for various estimations, to test various hypotheses, to detect trends, etc., as dictated by the objectives; comment on likely internal validity and external generalisability of the results, including the strategies for handling missing data, confounding, and biases.

Limitations — Conditions or groups to which the results would not apply.

Logistics — Arrangement of resources, assignment of duties, sharing of responsibilities, and training; feasibility of the study within the time frame and resources; various possible contingencies and how they would be handled.

References — Those cited in the text of the protocol and possibly a bibliography of other literature on the topic that could be of interest to the reader.

Appendix — Forms such as questionnaire, schedule, or proforma to be used: structured or open, precoded or not, and pretested or not; the consent form; letter of support; ethical clearance; etc.

In short, the protocol should be able to convince the reader that the topic is important, the data collected would be reliable and valid for that topic, and that contradictions, if any, would be satisfactorily resolved. Present it before a critical but positive audience and get their feedback. You may be creative and may be able to argue with conviction, but skepticism in science is regularly practiced. In fact, it is welcome. The method and results would be continuously scrutinised for possible errors. Protocol is the most important document to evaluate the scientific merit of the research proposal by the funding agencies as well as by the accepting agencies (the teaching faculty in the case of postgraduate research). Peer validation is a rule rather than exception in scientific pursuits. A good research is the one that is robust to such reviews.

Merits of a Protocol

A protocol should consist of full details with no short cuts yet should be concise. It should be to the point, and coherent. The reader, who may not be fully familiar with the topic, should be made absolutely clear about why, what, and how of the proposed research. To the extent possible, it should embody the interest of the sponsor, the investigator, the patients, and the society. It also is a reference source for the members of research team whenever needed. It should be complete and easy to implement.

Protocol is a big help at the time of writing of the thesis or a paper. Introduction and methods section remain much the same as in the protocol, although in an elaborate format. The objectives as stated in the protocol help to retain the focus in the report. Much of the literature review done at the time of protocol writing also proves handy at the time of writing a report such as MD/MS thesis.

Inclusion and Exclusion Criteria

Inclusion criteria — These are the characteristics such as age-group, type of disease, severity of disease, and comorbidity that are necessary for subject to be considered as eligible for inclusion in the study. Whether or not such a subject is actually included will depend on the selection procedure. Some of these may become ineligible when exclusion criteria are imposed.

Exclusion criteria — These are those conditions the presence of which will exclude an otherwise eligible subject from the study. Generally, these conditions are indicative of severe form of disease or complications that render a subject unsuitable for that research or are confounders that complicate the interpretation. For example, pregnant females are excluded in many studies.

Inclusion and exclusion criteria are part of the case definition that delineates the target population. The purpose is that only appropriate subjects participate, and they remain safe. Sometimes research requires that only very specific type of cases is included so that unadulterated results are obtained. But then the generalisability suffers. You will like that your results apply to patients seeking medical help of the type under study, but the results would not be applicable to such general class of patients because of inclusion and exclusion criteria. Nonetheless, investigation on such restricted class proves a point about, sch as the efficacy of a regimen.

9.2.2 STRUCTURE OF THE PROTOCOL

Different institutions require protocol in their specific format, but the general pattern as stated earlier is Title, Introduction, Review of Literature, Objectives and Hypotheses, Material and Methods, Data Analysis, System of Conclusions, and References. Protocol does not have a Discussion section, which is required for a thesis and a paper for publication. Many of these are already discussed in the previous section. However, some need more elaboration as follows.

Title and Introduction

Title specifies the topic of research and broad methodology without being long. For example, 'A case-control study of colorectal cancer risk in obese vegetarians in south India' says it all. It contains the topic of research, the broad methodology and the locale. There is no need to add any frills. Sometimes the title is framed after completing first draft of the protocol.

Introduction in a protocol should be short, say not exceeding one page, giving details of how the problem crossed your mind. Begin introduction by clearly identifying the subject area of investigation and the specific problem you want to investigate and why. Identify the gaps in knowledge. Use important words in your title if that is decided. The purpose is not to lose focus and to avoid a general discussion. Briefly state how you plan to approach the problem without discussing the actual technique. The details would be in Material and Methods section. Finish the introduction by clearly stating the purpose and/or hypothesis you propose to investigate, such as 'The purpose of this study is to determine the effect of enzyme concentration on its reaction rate in cases of benign prostatic hyperplasia'.

Review of Literature

Restrict the review to the literature directly pertinent to the topic of research. The review must support your contention about the gap in knowledge you wish to plug. Most efficient in this respect are review articles because they tend to highlight the lacunae. Latest articles are more helpful as they provide a recent picture. For details of how to review and what, see Chapter 3.

The review of literature should be balanced and impartial. It should include all recent literature and not selective in support of your hypothesis so that there is no bias. Include those also that are inconsistent with or opposed to the hypothesis. Justify the rationale of research with reasons that effectively counter the opposite or indifferent view. Remember that research is a step in relentless search for truth, and it must pass the litmus test put forward by conflicting and competing facts.

Objectives and Hypothesis

These have been discussed in detail in Section 9.1.

Material and Methods

Consider this as the most important constituent of protocol, particularly for a **PG thesis.**

Make no compromise and adopt the most suitable methodology that can directly achieve the stated objectives. If the most suitable is not feasible due to resource constraint, specifically say so and justify why you would not be able to use the most appropriate methodology. In this case choose an alternative methodology but explain why this not so optimal methodology can still provide valid results.

Beside methods for collecting and collating the evidence, comment about their validity and reliability. Identify the variables that would provide information on each specific objective. Do not collect data more than you need because that will divide your attention, deviate the focus, and unnecessarily load the patients under your study.

As far as possible, choose subjects by random method. If you do not have a big pool of cases for random sampling, include subjects that consecutively attend the participating clinics. They will of course be filtered by inclusion and exclusion criteria, and by the informed consent.

Most important statistical consideration will be the number of subjects you plan to investigate. This depends on a host of specifications as mentioned in a previous chapter, including reliability required and statistical power to be able to detect a medically relevant result.

Data Analysis

This is discussed in detail in a subsequent chapter. Your task at the protocol stage would be to visualise the data and identify the statistical methods. In case you are not confident, consult a biostatistician.

Never make innocuous statement such as 'results would be tabulated and statistically analysed'. In most cases, it is also redundant to say that continuous variables would be compared by *t*-test and categorical by chi-square.

System for Conclusion

It is important to realize the distinction between result and conclusion. Result is what your data tell you after it passes through the rigmarole of analysis. This is restricted to the aspect you specifically studied and pertain to the subjects included in the sample. This result is interpreted in the light of knowledge about peripheral issues and the environment in which the study was carried out. When such extraneous factors are given due consideration, you get the conclusion. For example, the result might tell you that yoga for 30 minutes a day, 5 days in a week for four weeks, reduces diastolic blood pressure by 7 mmHg in those who are borderline hypertensives. When you juxtapose this to the physiological and metabolic changes that yoga can make and support it with evidence from literature, you get a conclusion that yoga tends to reduce diastolic BP in borderline hypertension.

At the stage of protocol, see if you can anticipate and state the other knowledge and evidence that would be considered to draw a conclusion. Also state how you plan to resolve the conflict in case the results contradict the present knowledge, and if the results do not come up to your expectations.

Citing the References

Last wrinkle is about the system you follow in the text of the protocol for citations and for their listing at the end. Two systems are available. First is citing the reference in the text by last name of the first author and the year of publication such as Mehta et al. (2009). Et al. stands for 'and others' and used if there are three or more authors. For two authors, last name of both are cited. In this system, the listing at the end is done in alphabetical order of last name of the first author. This book follows this pattern.

Second system, followed in medical journals, is citing reference in the text by a number either in parentheses or as superscript in the sequence of their appearance, and listing at the end in the order of these numbers. Last name of the first author can also be cited. Thus, you can either say, for example, that 'risk of miscarriage is partly dependent on previous induced abortions (1), or that 'Sun et al.[1] observed association between risk of miscarriage and previous induced abortions'. But follow the same system uniformly throughout the protocol. Method of listing of references is discussed in a later chapter.

Do not confuse list of references with bibliography. All references in the list must have been cited in the text. **Bibliography** is a list of all related literature – cited or not.

9.3 INSTITUTIONAL CLEARANCES

Most institutions and organizations conducting medical research setup a layer of committees to review the protocol. The purposes of this are two-fold: (i) the research should be of required standard so that it does not bring bad name to the institutions – in fact, should possibly enhance its reputation; and (ii) the research is such that it does not harm the subjects of research if not be beneficial to them. Generally, two committees look after this work although in some cases both can be assigned to the same committee – first is to review the technical aspects and the other for ethical aspects.

Research Review Board

Sometimes called the Scientific Committee, this board mainly comprises internal members of the institution and reviews the technical aspects such as whether the topic is worth spending time and resources, it is feasible, the methodology is sound, and it is likely to yield the result of the type stipulated and it will give the required training to the PG student. In almost all medical colleges, such a committee under different names exists for reviewing post graduate thesis protocols and in the universities for reviewing the PhD dissertation protocols. Occasionally, an outside expert of the topic of research is co-opted to provide an opinion regarding the adequacy of the protocol. A qualified statistician is an integral part of this board.

The candidate presents the protocol and answers the concerns of the members. Supervisors and advisors are invited to the meeting so that they also can explain those aspects that the candidate could not, and the concerns of the board members are recorded and conveyed for rectification. The board chairperson approves the protocol after being satisfied that it has been adequately revised.

Institutional Ethics Committee

The responsibility of this committee is to ensure that the research is not going to harm the institution, the researchers, and the subjects. The members and the chair of this committee should be mostly outsiders not belonging to the institutions. The member secretary should be from the institutions. The chair should be a well-known researcher with established reputation. The committee may have 2 or 3 subject experts of which 1 or 2 can be from the institution. It is customary to incorporate at least one member from the legal profession who is primarily responsible to look after the interest of the subjects of research. A social scientist and one lay person from the community are also included. The total size can be 7 to 10 members. But none should have any conflict of interest. The committee examines the aspects of informed consent process, risks involved, potential benefits, compensations to the subjects, etc. Ethics committee may be different for human research than for animal research.

Both these committees are required to hold formal meetings at regular intervals so that the clearance can be given in a time-bound manner. In some unfortunate instances, these committees delay the process that causes much of heartburn among researchers.

Preregistration of the Protocol

Some journals provide the facility to submit a research protocol for review by the experts under, what is called, preregistration. If you are carrying out a study that you think is important for medical science, submit the protocol to a journal of the concerned specialty and get benefit of their expert comments before the study is executed. This can help in substantially improving the methods of the study and improve the chance of getting the paper accepted when the paper is sent for publication even if the results are negative. Preregistration is another way to ensure reproducibility and applicability of your research, and to enhance the transparency and trust of the medical community.

SUMMARY

Protocol is the chief architect of the study and provides support in case any confusion or doubt arises. Thus, it should be clearly worded and should be prepared with utmost care. Structure and contents of the protocol as described in this chapter would help you to formulate a protocol of a credible research.

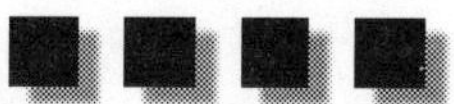

CHAPTER 10

How to Collate the Data

KEY TERMS AND CONCEPTS

- ✓ Master Chart
- ✓ Data Tables
- ✓ Graphs and Diagrams
- ✓ Infographs
- ✓ Standardized Rates

After the preparation of the protocol and its clearance by the authorities comes the step to execute the actual study and collect the data from the subjects by following the methodology outlined in the protocol. This includes the methods such as interview, examination, and investigation, and the responses are recorded on a predesigned questionnaire or schedule. Then comes the collation before the data are put to rigours of statistical analysis.

Collation of data refers to initial management so that the data are properly arranged for meaningful analysis. It includes activities such as preparing a master chart, arranging the data in intelligible tables, preparing the convincing graphs, calculation of the relevant rates, indexes and scores, and other related activities.

In an empirical research such as in medicine, there would always be some incomplete records. Collation of data starts with scrutiny for **missing values**. They should be treated according to the procedure outlined in the protocol. Subjects with incomplete records can be removed altogether if they are few and do not have potential to cause bias. If they are more, two options are available. First is that their records are used partially for adjustment, particularly if they tend to follow a pattern. Second is that the records are artificially completed by imputing missing values when they do not follow any discernible pattern. Use one of these methods as appropriate. If the missing values are far too many, use the data to draw lessons and plan another study.

Check for any sudden changes or breaks in the data. This can occur either due to changes in definitions or due to changes in data collection procedures. Such breaks are annoying, and statisticians can detect predictable and systematic patterns in the silence between the numbers. If the series lacks random variation or starts to show regularity, suspect that the reality in disguised, particularly if the improvement closely matches the target levels.

Beware also of the 'other' and 'unknown' categories of responses. They may be hiding important information such as cases that are adverse to the hypothesis of the investigators. The response in these categories should be very small – certainly not exceeding 10 percent of the responses.

Master Chart

Many new researchers, such as PG students, falter at the stage of preparing a **master chart**. This is generally prepared in an Excel format that collates the collected information on each subject in one row. This is called a record. Each record has different cells, called fields, for filling up the information. For example, the first cell may be patient ID, second age, third sex, fourth date of admission, etc. An example is in Figure 10-1.

Important is to realise that each cell must contain one piece of information and the cells in each column must be in a uniform format. Quantitative variable such as age (years) is to be entered in terms of numbers only so that mean and other calculations can be done. For example, do not write '45 years' but only '45'. All dates must follow the same format. Do not enter 'm 'for male at one time and 'M' at another time

Master chart is an excellent tool to provide an overview of the data and to begin further collation. Prepare this after coding wherever needed if not already incorporated in the form. Identify baseline and repeated measures, such as heart rate before, during, and 1, 5, 10 and 30 minutes after a surgery so that they can be properly analysed as repeated measures. Before preparing tables and graphs, do calculations (by computer

Study ID	Age (Years)	Gender	Date of admission	Date of discharge	Days in ICU	Ventilation (1= Yes, 0 = No)	RASHES (1 = Yes, 0 = No)	LOSS OF TASTE (1 = Yes, 0 = No)
PC0001	78	M	11-07-2020	20-07-2020	0	0	1	1
PC0002	1	F	06-07-2020	14-07-2020	0	0	0	0
PC0003	41	F	22-06-2020	29-06-2020	0	0	1	1
PC0004	5	M	02-06-2020	12-06-2020	0	0	0	0
PC0005	72	M	01-04-2020	10-04-2020	6	1	1	1
PC0006	91	M	24-07-2020	30-07-2020	0	0	1	1
PC0007	63	M	09-04-2020	20-04-2020	0	0	0	0
PC0008	35	M	30-06-2020	07-07-2020	0	0	0	0
PC0009	46	M	17-04-2020	29-04-2020	0	0	1	1
PC0010	25	M	15-05-2020	19-05-2020	0	1	0	0
PC0011	27	M	20-05-2020	25-05-2020	3	1	1	1

FIGURE 10-1: An example of a master chart

if needed) such as body-mass index from height and weight, and disease score from the signs and symptoms.

Although master chart should be prepared only after thorough scrutiny of forms, but it is generally at the stage of master chart that many errors are detected. In place doing these corrections in the original form, the changes are sometimes done in the master chart – wrong values are replaced, missing are inserted, etc. If so, make a note of these changes in the master chart itself in a separately defined comments column. You will probably forget about such changes if comments are not properly noted. These comments help in re-examining the data in case a doubt arises later. Take it from me that many such opportunities to re-examine the data would arise if you are true to your research.

10.1 TABLES

Tables are powerful tools to summarise a large dataset in an intelligible format. They are extensively used in reporting of research findings and help in providing structure to the results. They add variety and break monotony. Text adds meat but there should not be much duplication. Only the salient features or results emanating from the tables are described in the text. While preparing tables, the variability in the data must be preserved but it may be counter-productive to use too many categories in one table. Tables can become a source of confusion also when not properly drawn. Prefer tables over graph when display of exact values is important – graphs are for trends and patterns. Tables should be self-contained but should not be horrendous mess. The format of tables for qualitative data is slightly different from that of tables for quantitative data but in all cases the information in the tables must be consistent with the text. As much as possible all tables should be internally complete and self-contained. For publication, follow the guidelines of the concerned journal.

Frequency Tables for Quantitative Data

For summarising and collating quantitative measurements, data-intervals are necessary. If there are 450 subjects whose cholesterol level was measured, it is not feasible to present all 450 values. The table summarising this measurement will have data-intervals such as 100-149, 150-199, 200-219, 220-239, etc., and the number of subjects in each interval would be stated. As remarked earlier, do not make these intervals at the time of data collection. It is only at the stage of data collation that these may be needed. Even at this time, mean and SD can and should be calculated based on exact values rather than data-intervals. If there are seven subjects with cholesterol level between 100 and 149 mg/dl, making an interval before calculation would wrongly presuppose that levels of all seven subjects are at its mid-point, namely, 125 mg/dl. Thus, this should be avoided as much as possible. Nevertheless, the intervals would be necessary at the time of reporting of the results. At that time, the intervals should be so formed that conventional normal range can be easily marked out, and other intervals are easily labelled as below normal, above normal, serious, critical, etc. Such qualitative terms are very helpful in assessing the patients as well as the results of a study. The interval 100-149 mg/dl for cholesterol is useful since the conventional cut-off for normal range starts at 150 mg/dl. A level between 150-199 can be considered borderline without making any distinction that it is between 150-159 or between 170-179, etc. After the level goes beyond 200, smaller intervals are proposed because then increased level may have differential clinical significance. Generally, not more than eight categories are made. Too many categories are confusing and render the table clumsy.

Also note that cholesterol level is never measured to any decimal accuracy. Thus, there is no possibility of anybody with recorded level between 149 and 150 mg/dl. The data-intervals that we mentioned in the preceding paragraph are a global convention. For example, in case of age, a person may be of 39 years and 8 months but would still be counted in the age-interval 30-39 years since age is conventionally recorded in completed years (or, age last birth day).

Contingency Tables for Qualitative Data

Qualitative data are also collated in the form of tables that contain the count of subjects in different categories of one or more characteristics. The categories must be mutually exclusive and exhaustive. That is, each subject must belong to one and only one category. Contingency arises either because of fixed totals, or because the counts are restricted to specified categories.

EXAMPLE 10.1: A three-way contingency table

Prescott et al. (2003) analysed data from Copenhagen City Heart Study for risk of ischemic heart disease (IHD) in people with various degrees of vital exhaustion. They explain that vital exhaustion is a psychological measure of fatigue and exhaustion. Vital exhaustion score is the number of items present in a person out of a list of 17 such as 'feel dejected', 'lately have difficulties concentrating', and 'sometimes just feel like crying'. The authors found that as the vital exhaustion increased, the hazard ratio of IHD (as well as of all-cause mortality) also increased in both women and men, and suggest that this should begin to be implemented in risk assessment in clinical practice. The following is a three-way table adapted from their results.

Vital Exhaustion Score*	Women			Men			Both genders together		
	IHD cases	Others	Total	IHD cases	Others	Total	IHD cases	Others	Total
0	43	1307	1350	62	1360	1422	105	2667	2772
1-4	78	2255	2333	122	1670	1792	200	3925	4125
5-9	56	1016	1072	37	488	525	93	1504	1597
10-17	37	449	486	20	202	222	57	651	708
Total	214	5027	5241	241	3720	3961	455	8747	9202

*Number of items present out of a list of 17

Source: Adapted from Prescott et al. (2003)

A contingency table is called *K*-way when a group of subjects is cross-classified by *K* characteristics. The table in Example 10.1 is a three-way table: three characteristics being (i) vital exhaustion scores (ii) gender, and (iii) occurrence of ischemic heart disease (IHD). A higher-way table is difficult to read and interpret. If there are four or more factors under study, split them and prepare separate tables not containing more than three factors each. Also, the table becomes clumsy when too many categories of any characteristic are used. In this table, score has four categories, gender has two categories, and IHD also has two categories. If gender variation is not of interest, the last three columns of table that collapse gender for various scores is a two-way table. If the interest is only in distribution of scores and not IHD or gender, the last column provides the one-way table. This incidentally is a *frequency table* also since the score is quantitative. If vital exhaustion is relabelled as none, mild, moderate, and serious instead of 0, 1-4, 5-9, and 10-17, respectively, the last column would provide a one-way *contingency table* in true sense.

When all totals are excluded, the three-way table in Example 10.1 has 16 **cells**. These cells contain the number of subjects found in various categories and called **cell frequency**. The total number of cells corresponds to the number of possible categories. Since vital exhaustion score is in four categories, gender in two categories, and IHD too in two categories (IHD and no IHD), the **order** of this table is 4×2×2 that makes a total of 16 possible categories. No cell of the table should be blank – write 0, NA for 'not available' or 'not applicable' none, etc., as is applicable.

You will need these basic concepts to collate your data properly and to analyse them later. If collaborating with a statistical department, you will need these concepts to effectively communicate with a statistician.

Features of a Table

Each frequency table or contingency table must contain the total number of subjects—groupwise if groups are present. First confusion arises at the time of calculating percentages. The base for percentages should be a predetermined number. In a case-control study, the relevant percentage is of those possessing a particular disease out of the total cases and controls separately. If 28 out of 80 breast cancer cases, and 21 out of 80 matched controls report age at menarche <12 years, do not calculate percentage of 28 and 21 out of their total 49. Calculate this out of 80. In a prospective study, the percentage should be based on the exposed and unexposed cohorts that have been followed-up. In a cross-sectional study, the percentage should be calculated out of the grand total (and not row totals or column totals) because grand total is the prefixed number. For number of decimals in a percentage, use the rules that we describe in a later chapter. All percentages must add upto 100 except in the case of multiple response. Example 10.2 illustrates such percentages. The table in this example also illustrates the placing of explanatory matter in footnotes. Use symbols *, †, ‡, §, and ¶ in that order or superscripts a to z if there are many to link footnote with the table contents. If the text in the column is too long, consider using abbreviation. Codes, abbreviations, symbols, inconsistencies, obscure information, etc., should be explained in footnotes.

If the data are not original, give the source in footnote without using a connecting symbol.

EXAMPLE 10.2: Illustration of features of a table

Consider the following table containing hypothetical data from Anamika Hospital. See if the table is self-explanatory or not. Note that this is not a contingency table since multiple response is allowed – the complaints are not mutually exclusive: two or more complaints can be simultaneously reported by one patient.

Postnatal Complications*	Number of Women	Percentage
Excessive bleeding	30	7.25
Urinary tract infection	52	12.56
Convulsions	68	16.43
Foul discharge	56	13.53
Others	39	9.42
Total with complications	209	50.48
No complication	205	49.52
Total†	414	100.00

*Multiple response

† Total women are 427 but complication information is not available for 13.

Calculating percentage of 30 cases of excessive bleeding out of 209 women with complications would send a wrong message that excessive bleeding occurred in (30/209)×100 = 14.35%. This occurred in only 7.25% women. Exercise caution in choosing the base for calculating percentages.

While in a PG thesis you can have one table for one variable, journals prefer composite tables to save space. These tables contain information on many variables and replace many tables with one. For example, you can show number of participants in case and control group with age distribution, gender distribution, BMI categories and smoking status, all into one table. Such composite tables may require cut-in headings and indent for subheadings or categories. See Example 10.3 for an illustration, particularly for smokers. Note that text is left adjusted and numbers are right-adjusted. All percentages have same number of decimals. The numbers to be compared should be in column since English reads left to right. Thus, for comparing cases with controls, cases should be in one column and controls in the adjacent column as in the table in

Example 10.3. However, if you have many groups for comparison, consider splitting the table – generally table should contain no more than 7-8 columns. All column headings must be capitalized. The table titles should be brief yet descriptive to convey what the table contains. They are written as phrases rather than sentences and numbered consecutively in the order they appear. All tables must be referred in the text.

EXAMPLE 10.3: Features and layout of a composite table

Background characteristics of the participants in a trial centre

	Cases (n = 200)		Controls (n = 200)	
Particulars	**Number**	**Percent**	**Number**	**Percent**
Age (Years)				
20-24	32	16.0	40	20.0
25-29	51	25.5	57	27.5
30-34	76	37.0	63	31.5
35-39	41	20.5	40	20.0
Gender				
Male	103	51.5	95	47.5
Female	97	47.6	105	52.5
Smoking status				
Smokers				
Current	45	22.5	36	17.0
Past	23	11.5	24	12.0
Never smokers	129	64.5	140	70.0
Not available	3	1.5	0	0.0

Tables containing statistical results can have mean, standard deviation, odds ratio, confidence intervals, etc., but they basically have the same features.

10.2 GRAPHS AND DIAGRAMS

Figure is a generic term used for all illustrations that include graphs, diagrams, charts, photographs, and drawings. The purpose of graphs and diagrams is to collate the data and depict the pattern visually. There are nondata-based diagrams also such as spot maps as mentioned later in this section. The message borne by these data-based figures is easily grasped and tends to remain in memory longer than the numbers in a table. However, the depiction is approximate rather than exact in the sense that quantities 103.2 and 103.4 can be shown distinct in a table but rarely in a graph. Diagrams are even more approximate.

With the availability of a variety of software, visualisation of data has become much more effective, although more complex. You may have seen some interesting depictions on TV and print media. You may like to watch the video of Hans Rosling on YouTube of how 200 countries have progressed over the past 200 years about income and life expectancy. Some depictions can indeed be visually compelling. Corona pandemic has brought graphs into the centre stage of news reports.

Many graphs and diagrams are illustrated throughout this text. Particularly see Figure 4-1 on aetiology of myocardial infarction and Figure 4-2 on validity and reliability. Figure 5-1 in Chapter 5 on levels of evidence is an example of a chart, which is neither graph nor diagram. Graphs in Figure 6-1 in Chapter 6 on sampling methods cannot be classified into conventional names. The conventional ones are described in the following paragraphs.

Graphs

Numerical axis is a prerequisite for a figure to be called a **graph.** Generally, it has a horizontal axis called x-axis and a vertical axis called y-axis. But it can have three dimensions or just one dimension depending upon the number of variables shown. It can be based on polar coordinates also but those are not used in medicine.

Most appropriate graph for showing the frequency distribution of a quantitative measurement is histogram and, in some situations, polygon. These can be drawn for relative frequencies also, which are proportion or percentage of subjects in different categories. See Figure 10-2 for an example of these and other graphs. In a **histogram** the categories of the quantitative measurement under collation is generally shown on horizontal axis and the frequencies on vertical axis but they can be reversed also. A **polygon** can be smoothened into a **frequency curve.**

Use **line diagram** for showing trend over time, over age, or any such numerical characteristic. Figures 5-2(a) and (b) in Chapter 5 are line diagrams that illustrate interaction. Many lines (or curves) can be shown in one diagram. Visual study of relationship between two quantitative variables is best done by a **scatter diagram.** For inter-relationship among three variables, **scatter matrix** can be used as shown in Figure 10-2. Line diagram and scatter diagram are in fact graphs but are conventionally called diagrams. Log-scale can be used on either or both axes when the range of values to be shown is extremely large such as gamma radiation counts from 100 to 100,000. Units of measurement should be invariably mentioned. As far as possible, statistical

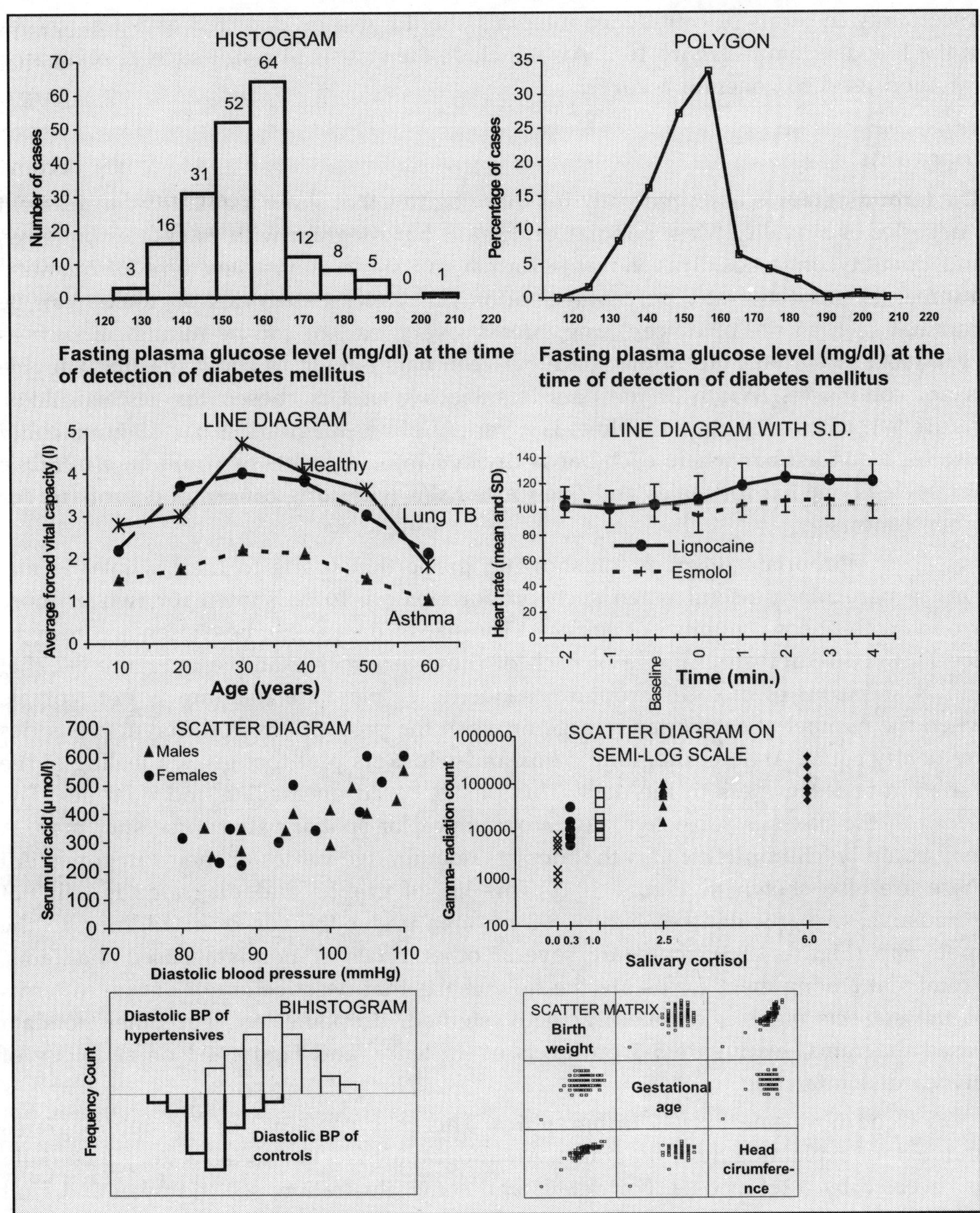

FIGURE 10-2: Some examples of graphs

uncertainty in terms of confidence intervals should also be depicted as SD as shown in the line diagram in Figure 10-2. Also, include the statistical result such as regression equation used to generate a curve.

Diagrams

The term **diagram** is used generally for those figures that show a quantity for different categories of a quality. Most popular of these is **bar diagram** with categories on x-axis and quantity on y-axis. This versatile format can show almost any type of quantity: number of subjects, rate, percentage, odds ratio, etc. Categories on x-axis can be nominal such as site of cancer: lung, breast, ovary, etc.; or can be numerical such as year 1950, 1955, 1960, etc. Some space between bars is kept to show that the variable is not continuous. Width of the bars is subjective and is chosen for aesthetic look. Figure 9-1, which depicts a timeline, is a variant of bar diagram. A bar diagram could also be a divided bar where each bar is divided into segments or could be a multiple bar such as one bar for males and one for females with lung cancer, and similarly for other cancers.

Most appropriate diagram for showing proportion (parts to their whole) is **pie**. This is particularly useful when such proportions are to be shown for two or more groups with unequal number of subjects. The size of the pie can be chosen accordingly. See Figure 10-3 for an example of each of these. Another example is Figure 8-2 that shows spectrum of disease through a sequence of pies. Pie diagram is not suitable when the number of categories is large or when the proportions in different categories are nearly equal. Another diagram is **box-and-whiskers plot** that gives a feeling of the variation and skewness in the data. This plot is based on median and quartiles. The width of the boxes is subjective. For geographical or spatial pattern use **spot map.** A map could be **choroplethic** also that depicts quantitative values or their categories. All these are also shown in Figure 10-3. This list of graphs and diagrams is still not exhaustive. In particular, see Figure 8-3 on area under the curve. In addition to the spot map (Figure 10-3), there are several other types of nondata based diagrams. Prominent among them for us are the flow charts that describe study design in terms of the subjects eligible, enrolled, actually studied, dropouts, etc. For other nondata based diagrams, see Figure 5-1 on levels of evidence, and Figure 4-1 on aetiology of myocardial infarction.

A trend now emerging is **infographics.** This may contain 2 or 3 graph/diagrams and text for explaining these diagrams. An infographic is a tool to tell a story pictorially as revealed by a set of data. For details and some illustration, see Indrayan and Holt (2016).

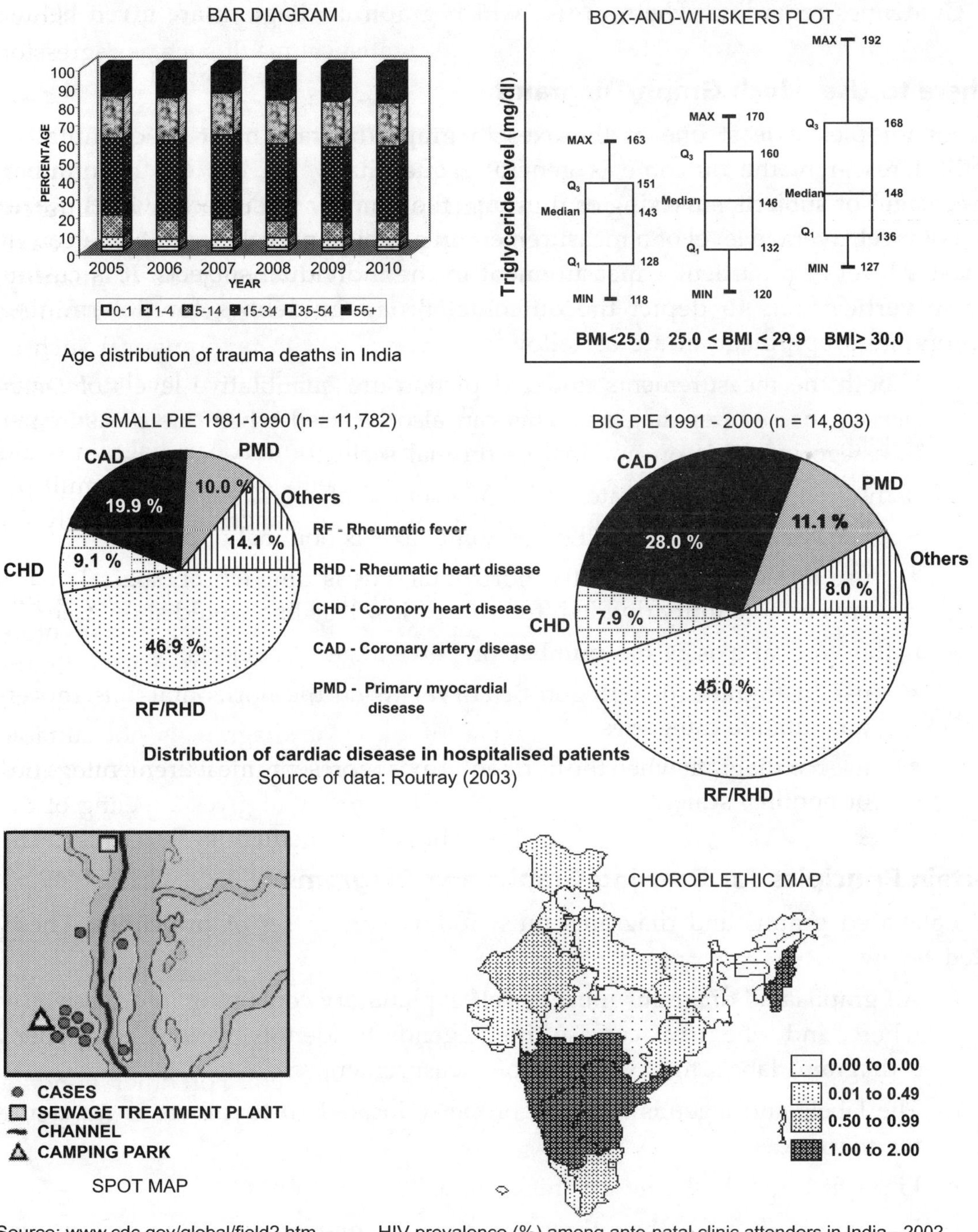

FIGURE 10-3: Examples of some diagrams

For a comprehensive account of various types of tables, graphs/diagram and other illustrations, see Christiansen (2007).

Guidelines regarding where to use which graph or diagram are given below.

Where to Use which Graph/Diagram?

Except for pie, at least one of the axes in graph/diagram must be quantitative. In medical research, the outcome is generally quantitative. It can be the number (or percentage) of subjects surviving in a group, the number of subjects with a particular kind of level, average level of a measurement in a group, prevalence rate of a condition, or just a level of a particular measurement in the individual subjects. It is customary to use vertical axis to depict the outcome. Broad guidelines for determining an appropriate graph/diagram are as follows:

- If both the measurements under depiction are quantitative levels of *individual subjects*, use scatter diagram. This can also be used when one measurement is in categories, or is on nominal or ordinal scale.
- If the vertical axis is a rate, ratio, or average of a *group of subjects*,
  - use bar diagram when the horizontal axis is nominal or ordinal.
  - use line diagram when the horizontal axis is time (chronological year, age, etc.) or a quantity divided into categories. This line would show trend.
- If the vertical axis is the number or percentage of subjects,
  - use histogram (or polygon or curve) when the horizontal axis represents quantitative categories.
  - use bar diagram when the horizontal axis represents measurements on ordinal or nominal scale.

Certain Principles for Drawing Graphs and Diagrams

All databased graphs and diagrams must follow certain set of principles. These are listed below:

- All graphs and diagrams must be self-explanatory containing informative (what, where, and when) yet concise title, legends to identify various components of a diagram, labels for axes, unit of measurement, etc.
- The labels and legends must be properly located so that there is no confusion for the reader.
- Lines in a graph should be thicker than the axis lines.
- Do not show more than three variables in one graph/diagram. Use distinct pattern of line or symbol for each variable. See scatter matrix in Figure 10-2 that is based on three variables but is still clumsy.

- Scale of calibrations should be clearly indicated. Choose scale that is suitable and does not exaggerate or attenuate the values. For comparing two or more groups, use the same scale.
- In case secondary data is being used to draw a figure, give source of the data. Also give reference of the source document in case the graph in copied, and also give the details of the permission to reproduce.

10.3 STANDARDISATION AND OTHER ADJUSTMENTS FOR DATA COMPARABILITY

In a clinical trial, patients are randomly allocated to the treatment and control groups. When the size of the groups is large, random allocation is quite likely to yield similar baseline of the two groups. But that is not a guarantee and it is unlikely in smaller groups. If posthoc comparison reveals that one group had predominantly serious patients relative to the other, the efficacy comparison will not be valid. An adjustment of results would be required.

Difference in two or more groups, or a relationship between two or more variables, can arise due to two types of factors. Those that are of direct interest for their effect, and those undesirably creep in and cause distraction. If the interest is to investigate effect of age at onset of dilated cardiomyopathy on survival in children of age upto 12 years, the undesirable factors are cardiothoracic ratio, duration of symptoms, left ventricular hypertrophy, etc. These are confounding factors since these can also influence the outcome. Any relationship between age at onset and survival would be clouded unless the effect of these confounders is filtered out. Good design cannot help in this situation since it is not possible to choose cases with uniform cardiothoracic ratio nor with same duration of symptoms. Methods are required that can give net effect of age at onset on survival without being influenced by such confounders.

Methods for making data comparable as well as those that compute net effect of a factor are essentially statistical. They commonly take a form of either standardisation or covariance analysis. A summary is given below. Take help of a statistician for this. Show him the methods listed next and let him choose the right method.

Some Methods of Standardisation and Other Adjustments

I. Standardisation

Standardisation is a procedure that brings the groups under comparison to a common base so that the influence of their differential structure on outcome is removed. It is generally used to control effect of only one factor.

Direct Method – Recalculate the rate by applying the observed subgroup specific rates on to a 'standard' composition such as applying observed age-specific prevalence rates of cataract blindness in diabetic patients to a standard age-structure of a population. Use this method when observed subgroup specific rates are reliable. Else use indirect method.

Indirect Method – Recalculate the rate by applying the 'standard' subgroup specific rates on to the observed structure of the groups, such as applying population-based age-specific prevalence rates of cataract blindness to the observed age-structure of diabetes patients.

II. Other methods of adjustment

These also are primarily of two types:

1. **Covariance analysis** – Includes regression, analysis of variance, and analysis of covariance. This allows simultaneous consideration of several qualitative and quantitative variables that helps to evaluate net effect of anyone keeping all others constant.
2. **Manual adjustment** – Common sense based simple calculations to adjust a factor suspected to undesirably affecting the outcome.

SUMMARY

The data are usually collected on a predevised form, where one form is filled up for each subject. Before the statistical analysis is taken up, these data have to be collated. First step is scrutiny of the data for their completeness and to rule out any aberration. Next is to put them into a maser chart that gives a comprehensive view of the data. Then come the tables and graphs.

Tables are mainly of two types. First are data tables that summmarise the cases in appropriate categories. Quantitative measurements such as the age and blood pressure levels may have to be categorised in small number but appropriate categories. This may require percentages out of an appropriate total. The second are tables on statistical results such as values of the logistic coefficients, confidence intervals, statistical significance. Both should be clearly formulated so that the message is clear to the reader.

Several types of graphs are available but choose the one that is suitable for the data to be depicted. You should be aware about different varieties of graphs so that a proper choice can be made.

Results sometimes cannot be used straightaway because of underlying aberration due to intervening factors. The results are standardised so that they become valid for comparison. Standardisation can be done by direct or indirect methods. Among other methods of adjustment, analysis of covariance that includes regression is very useful.

REFERENCES

Christiansen S. Visual presentation of data, Chapter-4 in AMA Manual of Style: A Guide for Authors and Editors (10th Edition). Oxford University Press, 2007.

Indrayan A, Holf MP, Concise Encyclopedia of Biostatistics for Medical Professionals, New York: CRC Press, 2016.

Prescott E, Holst C, Gronbaek M, Schnohr P, Jensen G, Barefoot J. Vital exhaustion as a risk factor for ischaemic heart disease and all-cause mortality in a community sample. A prospective study of 4084 men and 5479 women in the Copenhagen City Heart Study. Int J Epidemiol 2003;32:990-997.

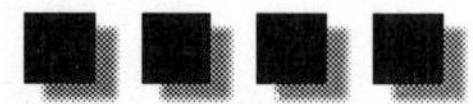

CHAPTER

11

How to Analyse the Data

KEY TERMS AND CONCEPTS

- ✓ Statistical Significance
- ✓ *P*-value
- ✓ Statistical Power
- ✓ Medical Significance
- ✓ Testing of Hypothesis
- ✓ Court Judgment
- ✓ Type-I and Type-II Errors
- ✓ Chi-square Test
- ✓ Student t-test
- ✓ Nonparametric Tests
- ✓ Confidence Interval
- ✓ Association and Correlation
- ✓ Cause-effect Relationship
- ✓ Linear, Logistic and Cox Regression
- ✓ Validation of Findings

The data collected at the time of executing the study is analysed to get an evidence-based answer to the research question initially proposed. The answer may be positive or negative depending on the responses obtained from the subjects and that should not matter. As mentioned earlier, the answer cannot be predicted because that is what the research is all about.

Most medical researchers around the world take help of a professional biostatistician to analyse their data as per the procedure set out in the protocol. They can do amazing things but remember that they cannot perform miracles. Getting professional help is a welcome sign for quality research because most medical researchers are not trained in choosing and applying a correct statistical method for the data in hand. Whereas intricate statistical methods such as logistic and linear regression, sensitivity and uncertainty analysis, and multivariate methods are best left to the expertise of a qualified biostatistician, a medical researcher must be familiar with elementary concepts and methods. These include the concepts of estimation and testing of hypothesis, statistical significance emanating from *P*-values, statistical power to detect a medically important effect, and elementary tests such as chi-square and Student *t*-test. Most medical colleges include these concepts and methods in their curriculum but not with emphasis required for research endeavours.

The meaning of statistical significance and *P*-value is explained in Section 11.1. Some statistical tests for qualitative and quantitative data are presented in Section 11.2. Only their practical implication and interpretation are discussed. Calculations are left on to the computer.

Many researchers prefer to work out confidence intervals for their results. This is the range within which a summary measure such as mean, proportion or odds ratio is expected to lie in repeated studies. Meaning and interpretation of such interval is in Section 11.3. The last section contains an outline of the complex statistical methods for which expert consultation should be sought.

11.1 STATISTICAL SIGNIFICANCE, *P*-VALUE, AND POWER

In an empirical research, statistical tests of significance are not just done but also talked about regarding what specific observations caused significance, how they are affected or not affected by confounders, what biological explanation is available, etc. It is necessary for this to understand the basics of statistical significance.

Statistical significance and *P*-values are commonly used terms in medical research literature. These arise mostly when two or more groups are compared and measurements in sample subjects are used to decide that the corresponding target populations are similar or not with respect to a medical parameter. For example, the difference apparently seen in average lipoprotein (a) levels in a sample of 30 male and

40 female hypertensives could either vanish if the study is done in another group of similar subjects or may be real that would recur in repeated samples. Statistical significance is decided by the probability that the difference will not vanish if repeated samples of the same nature are studied. But repeated samples are not actually drawn. Instead, statistical methods are used to evaluate the probability based on just one sample. For this a hypothesis is set up and tested for significance. Such a procedure is vital to analytical studies that aim to demonstrate existence of a difference between two or more groups. Many times, statistical analysis is considered keystone of analytical empirical research although it is not wise to depend too much on statistical results.

11.1.1 PHILOSOPHICAL BASIS OF STATISTICAL TESTS

Look at the following example. There are many references of sighting a Yeti, or at least big footprints in Himalayas. Does that prove that Yeti exists? The only conclusion made is that evidence is not sufficient yet that this exists. He may be there in hiding – who knows. But where is the conclusive evidence? Statistical tests are all about searching the evidence. The underlying philosophy is propelled by medical uncertainties and can be explained as follows.

Evidence is Sought Against a Null and Not for the Null

Ptolemy in second century AD propounded that sun revolves round the earth. It remained 'truth' for fourteen centuries when Copernicus came up with evidence against it in the 16th century and established a new truth that says that earth revolves round the sun. We earlier mentioned that peptic ulcer was believed to be caused by acidity until sometime ago when *H. pylori* were found to be a culprit in many cases. As of today, coronary heart disease is not considered caused by any infection, but this may soon become a topic of research.

Empirical strategy is to find evidence against a **hypothesis** that is stated in **null** form. If this evidence is sufficient, the null hypothesis is rejected, otherwise continues to be considered 'truth' by default. Transplanted to development of new regimen, it seems reasonable to demand evidence against that there is no effect at all. This process is difficult to conduct without recourse to setting-up a null hypothesis (Sterne 2003), which could be rejected in the light of the evidence provided by the observations.

Samples by their very nature are uncertain. The conclusion depends on what sort of data is obtained from the selected subjects. One sample differs from the other. Statistical tests are precisely meant to deal with uncertainties arising from sampling fluctuations. They provide the answer to the question: What is the likelihood of the sample values you got when the null is true. If this likelihood is exceedingly small, say less than 5 percent, the null is considered implausible and rejected. At the same time, it would be wrong to 'accept' a hypothesis whose likelihood of giving that sample is only 20 percent. Thus, the only conclusion drawn is that the sample fails to provide sufficient evidence to *reject* the null hypothesis. In this case the situation reverses to what it was before as though this study was never done.

Many would wonder that the sample values are searched for evidence against a null without finding what they are for—what do they support. We will describe alternative hypothesis soon that would clarify this dilemma but finding evidence *against* is widely followed in empirical setups as in a court setting.

11.1.2 TESTING OF HYPOTHESIS AND COURT JUDGMENT

It is customary in a court of law that the judge starts with the assumption of innocence—no crime has been committed by the accused. The burden is on to the prosecution to provide substantial evidence that can change his initial opinion and pronounce guilt. If the evidence is not enough, the person is acquitted even if the offence was committed. The judgment hinges on providing convincing evidence, and the responsibility is on the prosecution.

Null Hypothesis

Statistical methodology is completely analogous. We illustrate this with comparison of two groups such as cases and controls that commonly occur in a medical research setting. This starts with the assumption that any difference seen is a product of chance, and actually there is no difference between the groups. This is called a **null hypothesis.** This is equivalent to assumption of innocence in a court setting. Sample observations or the measurements obtained in the selected groups of subjects act as evidence. They must provide sufficient evidence that the groups are very likely to be different. If the sample evidence is weak, the initial assumption of no difference holds. We will shortly discuss about the methods to find that the evidence is weak or strong but understand for the time being that a large difference in samples should be construed as strong evidence and a small difference as weak evidence.

Errors in Testing of Hypothesis

It is quite common in court judgments that a real offender is acquitted because of weak evidence. This is not considered a serious error. But the other error also occurs. An innocent is pronounced guilty because there is a strong circumstantial evidence.

If there is no real difference between the groups but the data strongly indicate presence of a difference, the true null hypothesis has to be undesirably rejected. A false positive conclusion is reached. This is serious and called **Type I error** (Table 11-1) or *alpha error*. The seriousness of this error can be understood from the set-up of a trial on a new drug. This type of error occurs when an ineffective drug is proclaimed effective. Then the ineffective drug would be unnecessarily marketed, prescribed, and ingested, and side-effects tolerated. Imagine the cost and inconvenience caused by this error. Statistical procedure requires that this type of error be kept at a low level, generally within five percent.

TABLE 11-1: Errors in judgment

Court setting			Statistical setting		
Judgment	Assumption of innocence		Study results	Null hypothesis	
	True	False		True	False
Guilty	Serious error	✓	H_0 rejected	Type I error	✓
Not guilty	✓	Error	H_0 not rejected	✓	Type II error

Type II error is committed when the drug is really effective, but the trial results indicate that it is not. This leads to a false negative conclusion and called *beta error*. The society will be deprived of the benefits of this drug, but the situation will not be worse off than what it was before the trial. Also, the deprivation would be short-lived. If the drug is really effective, the manufacturer will not keep quiet and will conduct further trials till such time that the convincing evidence emerges in its favour. Then the drug could be rightly placed in the market. Thus, this error is not serious. The only loss is time. While discussing statistical power a little later, we clarify that Type II error must be associated with a *specified* difference between the groups.

EXAMPLE 11.1: Alpha and beta errors in comparing deliveries by active pushing and passive descent of foetus

Hansen et al. (2002) report an RCT for comparing active pushing vs. passive foetal descent in the second stage of labour in natal women. The outcome variables are rate of foetal descent, length of time of pushing, Apgar score for the infant, etc. They fixed an alpha error rate at five percent and **beta error** rate at 20 percent (although this has to specify the medically important difference, but the authors have not specified). This means that in this trial there could be 20 percent chance that a difference exists in the outcome of active pushing and passive descent but will remain undetected. The chance that presence of a difference is concluded when none really exists is less than five percent.

Alternative Hypothesis

Null hypothesis is only one side of the story. When the sample evidence is strong against the null, this hypothesis is discarded. What is adopted is called the alternative hypothesis. In a phase III trial for a drug against placebo, the null would be that there is no difference. Although it is not impossible that a drug is worse than placebo but considering this possibility would mean that there was something drastically wrong with the earlier phases of the trial including laboratory and animal studies on pharmacological properties of the regimen. Thus the plausible alternative hypothesis in this case would be that the drug is *better* than placebo. This is called **one-sided alternative** and leads to one-tailed tests. When both possibilities (better and worse) are admitted, it would be a **two-sided alternative** and leads to two-tailed tests. Most medical situations have two-sided alternative. Some researchers are of the view that a phase III trial result should be judged independent of previous phases and the alternative hypothesis should be two-sided for this phase also. In any case, if the objective is to judge equivalence of two regimens (i.e., the control too is an active regimen) than two-sided alternative hypothesis would be considered.

11.1.3 STATISTICAL SIGNIFICANCE

Basic statistical procedure for testing a hypothesis uses Gaussian properties to find the chance of obtaining the observed sample values when the null hypothesis is true. If this chance is small, the conclusion reached is that possibly null hypothesis is false. This is generally termed **statistical significance.** Obviously, this conclusion can be wrong and Type I error can occur. The details are as follows:

P-value

The probability of Type I error is called *P*-value. (We will soon describe some procedures to obtain this probability.) Thus *P*-value is the probability that a true null hypothesis of no difference is wrongly discarded. This could occur if the patients included in the trial by chance happen to exhibit a difference between the groups when actually there is none. Because of inter-individual variation, it is not an entirely unlikely scenario. *P*-value helps in increasing or decreasing faith in the results. *P*-value could be any value between 0 and 1 such as 0.72, 0.58, 0.37 or 0.02. This is the probability of Type I error and obtained after analysing the actual data set. If $P = 0.75$, concluding that a difference exists could be wrong three-fourths of the time, and if $P = 0.04$ the chances are only four percent.

Level of Significance

Seriousness of Type I error requires that a threshold for *P*-value is fixed in advance beyond which it would not be tolerated. This threshold is called the **level of significance.** This is denoted by α and called the alpha *level.* Note the distinction between alpha error mentioned earlier, and alpha level mentioned now. Generally, an alpha level of five percent (or $\alpha = 0.05$) is fixed. When this is so, a difference between the groups is considered statistically significant if the chance of it not being there is less than five percent. Omni-present variations and uncertainties do not allow this chance to be zero, and it is extremely difficult to reduce this to one or two percent. Five percent is an internationally accepted norm that is rarely breached although there is a discussion now to reduce it to 1% that would reduce the chances of reaching to a false conclusion. In situations where five percent error can translate into serious consequences, such as in missing a cancer diagnosis, a lower level can be fixed. Also, when *P*-value is marginally higher, such as 0.06, it may be appropriate to conclude that the results are on the verge of attaining statistical significance. Significance level could also be fixed at $\alpha = 0.10$ for behavioural research, or $\alpha = 0.01$ or any other level depending upon tolerance for Type I error for the problem in hand. Alpha level does not depend on the actual data set.

Statistical Significance

When the *P*-value for a difference in the samples is less than predetermined threshold level a such as five percent, the difference is called statistically significant. In other words, significance of *P* is in being less than 0.05. *A statistically significant difference does not mean that it is large or that it is medically relevant – it only means that the chance of no difference is smaller than the threshold.* The difference could still be small to be of any consequence in medical management. Also, a difference not statistically significant is not any assurance that the groups are equivalent. A difference of good stead would fail to be statistically significant if the sample size is small.

A researcher almost invariably tries to achieve statistical significance of his results. However, in some situations, nonsignificance should be welcome. When a test group is checked post-hoc against control group for matching regarding baseline characteristics, nonsignificance is considered a valid sign for adequate matching *provided* the number of subjects is large to have sufficient power as discussed next. When a low-cost test is evaluated against an expensive 'gold' test, nonsignificance may imply that it 'can' be equally good. Thus, the general feeling that statistical significance is a good result is not valid in some situations.

Statistical significance is just one aspect of the results and should not be given undue weightage. It "tells nothing about the quality of thought, planning, or execution in the work; nothing about the biologic or clinical meaning of the difference in numbers; and nothing about whatever has allegedly caused the difference" (Feinstein 1977). Nevertheless, *P*-values are in epidemiologists' air and cannot be fully eliminated from the 'corpus epidemiologicum' without unacceptable consequences (Lang et al. 1998).

11.1.4 MEDICAL SIGNIFICANCE AND STATISTICAL POWER

Type II is not a serious error but that should not be construed to imply that this can be ignored. In scientific pursuits, in fact anywhere in life, any error is tolerated to a limit and not beyond. Thus, there is a need to control Type II error also and increase the so-called power.

Statistical Power

Type II error occurs when a study fails to detect a real effect. Complementary to this is the ability to detect an effect. Measured as probability, the ability to detect an effect when present is called power and relates to a *prespecified* clinically relevant effect. Such an effect may not be easy to specify in some situations. Some subjectivity can creep in, and it is sometimes referred to in lighter vein as 'cynically' important effect. When this is specified, the trial should be conducted in a manner that it has adequate power to detect that kind of effect when present. Power measures the degree of assurance that the specified effect will be detected even when clouded by high variability in the measurements.

The literature strongly advises not to calculate power after the results are available. Indeed, the concept of power is meant to be used to plan a study and not do a post-mortem. Yet, it could be instructive in some situations to calculate power after the results are available. This can tell you what shortfall existed that caused statistical nonsignificance despite reasonably good effect. Thus, post-hoc power calculations are not as useless as generally made out in the literature. Also, such post-hoc calculations may also reveal if your initial guesses of the effect size and the variability were wrong. Both these aspects: (i) sample size, and (ii) effect size, could be helpful in planning the next investigation. Sometimes, the calculations are done while the study is going on, which help to confirm that the sample size is adequate, or you should increase the sample size. But such interim analysis and adjustment affects statistical significance.

Most important determinant of power is the number of subjects when all sources of bias and uncertainties such as lack of knowledge and inadequate design are in control. The best approach to achieve good power for detecting a medically relevant difference is to increase the number of subjects in the study. Formulae are available that can give this number for different settings and we have provided some in a previous chapter. Power calculation depends on whether the characteristic under assessment is quantitative or qualitative, the form of its statistical distribution in the target population, the variance across subjects, the minimum difference between groups that can be considered medically relevant, and the chosen level of significance. Most researchers aim to achieve a power of 0.80 or 0.90. For analogy with statistical significance, it is customary to term existence of a medically relevant effect as medical significance of results. In view of its importance, we explain this further.

Statistical Significance is Different from Medical Significance

Some medical professionals consider statistical methods notorious for discovering significance where there is none, and not discovering where one really exists. The 'difficulty' is that statistical methods give importance to the number of subjects in the sample. If a difference exists in 12 cases of chronic cirrhosis of liver and 12 cases hepatitis with respect to average Aspartate Amino-Transferase (AST) levels, it can be considered a fluke because of small size of groups. This is like weak evidence before the court of law. But if the same difference is exhibited in a study on 170 cases of each type, it is very likely to be real. The conventional statistical methods of testing hypothesis only tell whether a difference is likely or not. They do not say how much. The difference in average AST levels between cirrhosis and hepatitis cases could be only 3 units/ml that has no clinical relevance, but it will turn out to be statistically significant if this occurs in large groups of subjects. Medical significance of such a small difference should be separately evaluated using clinical criteria, and it should not depend exclusively on statistical significance. However, clinical criteria could be very subjective in many situations.

On the other side, a study on small groups of 12 subjects each may reveal a difference of 10 units/ml in mean AST level, which has a great medical relevance, but it would not be statistically significant primarily because the groups are so small. The other important contributory factor in achieving or not achieving statistical significance is the interindividual variability measured by the Standard Deviation (SD). If the variation among patients is large, an unreal big difference can arise due to inclusion of typical cases in the sample.

In the face of all this, we can still emphasise that the difference must be statistically significant for it to be medically relevant. If it is not statistically significant, nobody can be confident that it really exists. Thus, the first step is to assess statistical significance. If not significant and the statistical power is adequate, there is no need to worry about its medical relevance. If significant, further statistical test is used to judge if it reaches a medically relevant threshold. This threshold comes from medical acumen.

The correct strategy is to specify the minimum difference that would be considered medically relevant and conduct a study on reasonably large groups to be able to detect that level of difference.

EXAMPLE 11.2: Concern about statistical power in 'negative' trials

There is a growing concern among medical community regarding failure of many randomised controlled trials in detecting a medically relevant difference because they do not have sufficient power. The main driving force for power is the size of the trial and the interindividual variability. About half a century ago, Freiman (1978) observed after studying 71 'negative' RCTs on new therapeutic procedures that the sample size was too small in most of them for power 90 percent to detect a 25 percent improvement in outcome. In nearly three-fourths of these trials, the sample was inadequate to detect a 50 percent improvement. In other words, even if there is a 50 percent improvement in efficacy of the new treatment compared to the old, the trial results were still statistically not significant. It would have most likely become significant had there been bigger trial. Twentythree years later, Dimick et al. (2001) report the same for surgical trials. This once again underscores the need to be careful about the size of trial—the number of subjects must be adequate to inspire confidence that a medically relevant difference would not go undetected.

11.1.5 STATISTICAL ANALYSIS

After the data are collected, entered, cleaned, and collated, they are ready for the rigours of statistical analysis. This includes procedures such as generating correct estimates of various parameters (e.g., incidence and prevalence), building up confidence intervals, testing statistical significance, assessing the strength and type of relationship, etc. Actual methods depend on the nature of data, the type of hypotheses to be examined, and the theoretical conjectures that form the foundation of the study. The basic purpose of this analysis is to come to valid conclusions after minimising and quantifying the uncertainty level due to sampling. They are minimised by following techniques of adjustment that were discussed in a previous chapter and quantified by using the methods in this chapter. Remember however that statistical analysis, howsoever impeccable, is no substitute for a well-planned and carefully executed study.

Elements of Statistical Analysis

Statistical methods are useful tools but are sometimes abused. Help of a biostatistician or use of statistical tests does not divest a researcher of the responsibility of owning a conclusion. Interpretation of results should be guided by clinical and biological considerations. There is no escape from owning them if wrong. Ensure that you are not deceiving yourself by passing the buck. Do not torture the data to confess your belief.

A top-grade research restricts analysis to the protocol specifications unless mistakes are discovered. But do not hesitate to use the data to investigate new relationship encountered at the time of analysis. Report such incidental findings as hypothesis rather than as conclusion. Scientific ethics disdain using the same data for confirmation of hypothesis that generated it. New data focused on that hypothesis should be collected to check if it withstands scrutiny. Distracters cite Columbus accidentally discovering America when set out for India as an example against this paradigm. They forget that Columbus' discovery was not empirical—it was not based on collection of a series of observations that were subject to chance. The existence of the Americas was a hard fact with no probabilities attached. If such a discovery accidentally happens in your research that can be stated with complete confidence, go ahead, and report it with all the emphasis.

Steps in a Statistical Test of Significance

The argument of a statistical test goes something like the following. For quantitative data, the difference between a sample mean and the value expected under the null should be small if the null is really true. A large difference would indicate that the sample is not consistent with the null. How large is large enough is decided by comparing the difference by its Standard Error (SE). The SE depends on the SD and the ample size. Test criterion generally takes the form of ratio of difference and its SE. Specific steps are listed below. A computer package is almost invariably used to obtain the *P*-value after the test criterion is specified. For qualitative data, the criterion generally used is chi-square that is based on the difference between the observed frequencies in different categories and those expected under the null hypothesis.

For a one-sided alternative, **one-tailed test** is used that keeps all the probability of Type I error either on the left side or on the right side depending upon that the alternative is 'less than' type or 'more than' type. For a two-sided alternative, a **two-tailed test** is used that keeps half the probability of Type I error on the left side and the other half on the right side.

Steps for Carrying Out a Statistical Test

- Identify the variable, and determine that it is quantitative or qualitative.
- Identify the summary measure of interest: This could be a mean, a proportion, a difference in means, a difference in proportions, a regression coefficient, a

Relative Risk (RR), an Odds Ratio (OR), etc. The summary measure would partially depend on that the measurement is quantitative or qualitative.

- Set-up a null hypothesis that you would like to reject, and an alternative hypothesis that you would accept in case the null is rejected. Decide that the alternative is one-sided or two-sided.
- Assess the statistical distribution of the chosen summary measure for the sample in hand. If the sample size were large, many of such distributions would be approximately Gaussian. If the sample size is small, a nonparametric test or exact procedures may be needed.
- Determine the level of significance—five percent or whatever is considered appropriate.
- Identify the appropriate statistical test criterion based on the above-mentioned considerations. Consult a biostatistician if you are not too sure. Use computer package and obtain the *P*-value.
- Reject the null hypothesis and accept the alternative if *P*-value is less than the level of significance. If the *P*-value is more, conclude that the sample does not provide sufficient evidence against the null and the situation reverses to what it was before the study, except that it provides lessons for future studies.
- If necessary, calculate the power of the test for the specified medically relevant difference.
- In case several statistical tests are used on the same variable, use methods of multiple comparisons so that the Type I error remains under control.

11.2 TESTS FOR STATISTICAL SIGNIFICANCE

Statistical tests for significance in qualitative data are different than for quantitative data. This is analogous to saying that the 'diagnostic test' for hypertension is diastolic BP and for diabetes is glucose intolerance. The basic interest in qualitative data is in proportion of subjects possessing different characteristics, and the data are generally collated in the form of contingency tables. This includes categorical data also such as birthweight into -2500 gm, 2500-2999 gm, and 3000+ gm categories. The underlying measurement in this case is quantitative but since the number of categories is small, the interest is in proportion of births in different categories instead of average birthweight. Thus, such categories also are qualitative for statistical purposes.

11.2.1 ELEMENTARY TESTS FOR QUALITATIVE DATA

Basic criterion for evaluating statistical significance in the case of qualitative data is **chi-square** (χ^2). This is applicable for large *n*, no cell frequency zero or one, and not more than one-fifth categories containing less than five subjects. However, there is no requirement regarding shape of the underlying distribution—it could be Gaussian or nonGaussian. Different forms of chi-square help to find *P*-value in a variety of situations such as 'goodness of fit', association in contingency tables, and trend in proportions. Some of these are described in brief in this section. Logistic regression is a very powerful tool for qualitative data, and this is briefly described toward the end of this chapter. Logistic is specially used for evaluating statistical significance of Odds Ratio (OR) and Relative Risk (RR).

Chi-square is associated with a weird concept called **degrees of freedom** (df). This depends on the number of categories in which the subjects are divided. Just as people of different age have different levels of lung functions so is chi-square different for different dfs. In most situations the statistical software package will automatically decide df after looking at the number of categories. The package will also give *P*-value that could decide about statistical significance.

The objective of the present text is not to impart skills for carrying out these tests but only to impart the knowledge of what sort of basic methods are available to analyse qualitative data and to obtain the *P*-value. Since calculations easily come from computer-based statistical packages, the formulae are being avoided. If needed, many can be found in any standard statistical text such as by Indrayan and Malhotra (2018).

Goodness of Fit Test – One-way Table

After all what is 'goodness of fit'? Suppose it is believed that Down syndrome in children is in the ratio of 2:1 in males and females. This hypothesis can be tested with actual data that may not exactly follow this pattern. Goodness of fit would indicate whether the deviations from 2:1 are within the statistical tolerance or are beyond. If beyond, the ratio 2:1 in all probability does not apply to these cases. Chi-square is used as a criterion to test goodness of fit in such cases.

Two-way Tables with at least One Dichotomous Variable

Now shift attention to simultaneous consideration of two or more qualitative characteristics. The objective generally in this situation is to investigate if one characteristic has any association with the other—whether one is occurring more commonly with other than expected by chance.

The simplest of two-way tables is a 2×2 table when the study subjects are simultaneously divided by two binary variables. Most common of these is the division of subjects into case group and control group, and each of these as with and without a specific antecedent. Presence of association is concluded when the observed pattern of frequencies in various cells is substantially different from the chance-expected pattern. To check that this difference is 'substantial' or not, chi-square test is used. For small *n*, **Fisher's exact test** is used.

If a new regimen is found to have an efficacy of 78 percent against 75 percent of an existing proven regimen in a study on 40 cases and 40 controls, would you take the risk of using new treatment on the future cases? Two pertinent questions are (i) whether a rather small sample of 40 each is enough to inspire confidence, and (ii) whether this small difference of three percent in efficacy, even if real, is worth the efforts of switching from the existing strategy to the new one. If three percent is too small to take a risk, what minimum gain can be considered medically relevant for adopting the new regimen? This is a ticklish question for many researchers. But *the encumbrance of specifying a medically relevant minimum difference is on the researcher.* Suppose clinical considerations indicate that the gain must exceed eight percent for shifting to new treatment strategy for future cases. The alternative hypothesis in such a situation is one-sided that says that difference in efficacies is more than eight percent. The null hypothesis is that it is eight percent. Less than eight percent is also part of the null as default. Test to detect such a medically relevant difference in proportions is easy to do with the help of ***z*-test** for proportions instead of chi-square, provided the samples are large.

Sexually transmitted disease patients are often advised to use condoms so that they do not spread infection. The pattern of use of condom can be categorised as never, sometimes, often, and almost always. These are ordinal categories. For each of these categories, the information of interest could be whether the spouse is infected. Spouse infection percentage could be 32% among never users, 28% among sometimes users, 29% among often users, and 15% among always users. Whether or not this **trend in proportions** is statistically significant can be tested by another form of chi-square.

McNemar's Test

Consider average frequency of micturition in 80 cases of enlarged prostate before and after a specific treatment such as finasteride for six months. The outcome of interest in this situation is frequency of micturition. This outcome in fact is quantitative but can be categorized as six or less times a day and seven or more times a day. If 52 of the cases had higher micturition before treatment and this number came down to 36 after the treatment, it is not necessary that that all these 36 are out of the previous 52.

There is a possibility that some of the other 28, who had less micturition before treatment, experienced increased frequency despite the treatment. Suppose such cases are 8. This gives rise to the data in Table 11-2.

TABLE 11-2: Frequency of micturition in patients with enlarged prostate (Hypothetical data)

Before Treatment	After Treatment		Total
	6 or less	7 or more	
6 or less	20	8	28
7 or more	24	28	52
Total	44	36	80

The statistical test used in this setup too is basically chi-square but is calculated in a different manner. This is popularly known as **McNemar's test.** This test is based on the number of cases in the discordant cells: 8 and 24 in Table 11-2 that changed their category. If McNemar's test yields $P < 0.05$, the null is rejected. The conclusion is that the treatment is effective. However, in this example, significance can also arise if many with less micturition have more micturition after treatment. Check that this anomaly does not occur in your research.

Bigger Tables

Bigger tables could be either two-way that present cross-classification of subjects for two characteristics, each with more than two categories, or sometimes three or more characteristics are considered together.

Consider tables where both qualitative characteristics have multiple (three or more) categories each. Peptic ulcer cases can be cross-classified by occupation (as a surrogate for stress level) and type of milk consumed such as full fat, low fat, and skimmed. Strange as it may sound, the objective could be to explore relationship between occupation and type of milk in cases of peptic ulcer. If the occupation is in five categories, this cross-classification will give 5×3 table since type of milk is in three categories. The analysis of such a table for checking the association can be done by the usual chi-square using any standard statistical software.

When the number of subjects in the study is really small, you may have to collapse a big R×C table into a 2×2 table and use Fisher's exact test. If such collapsing is found unacceptable in the sense that medically important information is lost, use exact methods of analysis of bigger tables. For these, special statistical software may be needed.

11.2.2 TESTS FOR QUANTITATIVE DATA

Blood pressure, body-mass index, parity, and pain score are examples of quantitative measurement. As explained earlier, some of these are discrete that can take one of only small number of possible values, whereas others are continuous with theoretically infinite number of possible values.

The summary measure under scrutiny in case of continuous data is mostly mean. The objective could be to know (i) whether the mean of the target population from which the sample is drawn has a specified value; (ii) when there are two groups for comparison such as test and control, whether the respective population means are different, or have some specified medically relevant difference; (iii) when there are three or more groups, which specific group or groups is (are) really different from others with respect to their means, or whether they follow a particular pattern. For means in one and two groups, the statistical test of choice in most quantitative situations is Student's *t*, and for three or more groups (or subgroups) *F*-test is used. The latter is based on analysis of variance (ANOVA).

Remember that mean is an appropriate summary measure with quantitative data in most situations but is not appropriate in some. For example, when outliers are present, mean can be highly distorted value. Another criticism mounted against mean is that an average patient does not exist. Indeed, that is so but empirical evidence suggests that many patients revolve around the average. Empirical research is about groups of subjects and not about individual patients. Only presumption is that individuals *mostly* behave as the group suggests. Although each individual patient is managed on personal basis, that requires guidelines, and these guidelines are obtained by research on groups of subjects.

Student's *t*-Test

Student's *t* could be the next most used statistical test after chi-square. It is applicable in a variety of situations as described below. Again, the formulae are being avoided because the calculations easily come from statistical software.

The fundamental requirement for Student's *t*-test is that the sample values are independent of each other. In case of Blood Pressure (BP) measurements, for example, familial aggregation is well known, and if sample subjects include two or more members of the same families, they are not independent. Student's *t*-test cannot be used for mean BP of such a sample unless 'family-effect' is first removed. In most situations this contingency does not arise and the observations are independent—thus Student's *t*-test can be safely used.

The second requirement is that the sample mean follows a Gaussian distribution. This is easily met in almost all practical situations for large n because of **central limit theorem** that says that the sample mean tends to follow a Gaussian pattern as n gets bigger. For small n, though, this requirement is met only when the underlying distribution of the measurements themselves is Gaussian. Thus, the only situation when t-test is not applicable is when n is small *and* the underlying distribution is nonGaussian. Many measurements in diseased persons have nonGaussian pattern. For such measurements, use nonparametric test as described later in this section.

Consider a pharmaceutical company claiming that their new drug newspirin reduces arthritis pain by an average of more than three points on a 10-point visual analogue scale. If this claim is not suspected, there is no need to investigate it further. A test is required only if there is a doubt. The null hypothesis for rejection in this situation is that the pain reduction is only three (or less) points. There must be sufficient evidence to refute this. The obvious procedure for this is to measure the pain before the drug, give the regimen as prescribed, and measure the pain again. If the average difference in the pain score is three or less in the sample subjects, the claim is not tenable and there is no need to proceed further. The big question is that if the mean reduction in pain score in the sample patients is more than three, suppose 3.7, is it still sufficiently against the null. Hypothesis such as this are tested by Student's t-test, although it is generally referred to as **paired-*t*** because the measurements are on the same patients before and after the treatment.

Suppose now that the interest is in finding whether aspartate aminotransferase (AST) level is the same on average in liver cirrhosis cases as in hepatitis cases. Now there are two 'populations': cases of liver cirrhosis and cases of hepatitis. The objective is to find whether these two populations have same mean AST level in the long run. The null hypothesis is that they are same. Evidence against this, if any, would be provided by the samples. Suppose a random sample of 40 cases of liver cirrhosis and 60 cases of hepatitis is studied. The sample means are 54 IU/l and 62 IU/l, respectively. Is this difference of 8 IU/l in sample means large enough to be confident that the difference will not vanish when other similar samples are studied? The answer is given by two-sample t-test that considers not only the magnitude of mean difference but also the variability in individual values (SDs) in the two samples. Large variability tends to negate even a big difference in means. Use a statistical software to do the calculations and to find the P-value.

Some other Applications of Student's *t*-Test

If the average fasting blood glucose level is 93 mg/dl among a sample of habitual morning walkers and 87 mg/dl among a sample of evening walkers (who do not walk in the morning) from the same community, what factors should be considered to decide that this difference is of some consequence? Foremost is the biological plausibility. What postulations are available that can justify this difference? Second is the role of confounding factors. If the walkers come from the same social milieu and belong to the same age-gender group, the difference indeed deserves attention. Third is the statistical significance. This in turn depends on the sample sizes and the SDs in the two groups. If the number of subjects is large in each group and/or the SDs are small, be quite confident that a difference exists. Two-sample *t*-test would decide one way or the other. But this significance, when tested in the usual manner, would only be able to say that a difference is very likely to exist without saying how much. For translating into action, the crucial question is that the difference is enough or not to have medical implication. In this example, if the difference is small such as 1 or 2 mg/dl, that too on average, perhaps it is not pragmatic to disturb the routine of morning walkers. Advising them to walk in the evening instead is unnecessary since such a small difference may not matter in the long run. What difference can be considered enough to ask for a change in the routine of the morning walkers? Suppose a difference of more than 5 mg/dl in the average blood glucose level is considered medically relevant. Although the sample mean difference is 6 mg/dl between morning and evening walkers, it can still be 5 or less in another sample. Thus, the null hypothesis is that the mean difference is 5 mg/dl and the one-sided alternative to be accepted in case of discarding the null is that the mean difference is more than 5 mg/dl. See Example 11.3.

EXAMPLE 11.3: A small, medically irrelevant, difference can become statistically significant if the sample size is large

It is commonly believed that Tricyclic Antidepressants (TCAs) enhance appetite and may facilitate weight gain in depression patients with low body weight. Rigler et al. (2001) conducted a retrospective cohort study on 1157 cases on antidepressants including TCAs for at least 6 months. Thus, the sample size is large. The mean weight gain among TCA users was only 0.4 pounds but was statistically significant ($P = 0.046$). The authors rightly pointed out that this small but statistically significant gain in mean weight is largely a reflection of large sample size rather than of clinically important difference.

ANOVA Procedure – *F*-test

Analysis of variance (ANOVA) based *F*-test is a versatile procedure used in a variety of situations. The name derives from the fact that the total variance among subjects is broken down to various parts such as between-subjects and within-subjects, or so much is due to factor A and so much is due to factor B, etc. For example, ANOVA may reveal that 50 percent of variation in P3 amplitude in healthy adults is due to genetic differences, 20 percent is due to age differentials, 5 percent due to gender differentials, and the remaining 25 percent due to other factors.

Most common application of ANOVA is in testing equality of means of a quantitative measurement in three or more groups, called **one-way ANOVA**. The procedure requires that the variances in different groups are nearly same—called homogeneity of variances, and the values follow a Gaussian pattern. While running ANOVA procedure on a computer, ask the software to first check that the data meet these requirements.

If the checks show either lack of homogeneity of variances or lack of Gaussianity, or both, consult a biostatistician if needed. He might advise alternative methods of analysis such as transformation or nonparametrics, particularly if the group sizes are small.

If the group means turn out to be significantly different, the next question is where exactly this difference is. Each group is compared with each of the others. For this, multiple comparison procedure such as **Tukey, Bonferroni,** and **Scheffe** is used. For pairwise comparisons, Tukey is preferred. For comparing each group with control, **Dunnett** procedure is used.

Statistical procedures are available that would rank groups from minimum mean to maximum mean with an in-between possibility of nearly same means of two or more groups but different from others. Consult a knowledgeable biostatistician if the interest is in such ranking.

In some situations, subgroups are obtained by further classification of cases and control groups by characteristics such as age, sex, and severity. This would give rise to **multi-way ANOVA**. In this situation, interaction between, for example, the effect of dose and effect of severity can also be examined. It is possible that dose-2 is effective in serious cases and dose-1 in mild cases. This differential would surface only when the interaction is examined. However statistical test may lack power to detect interaction if the sample size is based on the size of factor effects and not adequate to examine the interaction.

ANOVA requires that the values are independent of each other. This is lost when the same subject is repeatedly measured at different points of time. If motor function level is low in cerebral palsy patients before surgery, it probably will not improve as much at 1, 2, 6 and 12 months after surgery as of patients with good level initially. Thus, subsequent levels depend on the initial level. Because of this dependence, the usual ANOVA cannot be applied, and a special procedure called **repeated measures ANOVA** is used. If your research is giving rise to this kind of data, be careful in using a correct statistical programme. Perhaps it would be sensible to take help of a biostatistician who can choose the right procedure after he is explained the entire procedure of conducting the study.

Nonparametric Methods

Notice that Student's t-test and ANOVA F-test require Gaussian distribution of the means. This is likely if the sample size in each group is large. There are several other advantages of conducting a study on reasonably large number of cases as described below. If the sample size is small, these procedures can still be applied if the distribution of underlying measurements is not different from Gaussian. The problem arises when the sample size is small, and the underlying distribution is nonGaussian such as highly skewed. The methods of choice in this situation are, what are called, nonparametrics. The name arises from the fact that these methods do not compare any parameter such as mean, median, mode, or percentile but compare the location of the entire distribution. Nonparametric methods do not depend on the pattern of the distribution (a nonGaussian distribution is acceptable) and thus also called distribution-free methods. The only requirement is that the shape of the distributions is the same in different groups such as in Figure 11-1 though they can differ in location.

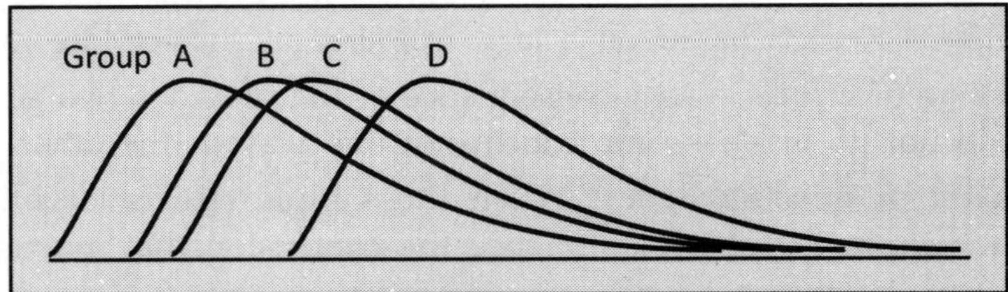

FIGURE 11-1: Example of distributions that have same shape but have differing locations

Most popular nonparametric method is Mann-Whitney test, also known as Wilcoxon test. This is nonparametric equivalent of Student's t-test. The other is Kruskal-Wallis test corresponding to F-test for one-way ANOVA. Friedman test is used for two-way ANOVA with one observation per cell.

All tests based on chi-square are also distribution-free. They do not require Gaussianity or any other specific shape of the distribution.

EXAMPLE 11.4: Mann-Whitney test for IFN-gamma levels in women with recurrent pregnancy loss

IFN-gamma is a Th1 cytokine that seems to play a critical role in unexplained Recurrent Pregnancy Loss (RPL). Daher et al. (2004) measured levels of IFN-gamma (and several other cytokines) in 29 women with RPL (at least three consecutive spontaneous abortions) and 27 control women with successful pregnancies. It is known that IFN-gamma levels have a highly skewed distribution, and the number of subjects in the two groups is not large. Thus, **Mann-Whitney test** was used to compare the two groups. Significantly (P = 0.01) higher average of IFN-gamma (355.8 pg/ml versus 98.0 pg/ml) were seen in RPL women compared to controls. Thus, the study supports the contention that Th1 cytokines are involved in the pathogenesis of RPL.

Side note: Although the authors described results in terms of higher average but nonparametric tests are not for means. The right result from Mann-Whitney test in this case is that IFN-gamma levels are significantly higher in RPL women.

Importance of a Reasonably Large Group of Subjects for Statistical Significance

Large sample is a wastage of resources when a reliable conclusion can be drawn by studying a small sample. Sometimes large sample aggravates bias and cost also increases. But there are several advantages of a study on a large sample.

- **Power** – Large number of subjects substantially raises the chance of detecting a difference of medical relevance if present.
- **Reliability** – Results based on a large number of subjects are more reliable.
- **No wastage of efforts** – As a consequence of the previous two advantages, the efforts do not go waste—some conclusion one way or the other is drawn.
- **Less effect of missing data** – When the sample size is large, few missing observations are not able to influence the conclusion that much.
- **Distribution advantage** – There is no need to worry about the underlying distribution of the measurement when the sample size is large—Gaussian methods can be applied with confidence in practically all situations.
- **Easy computation** – Exact statistical methods for small samples are complicated and the computer packages for these are rare – large samples are easy to handle.

11.3 CONFIDENCE INTERVALS FOR MEDICAL PARAMETERS

Suppose a research finds that the positive predictivity of a new diagnostic procedure is 74 percent. How confident one could be that a similar study on another sample of subjects would not give predictivity less than 70 percent? Just as individuals differ from one-another, so do the samples. It is useful to find how different the results are likely to be in different samples. However, repeated samples are not actually studied. Statisticians have developed a method that would provide an interval within which the actual result is likely to lie in repeated samples. This interval can be obtained by using the data of only one sample when randomly drawn. The likelihood of the interval containing the actual value is called confidence level, and the interval is called **Confidence Interval (CI)**.

Because of profound medical uncertainties, particularly the sampling fluctuations about which we have been talking from time to time in this text, it is never possible to work out an interval with 100 percent confidence. Generally, a confidence level of 95 percent is used. A 95 percent CI has probability 0.95 that it will contain the actual value of the parameter. More correctly, the chance is small—five percent—that it will **not** contain the actual value.

Any standard statistical software can obtain CI for any of the popular summary measures. Thus, we are not giving any formulae. The emphasis in this text is on the concepts so that situations where a CI would be useful could be identified, and properly interpreted. A different kind of explanation is in the following paragraphs to convey this concept and its interpretation.

11.3.1 CI FOR PROPORTION AND MEAN

Proportion of subjects with a specified characteristic such as with a particular sign or symptom, or those responding to a therapy, is just about the most common summary measure used in medical research. For quantitative measurements, the most common summary measure is mean such as of urinary creatinine in cases of a particular kidney disease and mean forced vital capacity in asthmatic children of age 6 to 10 years. Confidence intervals for these two types of indicators have the following implications.

CI for Proportion

Suppose a new procedure of kidney stones is successful in all 10 cases on which this was tried. Can it be concluded that failure rate would continue to be zero for all such operations in future? Statisticians have worked out that the failure rate in the long run can still be 25 percent! If none failed in a string of 50 operations, statistical methods suggest that the failure rate in the long run may not exceed six percent. This underscores the importance of the size of the trial. Such information is obtained by confidence intervals or confidence bounds. The following example explains them further.

EXAMPLE 11.5: CI for difference in the rate of Caesarean delivery in two types of analgesia

Wong et al. (2005) randomly allocated 750 nulliparous US women in spontaneous labour at term to receive intrathecal analgesia at early stage or systemic analgesia at late stage. They report that the rate of Caesarean delivery was 17.8 percent in intrathecal analgesia group and 20.7 percent in systemic analgesia group. The 95 percent **confidence interval** for the difference in these percentages was (–9.0%, +3.0%). The difference in this particular group was 17.8 – 20.7 = –2.9 percent but, according to the CI, it can be anywhere between – 9.0 percent and +3.0 percent in repeated studies. More correct interpretation is that there is exceedingly small chance that the difference in repeated studies of this type would be either less than –9.0 percent or more than +3.0 percent.

Side Note: The CI: (–9.0, +3.0) contains zero, and thus the other information obtained from this CI is that the rate of Caesarean delivery in the two groups could well be zero. Thus, difference is not statistically significantly different ($P > 0.05$).

Further points regarding CI for a proportion are as follows:

1. Where the study group size is small and the proportion of interest too is small, use exact methods based on binomial distribution. Gaussian approximation is not valid in this situation. Use appropriate software that can give exact CI.
2. When the observed proportion in the study group is extreme—nearly zero or nearly one—use exact method again even if n is large. If needed, consult a biostatistician.

CI for Mean

Consider a new herbal drug tried on 50 coronary disease patients that reduced lipoprotein(a) level by an average of 9 mg/dl in a 3-month time. The mean reduction obtained in this group is just one of many possible values in different samples. For this reason, this is called an **estimate**. Another group may give an average reduction of 8 mg/dl and a third an average of 11. CI quantifies the likely values. If the trials were large, the difference between the results of one trial from the other would be minimal. A large n leads to small CI that tells that the information from the sample is precise.

CI for mean, or for difference in means in two groups, is easy to calculate manually but is best obtained with the help of statistical software. In our example on improvement in lipoprotein(a) level, suppose the 95 percent CI is (3, 15) mg/dl. Chance is small – five percent – that the mean reduction in repeat studies would be either less than 3 mg/dl or more than 15 mg/dl. In individual cases, the reduction could be much larger or much smaller—even increased Lp(a) in some cases. Medical empiricism is about averages rather than individual values.

Both in the case of proportions and in the case of means, one-sided confidence bound can be obtained where needed. For example, for noninferiority trials, one-sided bound should be calculated. In equivalence trials, two-sided CI is used, and the entire CI should fall within the prespecified equivalence margin.

11.4 SOME COMPLEX STATISTICAL ISSUES

Biostatistics is a versatile science with extensive applications in empirical research, particularly in medical research where enormous uncertainties occur. The methods of biostatistics can help answer a range of issues starting with planning a quality research and ending with valid and reliable results. This book on research methods cannot discuss all of these but you should be aware of the methods commonly used in medical research. We give an outline of these methods in this section. For details, see Indrayan and Malhotra (2018).

11.4.1 RELATIONSHIPS BETWEEN MEDICAL FACTORS

Relationships have always fascinated researchers, and their understanding has contributed a lot to the advancement of medical science. Only the plausible relationships are investigated. Perhaps nobody would spend time in finding the relationship between prothrombin time and size of femur, although a hidden relationship can exist. Who knows! Establishing new relationships that can stand the test of time across different populations is a challenge that some researchers cherish to grab. Variation and uncertainties dampen optimism, yet an emerging trend can be revelation is some cases. The purpose of obtaining relationship is to (i) predict an outcome on the basis of the known factors, (ii) identify direct and indirect factors that contribute to the outcome, and (iii) get better understanding of the underlying mechanism.

Relationship is studied in two ways: (i) the strength of relationship and (ii) the nature of relationship. The first is measured in terms of correlation and association and answers how much, and the second is studied in terms regression equation and answers what is the nature of relationship.

Correlation and Association

The strength of relationship between two quantitative variables, such as albumin level and bilirubin level in cases with liver disease, is measured by the **correlation coefficient**. This is measured on a –1 to +1 scale with zero in between saying no relationship. Negative value indicates that increase in one is generally accompanied by decrease in the other, and the positive value indicates that both the variables are moving in the same direction. The correlation between vitamin D level and triglyceride level may be negative and between vitamin D level and bone mineral density positive.

The most used coefficient of correlation is the Pearsonian correlation. It measures only the linear component of the relationship. Lung capacity increases in the childhood, remains stationary in the adulthood, and declines at the old age but the Pearsonian correlation between age and lung capacity would be nearly zero. Positive relationship at the young age cancels out with negative relationship at the old age. Thus, use this correlation only where the relationship is expected to follow an increasing or decreasing trend in a line.

For qualitative characteristics such as blood group and hypertension, the relationship is measured in terms of **association**. Many researchers still call it correlation. The degree of association is measured by chi-square-based indicators. More common and more appealing is the **Odds Ratio** (OR). This is generally used for binary variables or after collapsing polytomous categories to dichotomous categories. This is calculated as a ratio of ratios. The numerator is a ratio of chance of occurrence of an event in the presence of a factor and chance in the absence of that factor in one group and the denominator is a similar ratio for the other group. In prospective studies, **Relative Risk** (RR) is used as a measure of association which is the ratio of incidence of disease in one group (such as the one exposed) to the incidence in the other group (such as nonexposed). The value of OR or RR < 1 indicates negative association (such as protection from a disease with increasing level of the risk factor) and OR or RR > 1 indicates positive association.

There are other kinds of correlations such as Spearman and biserial, and it is better to leave this to the wisdom of the biostatistics professionals.

Regression – General Concepts

Perhaps due to cumulative effect of salt intake or due to natural hardening of arteries, it is seen in many healthy adult populations that Blood Pressure (BP) rises with age. Suppose that this relationship for systolic BP can be expressed as sysBP = 110 + ½(Age in years). Such an equation that expresses one characteristic or measurement in terms of the others is called a **regression** model. It specifies the nature of relationship and is applicable to the *average* of a group and not to the individuals. This particular equation says that average sysBP at age 30 years is 110 + ½×30 = 125 mmHg, and at age 60 years is 110 + ½×60 = 140 mmHg. The multiplier ½ is called the **regression coefficient** of Age. If this equation is to be believed, change in Age by one year raises sysBP by ½ mmHg on average in healthy adults. Consider the power of this message in understanding this phenomenon. In some situations, regression equation can provide deep insight into what is going on, besides providing an effective tool for prediction.

Among many types of regression, the most common in medical research is the logistic regression. The others is linear regression. To obtain these for any data, the first step is to understand the concept of dependent and independent variables.

Dependent variable is the actual outcome of the interest. It is determined fully or partially, directly or indirectly, by one or more of the other variables under consideration.

If the primary focus of a research is to investigate how birthweight is affected by weight of the mother and father, opposed to the haemoglobin level of the mother, the dependent is the birthweight. This is a quantitative measurement. In a study of development of diabetic retinopathy based on duration of diabetes, nutrition level, regularity of treatment, and age, the dependent is the development of diabetic retinopathy. This is a dichotomous variable with yes/no categories. If the interest is in the grade of diabetic retinopathy (none/ mild/ moderate/ proliferative), the dependent is still qualitative. The statistical method of finding the regression equation is different for qualitative outcomes than for quantitative outcomes.

Antecedents that can affect the outcome are called the **independent variables** in a regression setup. In birth weight example in the previous paragraph, mother's weight, father's weight, and haemoglobin level are the independent variables. They can be manipulated in the sense that you can choose parents of different weights and of different Hb levels to see how these variations affect the birth weight. In the diabetic retinopathy example, independents are duration of diabetes, nutrition level, regularity of treatment, and age. They can be quantitative or mixed. (If all of them are qualitative, and the dependent is quantitative, the situation reverses to ANOVA discussed earlier). Independent variables are known by several other names: Regressors, factors, determinants, explanatory variables. Use the term that looks most appropriate for the measurement in hand. This text uses these terms interchangeably.

Medicine is an intricate science, and an outcome is generally affected by several factors. Thus, many candidates would be available as independent variables. A good research filters out the unimportant ones and concentrates on a few that can really affect the outcome. Regression results intimately depend on the proper choice of the regressors.

Linear and Nonlinear Regression

The concept of linear regression can be easily illustrated with the help of the hypothetical equation that we started with: sysBP = 110 + ½(Age in years) for adults. As an exercise, calculate sysBP from this equation for different ages and plot them on a graph. You will get a line. Hence the name 'linear'. The constant in front 110 is called the intercept and the regression coefficient ½ for Age determines the slope of the line. The regression is **'simple'** because there is only one independent in this regression. If there are more, it is called **multiple regression.** In sysBP example, BMI as well as physical exercise (hours per week) can be included as possible predictors. In that case, the equation can take the following form:

$$\text{SysBP} = 107 + \tfrac{1}{4}(\text{Age}) + \tfrac{1}{2}(\text{BMI}) - \tfrac{1}{3}(\text{Exercise})$$

A positive sign of a regression coefficient indicates that the concerned variable has positive effect, and the negative sign indicates that the effect is negative. The regression coefficient represents the average effect of that independent variable, duly *adjusted* for the effect of other independents in the equation. In this example, the effect of one unit increase in BMI is increase in sysBP by an average of ½ mmHg (or increase in BMI by 2 units increases sysBP by 1 mmHg on average) and it is adjusted in the sense that it is independent of the effect of age and exercise. This has special meaning when BMI decreases with exercise. If BMI is 22 in one group and 28 in the other group, and both groups happen to exercise 8 hours per week, the difference of 6 in BMI changes the average sysBP by (6×½=) 3 mmHg.

Other variables such as smoking are not in this equation and they can still confound the relationship. Thus, the coefficient still does not really represent the 'net' effect that some researchers erroneously make out of a regression equation that does not incorporate all the factors.

The two types of regression (simple linear and multiple linear) discussed above do well when the relationship can be expressed by a line. A regression becomes curve when terms such as square, cube, logarithm, exponential and reciprocal are included. For example, the relationship between FVC(l) and Age (years) can be expressed as

$$\text{FVC} = 0.8564 + 0.2104(\text{Age}) - 0.0028(\text{Age})^2.$$

Although not obvious, statisticians can tell from this equation that average FVC is maximum at age 37 years and declines on both the sides of age.

Logistic Regression

The dependent variable in logistic regression should be the probability of positive outcome. This is estimated by the proportion (p) observed in the study group. If 72 percent of critically ill patients survived in a hospital, $p = 0.72$ for that hospital. However, the number of patients with the positive outcome follows the binomial distribution instead of Gaussian. Thus, a transformation called **logit** is needed which gives rise to the name logistic. In a logistic regression this is obtained as a function of the independent or predictor variables and tells us how far the outcome can be predicted, and which predictors are more important than others.

When a logistic regression is obtained with only one independent, it is called univariate, and when the number of independents is more, it is called **multivariable**. A very useful property of logistic regression is that the regression coefficients of independent variables estimate the logarithm of respective relative risks (lnRRs) in prospective studies, and of the logarithm of odds ratios (lnORs) in retrospective studies. If this for Age in a logistic regression is –0.013, its exponent gives RR = 0.99. This is close to one and indicates that patients with different ages have the same survival rate.

In other words, age by itself has no role in increasing or decreasing the survival. By keeping other predictors in the logistic equation, an adjusted value of RR can be obtained. Statistical significance of each logistic coefficient can be tested. Most useful application of logistic is in case-control studies where the outcome of interest is the proportion of subjects with disease (or any other outcome) having specific antecedents. The logistic coefficients in this setup are lnORs.

Cox Regression

Cox regression is used when the outcome is survival. This is time dependent in the sense that survival at age 60 years is different from survival at age 80 years. In place of logit, now hazard ratio is used as the dependent variable where hazard is for death but is generically used for the occurrence of any event of interest. The independent variables are the risk factors that are expected to affect the survival.

Hazard in the absence of risk factors is called baseline hazard. This is like the hazard of death of a 70-year old who is otherwise a healthy person and not exposed to any specific risk factor. The focus of research could be the effect modification by the presence of one or more risk factors. Cox regression generally premises that the *ratio* of actual hazard to the baseline hazard remains same over the follow-up period for fixed regressors, although hazard itself can change over time. For this reason, it is called **proportional hazards model**. This has been found applicable to many practical situations in medical research.

In Cox regression, logarithm of the ratio of actual to baseline hazard is regressed on a linear or any other combination of the level of various risk factors. If the hazard ratio is 2 for a particular risk factor such as angina for MI, at every point of time during the follow-up, the interpretation is that persons with angina have twice the hazard of MI of that of persons without angina. The contribution of various risk factors to the hazard can be obtained by Cox regression.

11.4.2 CAUSE-EFFECT RELATIONSHIP IN MEDICAL RESEARCH

Incidence of cardiovascular diseases in India is increasing whereas birth rate is decreasing. They are inversely related. The correlation coefficient between these two entirely unrelated measurements could be around –0.6. This is an example of **spurious correlation** that arose because both are related to the process of development. If the interest is in biological relationship, the 'development' is a **nuisance variable** in this example because it is playing a spoiling game. The example is extreme but aptly illustrates difference between correlation and cause-effect relationship. Another interesting example is the strong correlation between age at onset of disease and survival duration. Older people tend to die quickly anyway and high negative correlation in these two measurements is trivial. However, coincidences can have some role in learning causality.

Evidence of Cause-Effect

Although the term factor is used for any characteristic of interest but in aetiological context a characteristic is a factor for an outcome only if it is a contributor or suspected to be a contributor in some respect. It can be either directly responsible or indirectly responsible for that outcome; it can be wholly responsible or partially responsible. For example, obesity is a factor in diabetes and coronary disease but not in typhoid.

Cause is a stronger term. Although the usage is not uniform, cause is generally used for a factor that is directly responsible for the outcome. Smoking is considered a cause of lung cancer even though its affect is also mediated either through nicotine deposits or cotinine level, both of which have potential to alter cell structure. Smoking causes atherosclerosis that causes hypertension. Thus, smoking has indirect role in hypertension. Ideally it should not be called a cause of hypertension. It is just a factor. Such distinction is rarely made in research literature but there is a gradual realisation that all factors are not causes.

It is sometimes argued that a factor is a cause if it is both necessary and sufficient for the effect to appear. This is too strict a condition in medical context. Smoking is neither necessary nor sufficient to cause hypertension. Yet it is considered a cause. Statistically, if presence of a factor A raises the chance of occurrence of B and its absence reduces the chance, A can be considered one of the many causes of B.

Criteria of Cause-effect

Just how much evidence is needed to accept cause-effect relationship? In medical research, cause-effect relationship is assessed by evidence regarding the following criteria.

1. **Temporality** — An elementary feature of cause-effect relationship is that prospective study should establish time sequence with the factor preceding the outcome. This is easily established in most situations but the relationships among concurrent factors such as between blood group and gender are difficult in this respect.

   Also, the relationship must stand the test of time. A cause-effect relationship would be true in the year 1950 as much as in the year 2022.

2. **Experimental evidence** — Since an experiment is conducted in controlled conditions, it can provide convincing evidence for or against enhanced chance

of outcome in the presence of the purported cause, and reduced chance in its absence. However, as mentioned in an earlier chapter, experiment on human beings could be conducted only for potentially beneficial factor, and not for potentially harmful factor. Thus, this criterion is not assessed for harmful factors except for specificity as explained in item 6 in this list.

3. **Dose-response relationship** — For cause-effect, presence of cause in greater magnitude should be able to produce greater effect. BP level and coronary events have dose-response relationship in the sense that the chance of coronary events is higher if BP is 130/85 mmHg than if it is 120/80, and still higher for BP 160/95. In some situations, the minimum and the maximum limits of the magnitude of the causal factor can be specified within which the gradient exists. Salt intake below the minimum physiologic need may give rise to other health problems – thus there is a minimum beyond which the relationship between salt intake and hypertension occurs.
4. **Consistency** — This has two facets. One, specific magnitude of the cause should always produce nearly the same effect when there are no confounders to subvert the relationship. Two, the relationship must occur across different populations where the cause exists. Several researchers under different settings should report similar relationship. The relationship between homocysteine level and coronary disease, after initial hysteria, has now been observed to lack consistency.
5. **Biological plausibility** — Plausible mechanism must exist to explain the relationship. Altitude and endemic goitre may be related but no mechanism can be conjectured unless iodine deficiency occurring in high altitude areas is brought in. As remarked earlier, any such explanation depends on the current knowledge. If this is not adequate, the relationship is relegated to mere association. Association of addition of vitamin A to the treatment of iron deficiency for correcting anaemia is an example for which an adequate explanation is still under investigation.
6. **Specificity** — Absence of the factor must be accompanied by the absence of the outcome: at least diminish it. Reduced exposure must reduce the chance or magnitude of the outcome. This is just another aspect of dose-response relationship, but the emphasis now is on negativity. Intervention trials that eliminate or reduce the exposure can establish specificity. If tension and stress are reduced by counselling or otherwise, does it lower the frequency or severity of depression? If reduction in contamination in water reduces diarrhoeal episodes, the relationship is specific, and a candidate to be called causal.
7. **Statistical significance** — As mentioned earlier, no medical significance can be attached to the results that fail statistical significance although statistical significance by itself is not enough to conclude medical significance. The same can be reiterated for casual relationship. A factor cannot be a cause unless its

statistical significance is demonstrated that rules out sampling fluctuation as a reason for the relationship.

A weak relationship can be statistically significant if *n* is sufficiently large. Strength of relationship is not an issue for deciding causality—thus, mere statistical significance is enough to suspect causality. Hereditary role in breast cancer may be small but it is there as a cause. Much of the medical literature wrongly includes *strong* association as a requirement for cause-effect relationship. Weak association can also be causal although that would indicate one of the many causes.

Assessment of Cause-Effect in Research

Judging causal relationship is central to human cognition. The procedure to investigate cause-effect relationship in empirical research is slightly different. See Figure 11-2 for a schematic presentation of the steps. The starting point would be to establish that a relationship does exist. This is done by showing statistical significance of the association, correlation, regression, or just a difference between two groups. If this significance in

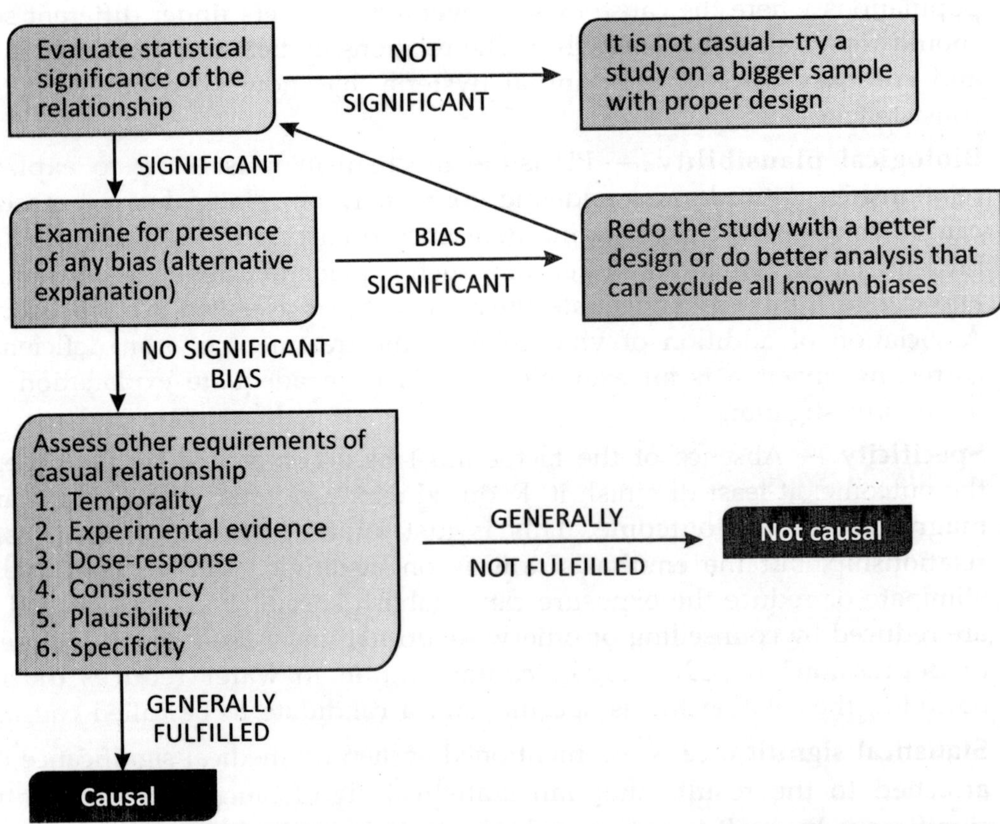

FIGURE 11-2: Procedure to establish cause-effect relationship

lacking, there is no point in proceeding further except to carry out another study, possibly on a bigger sample with proper design to rule out sampling fluctuation and other confounders.

After statistical significance, examine if any alternative explanation is available for that relationship. This exercise helps to rule out various sources of bias such as improper selection of subjects, faulty information or measurement, and inappropriate design, and possible role of confounding factors. When no alternative explanation is available, a causal relationship is strongly indicated.

The role of the first six features of cause-effect relationship discussed in the preceding pages comes after all known sources of bias and confounding are eliminated. Strictly speaking, all the six criteria (temporality, experimental evidence, dose-response, consistency, plausibility, and specificity) must be fulfilled. In practice, though, relaxation is allowed, and a cause-effect relationship is concluded even when one or two of these criteria are not fully met.

These steps indicate that causal relationship is difficult to establish. Caution should be adopted before concluding cause-effect. In most situations, the relationship would be associational that would require additional evidence to qualify as cause-effect.

11.4.3 VALIDATION OF FINDINGS

Although statistical significance implies that the results are replicable yet a study on another group of subjects is desirable to confirm the findings. To examine this kind of robustness, the first step is to test results on another group from the same target populations. If found valid, the next step is to test them on a group of subjects from a different but similar population. This is called external validation. Different samples can be taken in a variety of ways.

Split-sample Method

This method requires that the information is collected on all subjects, but only random half is used for statistical analysis. If the result fails statistical significance, just use it to draw lessons for another study and do not draw any substantive conclusion regarding the question under research. If significance is achieved, use the second half group of subjects, and examine if the results validate. However, this method can be applied when a large number of eligible subjects are available for the study so that even the half part is also adequate.

Suppose the interest is in developing a model to predict the gestation age on the basis of anthropometric measurements at birth. These are obtained for children born to women with known gestation age. If a large sample such as 1200 is available, random 600 of them can be used to develop the model (called the **training sample**), and the other 600 to test it (called the **validation sample**). If testing gives correct gestation such as within ±1 week in at least 80 percent cases, the model can be considered robust for application.

Validation by Another Sample

When the currently available group is not large for splitting into two halves, take a new sample at another point of time, possibly in other setting. If the result turns out true for a such a sample, its utility increases tremendously. In gestational age example in the preceding paragraph, the validation sample can be taken from some other hospital located in the same area or in some other area. Many researchers leave validation onto the future researchers. McGill pain score has been validated in a variety of settings by different researchers yet its utility in largely illiterate population remains questionable.

EXAMPLE 11.6: Validation of automatic scoring procedure for discriminating between breast cancer cases and controls

Medicine is largely a science of prediction—prediction of diagnosis, prediction of outcome

Micronucleus assay (MNT) in human lymphocytes is frequently used to assess chromosomal damage. Varga et al. (2004) developed MNT on the basis of computerised image analysis. In a test sample of 73 persons (27 breast cancer cases and 46 controls) in Germany, the automated score gave OR = 16. This is a substantial improvement over OR = 4 for the conventional score based on visual counting. The improvement was confirmed in a **validation sample** of 41 persons (20 cases and 21 controls) that gave OR = 11.

There are several other methods such as Bootstrap, sensitivity analysis, and uncertainty analysis that we have not discussed in this book. If interested, consult any good book on statistical methods.

SUMMARY

Statistical procedure of testing a hypothesis is similar to a court trial. The null hypothesis is set up to say that there is no difference between groups—equivalent to no guilt. Observations on sample subjects provide the evidence to decide to discard the null or not. Wrong rejection of a null hypothesis is a serious error and called Type I. The probability of this is called *P*-value. The maximum threshold tolerance of this error is fixed in advance, generally at five percent. This is called the level of significance and denoted by α. Type II error is not rejecting a false null. The probability of this is denoted by β. This is linked with the difference between groups, which is specified as medically relevant. The probability of correctly rejecting a null when the specified difference is indeed present is called statistical power. This is $1 - \beta$. Power can be increased by appropriately increasing the sample size of the study.

The test of statistical significance for categorical data where the interest is in proportions is chi-square. It is utilised to test, among others, goodness of fit to a prespecified pattern, presence of association between two or more characteristics, and trend in proportions when the categories are ordinal.

When the interest is in average level of a quantitative measurement in one or two groups, the statistical test of choice in most situations is Student's *t*. For three or more groups and for cross-classification of subjects by two or more factors, ANOVA-based *F*-test is used. A separate method is available for repeated measures although this also uses ANOVA and *F*-test.

Nonparametric tests such as Mann-Whitney and Kruskal-Wallis are used when the underlying measurement is suspected to follow a nonGaussian pattern such as skewed and the number of subjects under research is small.

Confidence interval provides a plausible interval within which the result can lie when repeat studies are done. This however takes care of only the inter-sample variability. Other sources of variation are not considered.

Robustness of results is tested by (i) carrying out the analysis in two stages – one on a training sample and the other on a validation sample, and (ii) actually carrying out another study on a similar group. There are other methods such as uncertainty analysis and sensitivity analysis that we have not discussed in this book.

REFERENCES

Daher S, de Arruda GDK, Blotta MH, et al. Cytokines in recurrent pregnancy loss. J Repro Immunol 2004;62:151-157.

Dimick JB, Diener-West M, Lipsett PA. Negative results of randomized clinical trials published in the surgical literature: equivalency or error? Arch Surg 2001;136:796-800.

Feinstein AR. Clinical Biostatistics. The CV Mosby Company, 1977:p11.

Freiman JA. The importance of beta, the type II error, and sample size in the design and interpretation of the randomized control trial: a survey of 71 "negative" trials. New Engl J Med 1978; 299:690-695.

Hansen SL, Clark SL, Foster JC. Active pushing versus passive fetal descent in the second stage of labor: a randomized controlled trial. Obstet Gynecol 2002;99:29-34.

Indrayan A, Malhotra RK. Medical Biostatistics, 4th ed. CRC Press, 2018.

Lang J, Rothman K, Cann C. That confounded P-value. Epidemiology 1998;9:28.

Rigler SK, Webb MJ, Redford L, Brown EF, Zhou J, Wallace D. Weight outcomes among antidepressant users in nursing facilities. J Am Geriatr Soc 2001;49:49-55.

Sterne J. Commentary: Null points—has interpretation of significance tests improved? Int J Epidemiol 2003;32:693-694.

Varga D, Johannes T, Jainta S, et al. An automated scoring procedure for the micronucleus test by image analysis. Mutagenesis 2004;193:391-397.

Wong CA, Scavone BM, Peaceman AM, et al. The risk of Cesarean delivery with neuraxial analgesia given early versus late in labor. N Engl J Med 2005;352:655-665.

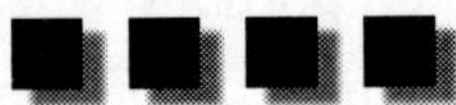

CHAPTER 12

What are the Principles of Scientific Writing

KEY TERMS AND CONCEPTS

- ✓ Ten Principles of Scientific Writing
- ✓ Text Style
- ✓ Format of Tables
- ✓ Graphs and Diagrams
- ✓ Who could be the Authors

After toiling hard for completing a research, it is time to share the excitement. Let the world know what new has been achieved or could not be achieved. You have a duty to disseminate the results regardless of achievement. No research is complete unless it is read, discussed, and evaluated. Medical colleges generally marginalise presentation skills and many emerging researchers find effective presentation a difficult proposition. Successful researchers are skilful biomedical communicators too. The dissemination could be in a conference through PowerPoint or other kind of presentation, but most medical research culminates into a written report that could take a form of a paper, a thesis, a dissertation, or a full-fledged project report. We discuss oral and poster presentation in a subsequent chapter and restrict for the time being to writing because that is the most dominant mode of communicating a research. The present chapter is on the principles of scientific writing. The next chapter is on the structure and the contents of a paper or a thesis.

Written is the predominant mode of communication of medical research. More than twenty thousand medical journals thrive around the world on this type of communication. In addition, scores of theses, dissertations, and project reports are prepared every year. Following are some guidelines on the principles and style of preparing a written communication, particularly for a paper to be sent to a journal for publication.

Backbone of research is described by reports based on original data or review articles. However, other forms of written communication, such as descriptive articles, clinical practice guidelines, opinions and commentaries, letters, news, and conference reports, are also published by many journals. You may like to consider other modes of publication. For example, if your work is voluminous and in-depth coverage of a specialised topic, you can publish a **monograph** yourself or as part of a series published by your institution. Think of publishing your work or its summary in a suitable website including your own. Many institutions provide a page for each staff where you can place your work. This will show up in Google search for anybody to access. There are dedicated websites who will accept your work for publication. In addition, there are many pre-publication archiving sites such as medrXiv, SSRN, Research Square, and Collection Of Biostatistics Research Archive (COBRA) maintained by Berkeley Electronic Press. Researchers across the world download article of their choice from such websites.

12.1 WRITING PRINCIPLES

Many researchers find themselves at cross-roads while trying to prepare a succinct and comprehensive yet concise paper despite completing a successful research. At the same time, some researchers may not have done excellent research but are able to communicate in an impressive manner and make an impact. A medical researcher is expected to follow the principles described next.

12.1.1 TEN PRINCIPLES

For our advice for preparing an impressive manuscript, we largely go by the ten simple rules provided by Zhang (2014). These are as follows.

1. Consider writing a research paper as an integral part of the research endeavour. Keep in mind that a full report or a paper based on your finding will be

prepared by you and your team for discussion by others while choosing a topic, at the time of framing your objective, for selecting a design, for choosing the method of measurements, for deciding about the method of analysis, and at the time of interpreting the data. When writing of the ultimate paper is in focus, you will see how various steps of your research automatically refine and improve its quality.

2. Keep a sharp focus at the time of writing. That is, do not try to cover too many hypotheses in one paper. This can dilute the findings and may confuse the reader. In case needed, split the paper into two or more papers on different hypotheses but mention in each that this is what you are doing. It does not mean that you leave out gaps – all aspects of one particular hypothesis must be comprehensively covered in each paper. This could mean some duplication when another paper on a different topic is prepared based on the same work but much of the duplication can be avoided by referring to the previous paper.

   Having said that, many journals, particularly those online with no space constraints, may like to have one comprehensive paper that includes all hypotheses discussed in a single paper. Consult the journal website about the limitation on the number of words for each type of article. Most journals prescribe a limit of 4000 words for an original research.

3. Pick the right journal. This is not as easy as it sounds but consider whether the right audience for your paper is the general physician, people of particular specialty, or even super-specialty. The organization and content of the paper is decided accordingly. The main finding can help to decide the right audience.

4. The draft should be logical and should be arranged to give a smooth reading. Logical does not mean IMRaD format but refers to how the ideas in the Introduction section should be arranged, how various Methods should be arranged, how different findings should be arranged in the Results section, and how arguments in the Discussion section should be arranged. This can help in avoiding duplication. Try if you can prepare an outline of the structure of each of these components before beginning the actual writing.

5. The manuscript of the paper should reflect the thoroughness with which the research was done and present it in a manner that the reader is convinced that a thorough work has been done. Include appropriate tables and figures and state what each figure and table conveys. Well known statistical methods such as logistic regression need not be described but specialized methods such as sensitivity and uncertainty analysis, in case used, should be briefly described and give reference for any reader needing more details.

6. Be concise. Journal space is precious, and most journals would want a concise report. This may sound like contrary to our earlier advice for complete and comprehensive paper but that is not so. The challenge is to draft the manuscript which describes the complete research in a concise manner. After finishing the draft, review it and examine what can be deleted without compromising the quality.
7. Weave your paper into a story so that the next follows from the previous description. Being professional does not stop you to be an entertainer. Some journals hate entertaining phrases, some welcome. Perhaps one or two anecdotes can make your manuscript lively for the audience.
8. Leave the first draft of the manuscript in a drawer for a while and read again. Consider that you are a reviewer and see what faults and qualities you can discover in the draft. Revise it accordingly. A manuscript is generally revised 3-4 times before it becomes appropriate for submission to a journal. This is an arduous task but is extremely desirable for producing a worthwhile paper that can attract attention.
9. Anticipate the questions the readers may raise about this work. Many readers are skeptical by nature and raise questions about even the most meticulously reported research. The manuscript can rarely be foolproof but anticipating such questions will help in improving the draft accordingly.
10. Work hard on manuscript as much as you did for conducting research. The method you used for research remains in the background and it is the paper that the world sees. Do not feel tired at this stage because this is how your research will be known.

12.1.2 BROAD CONSIDERATIONS

Much of how a manuscript should be prepared should be clear from the details provided in Table 4.2 in Chapter 4. That also gives some pointers about reporting. Excellent texts such as by Ray et al. (2016) are available that can help. In brief, the manuscript should contain the following. The details are in the next chapter.

- Do not delay in publication. With medical science rapidly developing and availability of a plethora of online journals, including preprint archives that publish in a few days, a research is published fast. We have seen how researchers were racing against time to publish their work quickly on COVID pandemic.
- Before starting the draft, prepare a short list of what you propose to communicate. This will help in retaining the focus and not miss out any important finding.

- Keep your terminology constant throughout the paper or thesis. Do not write COVID at one place and corona disease at another place.
- Convince the reader that the research question is such that its answer will help improve health in one way or the other. A novel question attracts widespread attention. The statement of research question should be unambiguous and accompanied by a full justification of the choice of topic with citation of the literature pointing to the lacunae. The lacuna could be in terms of conflicting or inconsistent reports or near complete absence of the kind of thinking you are now exploring.
- Crucial for the credibility of the results is the methodology. This should be described in detail so that nothing is left to the imagination of the reader or reviewer. Convince yourself and the reader that you have used appropriate tools to obtain correct data. The method of analysis should be focused on the stated objectives. The methodology should be stated in a manner that anybody with sufficient resources can replicate.
- State the result with complete clarity and all the results should be supported by the evidence collected during the study. Make sure that the results are reproducible. A recent BMJ Open Science (Amaral 2020) gives details of how reproducibility has become an overriding consideration. For this, demonstrate reliability and validity of the findings (reliability and validity are two different aspects of quality and should not be mixed). Demarcate the medical significance of the results from their statistical significance. State any coincidental findings as hypotheses and not as results of the study.
- Discuss the findings honestly in the light of the findings of the others without leaving out inconsistent or conflicting reports. Resolve such conflicts by providing holistic arguments. Do not gloss over the errors and limitations but, instead, state them frankly. That will increase the credibility of the paper.
- Make a distinction between results and conclusions. Results are what your data say whereas the conclusion is based on the results plus other evidence available in the literature and a plausible biological explanation of the results. Results tend to give too much importance to the statistical *P*-values, sometimes even ignoring the multiple *P*-values that compromise statistical significance. There is a great discussion going on these days regarding the validity of the results based exclusively on *P*-values (Wasserstein et al. 2019).
- Ask your research team to review each sentence of the manuscript and encourage them to suggest changes. Helpful colleagues not connected with your research can also be requested to read and provide comments. To encourage feedback, tell them to find errors so that they can provide fearless feedback.

- Take no chance with spellings and grammar. Many journals will send you the manuscript for proof reading. Do this carefully and make minor changes as needed. You may not be allowed to make any major change at this stage.
- Last is the typographical error that can happen even with most reputed journals. Vickers (2006) describes two such instances with British Medical Journal (BMJ). One article stated that the objective was to detect that the drug improved pain by 16 points when the SD is 8 points. It is unusual to power a study to detect such a large difference as 2SD. The authors admitted that the SD was 18 and not 8, and that was a misprint. Another article reported that anxiety, depression, and fatigue improved in the treatment group but quality of life worsened. It turns out that the minus sign was missed in the table of results. These are examples of internal inconsistencies and should have been detected at review stage. You as writer also have the responsibility to keep your windows open and examine the findings with sufficient alertness so that such inconsistencies do not go unchallenged.

12.2 STYLE OF WRITING

Style is the mannerism and dictated by the interest of the reader. This is as important as the statement of facts. The basic ingredient is that a manuscript should be effective in conveying the meaning. Put yourself in the position of an indifferent reader and write in a manner that it communicates. Scientific writing sans digression and calls for focused exposition. In any case, the message in any research presentation must be new and original that can evince interest. The text must contain all the details of the decision you took at every step, such as the choice of the topic, specification of the objectives, identification of variables, method of their operationalisation, choice of instruments, control of bias, contents of design, sample size and its justification, method of assessing data quality, and statistical methods. A good manuscript is clear and concise, flows from section to section and is free from errors of spelling, syntax, and grammar. We begin with general tips for writing a research paper.

Some Tips on Style of Writing a Medical Research Paper

- Write in logical sequence with proper linkages between paragraphs and sections. Use simple language without sacrificing the emphasis.
- Paper should be as short as possible but should contain enough details for reader to replicate the study. Thesis, dissertation, and project report should contain full details. However, these too should not contain unnecessary details because they can add to confusion in place of clarity.

- Summarise the data in tables and use illustrations to make a visual impact. Use them sparingly in a paper and liberally in a thesis. But there should be no duplication. Diagrams should be appropriate for the data in hand.

12.2.1 TEXT STYLE

The text of a communication should be as short as possible without compromising the quality of exposition. Brevity is a virtue that should not be compromised. Do not expect editors and reviewers to devote time for suggesting specific cuts. Examine your manuscript at least three times and delete any superfluous or duplicate material detected each time. Also plug appropriate words and sentences where holes are detected. Connect the dots and draw links between different ideas.

Writing process can be frustrating for beginners and difficult for many others. If so, perhaps the best course is to begin writing whatever comes to mind and edit it later. The finished manuscript must follow a logical sequence. Organise it in a manner that your enthusiasm and confidence in the work is clearly visible. Although scientific writing is not story telling, but a narrative format with events flowing from the previous occurrences may be more friendly to the readers. Weave it nicely so that paragraphs and sections present a coherent picture. Be prepared to do brainstorming to achieve clarity where needed. Use a judicious mix of text, tables, figures, and bullets to break monotony. Do not use pompous language as is used in some literary writings but also do not shy from using punch words that convey the meaning forcefully. Use proper words at proper place. Although figures of speech and idioms are not favoured in scientific writing but sometimes they provide a very apt description. Always quest for the right words and phrases. Do not use inappropriate words or controversial vocabulary. Request your colleagues and supervisors to read the manuscript and provide a feedback. Do not take their critique personally. Improve accordingly. As mentioned earlier, we have found that leaving a manuscript in a drawer for a couple of days, and then a self-review is very effective in detecting both technical and language deficiencies.

Science is complex but it needs to be explained in a manner that can be understood by a reader. The writer must understand what the reader needs, and the style should be such that the reader accurately perceives what the author has in mind. The key word for this is articulation. The following guidelines might help.

1. Use titles and subtitles to identify the contents. In theses, you may like to number each paragraph also that would make it easier to refer back and forth in the text. Do not have unlinked ideas in the same paragraph. Each paragraph must have at least two sentences.

2. Avoid nontechnical use of technical terms such as 'normal', 'significant', 'interaction', and 'correlation'. They might confuse the reader.
3. Text description must match the numbers and percentages given in accompanying tables or figures. Editors and other assessors are not kind to such discrepancies.
4. Check that there are no contradictions. If there is any, explain it fully.
5. Some repetition is allowed when necessary in the context but not much.
6. A written scientific communication is a formal prose. Thus, colloquial language should be avoided. Words with uncertain meaning such as 'soon', 'a lot of', 'something like', and 'seem', should be replaced by their exact counterparts as much as possible. For example, instead of 'soon' specify how many hours or how many days. Also avoid terms such as 'very', 'extremely', 'enormous'. These terms are fine for books.
7. Avoid unnecessary phrases such as "It is interesting to note that ....." In a paper, see if sentences in the beginning and at the end of big paragraphs can be deleted.
8. In a paper particularly, in place of saying that 'comparison is in Table X', say, for example, that 'cases had higher obesity (Table X)'.
9. Introduce only one new idea per sentence.

Explain all abbreviations when used first. Do not use too many abbreviations. Try to restrict to the popularly known ones.

12.2.2 TABLES

Tables are powerful tools to display the data in an intelligible and precise format. They tend to condense and summarise the information and sometimes communicate the intricacies better than text. Readers can explore the data for several combination of comparisons. Tables give structure to the answer and provide concrete evidence as large set of summary statistics can be recorded. But they can be source of confusion too when not properly drawn. Some tips on how to prepare various types of tables are in Section 10.1. Tables containing number and percentage of subjects in different categories have very different format than tables containing statistical results (such as odds ratios, confidence intervals, or *P*-values). Percentages should be based on appropriate total as described earlier. Number of subjects in each group should be mentioned, preferably in the column heading. Ensure that the numbers in different tables are consistent with one-another. Specify the unit of each measurement. Each table must be referred in the text.

Data on groups you want to compare should be in columns. For example, if your objective is to compare cases with controls, data on cases should be in one column and on controls in adjacent column. If you want to compare males and females, data on these two groups should be in columns (and not two rows). When two or more tables present results on the same set of variables, the order of variables should be the same.

Tables on statistical significance should contain exact *P*-values that give more insight to the reader than just saying $P<0.05/P>0.05$ or significant/not significant. But $P < 0.001$ is OK. Customarily only 3 decimal places are used in values of *P*. Use capital *P* since lower-case *p* is used to denote proportion in the sample. When feasible, also give the name of the statistical test on which *P*-value is based. But do not give value of the test statistic such as *t*, *F*, and χ^2 in a paper unless required by the journal. On the other hand, in a thesis, it is desirable that these test statistic values are also given. State the confidence intervals (CIs) wherever applicable.

Presentation of statistical results for repeated measures and Tukey test can be very difficult. Table 12-1 illustrates the problems encountered in this presentation and suggest one way of presentation. You might be able to devise a more ingenious way of presenting such results. The table contains mean and SD of quality-of-life scores in physical and mental domains in peritonitis patients at baseline, and 1, 2 and 3 months after two types of surgical intervention.

Sometimes it is not feasible to explain all column and row headings in a proper manner, or sometimes numbers are inconsistent that require additional explanation. For readers to understand the table in one shot, add footnotes to the table where necessary. Also, you may have to explain abbreviation in a footnote. For these and other details regarding content, structure, and style of tables, see Section 10.1.

12.2.3 ILLUSTRATIONS

Photos, graphs, and charts sometimes make a tremendous visual impact that text fails to make. Carefully examine when it would be more effective to insert an illustration instead of a text. If they do not reduce the text, they are not worth including in the report. Line drawings are sometimes very effective in depicting complex relationship among quantitative variables. For qualitative data, tables may be better.

Only an appropriate diagram for your data as described in Chapter 10 should be drawn. Do not draw a bar diagram where pie is more appropriate (e.g., for proportions), or where a line diagram is more appropriate (e.g., for trend). Bar is a versatile diagram, but it is overused too. Use scatter diagram sparingly only for showing special features such as trend, regression, outliers, and differential variance. Stating correlation coefficient in the text or a table would suffice in most situations.

FIGURE 12-1: Scores of peritonitis patients in physical and mental domains of quality of life at baseline and 1, 2, and 3 months after two types of surgeries

Domain and time	Surgery-1					Surgery-2				Differences in the two surgeries	
	n	SD	Mean score	*P*-value for time differences (*F*-test)	Tukey test for time differences*	SD	Mean score	*P*-value for time differences (*F*-test)	Tukey test for time differences*	*P*-value (*F*-test)	Tukey test*
Physical											
Baseline	20	2.90	10.25	<0.001	(a) Baseline is sig. different from 1, 2, 3 months (b) 1 month is sig. different from 2, 3 months (c) 2 months is sig. different from 3 months	2.62	10.30	<0.001	(a) Baseline is sig. different from 1, 2 months (b) 1 month is sig. different from 2, 3 months	0.085	NS
1 month	20	2.48	12.20			2.21	12.35				NS
2 months	20	2.56	13.05			2.21	11.15				NS
3 months	20	2.49	14.30			2.27	10.70				NS
Mental											
Baseline	20	2.39	9.95	<0.001	(a) Baseline is sig. different from 1,2,3 months (b) 1 month is sig. different from 3 months (c) 2 months is sig. different from 3 months	2.68	10.15	<0.001	(a) Baseline is sig. different from 1, 2 months (b) 1 month is sig. different from 2 months (c) 2 months is sig. different from 3 months	0.167	NS
1 month	20	2.23	11.65			2.56	11.60				NS
2 months	20	2.18	11.70			2.31	11.25				NS
3 months	20	2.23	13.65			2.20	9.90				NS

NS : Not Significant

*At 5% level of significance

A diagram should be self-contained for independent reading without reference to the text. Title, labels, and legends should be clear and appropriately placed. The size of the labels and legends should be proportional to the size of the diagram keeping in mind that it could be drastically reduced at the time of printing in a journal. As far as possible, provide direct labels to categories, lines, etc., to make legends redundant. Fonts and symbols should be big enough to remain legible after reduction. Diagrams must be high-resolution (at least 600 dpi). Avoid colour graphs.

No hard rules can be laid but it is rare for a medical paper to contain more than three diagrams. And it is rare for a medical thesis to have only three. A thesis may contain 10 to 15 illustrations including photographs. Use them sparingly in a paper but profusely in a thesis although not as repetition of tables or text. For accurate description of results, use tables instead of graphs because the numbers in tables can be written to decimal places that cannot be so accurately depicted in a graph. Graphs are good for depicting patterns but not exact values. The graph of value 2.1 to 16.0 may look similar as of value 2.0 to 15.8.

Each figure must be referred to in the text. It must be placed as close as possible to the text containing first reference to that figure. Try that a reader does not have to flip page either way to see the figure.

Photographs should be absolutely clear without digitally enhancing. If they are of patients, it is essential to obtain written permission. Even then suppress the identity by covering eyes and other distinguishing features. Digitally enhanced images (CT, MRI, ultrasound images, etc.) should be clearly identified as digitally processed, and indicate the method of digital enhancement. Photo micrographs should have internal scale markers. Mention the method of staining in photo micrographs. If colours are essential, ask the journal about the format of submission of colour illustrations. Some journals charge heavily for colour reproductions. In a thesis, dissertation, or a report, use colour photographs liberally so long as they are not repetitions and relevant to the text.

See the next chapter for details of what to write in a paper and a thesis.

12.3 AUTHORSHIP CREDITS

The practice 'I give your name and you give mine' as author is absolutely unethical for any research, least for medical research. Reputed researchers do not allow their name to be associated with work to which they have not sufficiently contributed. Only those can be authors who have substantially contributed to *all* of the following: (i) conception of the study or design of the study, (ii) acquisition of data or their analysis and interpretation, and (iii) drafting or revising the report for its intellectual content. Each author must take public responsibility of their contribution. These requirements are slightly different from Vancouver guidelines. Thus, those who have participated only in collection of data, those who have provided support as part of their duty such as those who carried out radiological or laboratory investigation or data analysis that they are expected to do any way, those who have helped only in acquiring funding, or those who have been merely general supervisors, cannot claim to be authors. Authorship inflation is not allowed. Also, no person contributing significantly should be omitted howsoever 'junior' he is. Usurping work of the disadvantaged and the vulnerable gives rise to **ghost authorship.** This is considered a gross misconduct. To avoid such instances, some journals now require a signed declaration that specifies the contribution of each author. Also, now all authors are required to take the responsibility for the integrity of the work as a whole.

Multiple Authors

The tendency to give the name of the head of a unit or a department just to secure his 'blessings' is abhorred in scientific circles. Sometimes this is done under coercion. All authors must be familiar with the entire manuscript and should accept public responsibility of the contents. None of them can say later when a deficiency is detected that the other author is responsible for that error. This in a way underscores the need to limit the number of authors to a few who are really eligible. Papers based on complex study can have several authors if all of them have contributed and accept the responsibility of the contents. Possibly for increased complexity, the papers in medical journals with higher number of authors is steeply increasing. With multicentric studies now common, the number of authors has naturally increased. Reverse can also happen when somebody contributes substantially but is omitted among the authors. Professional writers, who are paid for their service, are excluded from the list of authors.

No guidelines are available to name the first author. The authors themselves decide the order or authorship. It is natural to expect, however, that the one who has contributed most, or has been the driving force all through the research endeavour, would be the first author. But he must qualify to be an author first before being named as first author. For issues such as group authorship, consult Uniform Requirements of the International Committee of Medical Journal Editors (2021).

Authorship for Theses

The question of authorship for a thesis or dissertation cannot be debated. The author has to be the candidate himself. However, it is necessary in this case also that the candidate has actively participated in conception and design, has collected and analysed the data himself, and has drafted the report. Thesis supervisors can help in interpretation of results and may critically review the manuscript. Doctoral dissertation is mainly a candidate's enterprise whereas Master's thesis draws substantially from intellectual resources of the supervisors. Remember that the objective of a Master's thesis is training in research methodology rather than research itself, but doctoral dissertation describes frank research.

Many universities require that at least one paper based on the thesis work is published. This is desirable otherwise also to get a feedback of the subject specialists on the thesis work. If it is a Doctoral dissertation, the primary responsibility lies with the candidate and he will be the first author. Supervisor and others who helped will be the other authors. However, in the case of Master's thesis, the supervisor may have to contribute substantially and be the first author of the paper based on the thesis. If the candidate writes the paper himself with the assistance of the supervisor, he should be the first author.

Report of a research project is prepared by the Principal and Co-investigators, and they can claim to be the authors. However, it may be necessary to comply with the requirements of the funding agency.

SUMMARY

The principles of scientific writing require clarity, brevity without sacrificing completeness, truthfulness, and logic. Revise the manuscript 3–4 times and take feedback from your colleagues and supervisors. Insert tables and figures for clarity and brevity but should be drawn in a manner that they convey right and unambiguous message. Authors should be all those who substantially contributed, and none should be left out.

REFERENCES

Amaral OB. Can we predict the reproducibility of biomedical studies? BMJ Open Science 2020 (Blog). Available at: https://blogs. bmj.com/openscience/2020/01/22/can-we-predict-the-reproducibility-of-biomedical-studies - Accessed 6 April 2020

International Committee of Medical Journal Editors. Recommendations for the Conduct, Reporting, Editing, and Publication of the Scholarly Work in Medical Journals. 2021. https://www.icmje.org - Accessed 11 January 20121

Ray S, Fitzpatrick S, Golubic R, Fisher S, Eds. Oxford Handbook of Clinical and Healthcare Research. Oxford University Press, 2016

Vickers AJ. Look at your garbage bin: it may be the only thing you need to know about statistics. November 2006. https://www.medscape.com/viewarticle/546515 – Accessed 15 January 2021

Wasserstein RL, Schirm AL, Lazar NA. Moving to a world beyond "p< 0.05". Am Stat 2019;73(51):1–19.

Zhang W. Ten simple rules for writing research papers. PLoS Comput Biol. 2014 Jan 30;10(1): e1003453. doi: 10.1371/journal.pcbi.1003453.

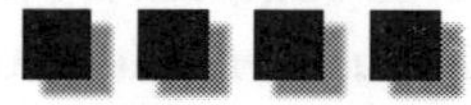

CHAPTER 13

How to Write a Thesis or a Paper and What are the Contents

KEY TERMS AND CONCEPTS

- ✓ Framing an Inclusive Title
- ✓ Impressive Abstract
- ✓ Choice of Key Words
- ✓ Features of Introduction
- ✓ Details of Material and Methods
- ✓ STROBE, CONSORT, and STARD Guidelines
- ✓ Presenting the Results
- ✓ Understanding the Interpretation
- ✓ Elements of Discussion
- ✓ Conclusions Different from Results

Manuscript writing is both an art and a science. It reflects a creative process that depends on the quality of thought (Brand 2003), and imagination is required in putting thoughts together in an interesting and lively manner. This requires a systematic step-by-step approach for achieving coherence. Your writing should enable the reader to find a way through a labyrinth of ideas by following a thread of thought. You should be able to organise any chaos and emphasize the relevant ideas while discarding the irrelevant ones.

A scientific manuscript can have one of many possible formats and you need to decide before hand the type of manuscript you wish to prepare. The dominant format is a research paper based on investigation of primary or secondary data, called original article. Adequate presentation of data is crucial for this format. The second, perhaps scientifically more valuable, is the systematic review. This is not based on primary data but is based on the compilation of results reported in different articles with meta-analysis occasionally thrown in to come to a unified conclusion with higher reliability. Choice of relevant articles is crucial for this kind of article. The third is a technical note that mostly deals with methodological issues and possibly to suggest a new methodology or a new way of collection, analysis and interpretation of data, or a new instrumentation or laboratory method. The fourth is a case study or case series of interesting cases about which we mentioned in an earlier chapter. The fifth is editorial, which mostly in written by one or more editors of the journal, or by an invited expert. The sixth are letters to the editor, book reviews, comments, obituary, etc. We have not included thesis/dissertation in this list that also follows the same format as an original article although in an elaborate form. Many research projects produce voluminous reports with chapters devoted to specific topics. In this chapter of this book, we primarily focus on thesis/dissertation and the original articles, both of which have nearly the same format but of different size.

This chapter has three sections. The first is on contents of various components of a preliminary of a research report such as title, authors, and abstract. Second section is on how to write introduction, methods, results, and discussion. Third section is on end feature such as acknowledgment, references, and appendices.

An important resource on manuscript preparation, particularly for journals, is the Recommendations of the International Committee of Medical Journal Editors (2021). This Committee represents more than 500 journals around the world and was earlier popularly known as Vancouver Group. In addition, consult websites of popular journals such as British Medical Journal and Journal of American Medical Association. They also discuss many issues not covered in this chapter such as writing a case report, a letter, editorials, practice guidelines, news items, and book reviews. Some of the ideas presented in this chapter are based on these sources and restricted mostly to reporting research results in the form of original article.

If your research is complex, consider if the results can be reported into two or three or more parts that are nearly independent of one-another with, minimal overlap. In this case, always acknowledge previously reported results as advised earlier.

For the primary medical research that we are discussing in this book, it is customary to divide the report in **I**ntroduction, **M**ethods, **R**esults, **a**nd **D**iscussion (**IMRaD**) format. If Abstract is also included, this becomes AIMRaD. Whereas most papers published in medical journals follow this format, theses and particularly dissertations, may choose to follow topic-by-topic approach. Results can be described in multiple chapters in a thesis. For research on kidney transplants, for example, these chapters can have titles such as 'Choice of Donors', 'Preparation of Recipients', 'Surgical Procedure', and 'Post-surgical Management'. Theses and dissertations are sometimes later apportioned into two or three papers for publication in medical journals where again IMRaD format would be required.

In a 3000-word article, which is sometimes considered standard for a research paper, Introduction would generally occupy 500 words, Methods 1000 words, Results nearly 500 words, and Discussion another 1000 words. Note that Results section does not occupy much of space. Introduction should contain the questions and Results their answers. Discussion is a coherent mix of questions and answers in the context of the observations reported by other authors and any other evidence. It also contains an explanation of how the findings are believable and not artifact due to methodological issues and how the results are useful in application.

Subsequent sections in this chapter give details of what each component of a research report is expected to contain, and how to prepare a good manuscript. Consider them as guidelines only. Consult the Instruction for Authors of the concerned journal for papers, or university guidelines for thesis and dissertation. Go to a reputed medical library and see some successful theses. For help in writing thesis and dissertation, refer also to Gladthorn (1998). For papers, see a series of articles by Peh and Ng (2008). However, remember that good writers are not born but made. Writing skills come with practice. Do not worry if your first draft is terrible — most of us have. Prepare first draft as early as you can – even possibly before the results are known so that you can anticipate the problems. Plan for several revisions and notice yourself how the manuscript improves.

IMRaD is only for the main body of a paper. There are always some preliminaries such as title and authors, and end features such as acknowledgements and references. All of them are important components and deserve a careful consideration. A brief description is given next.

Elements of Contents of a Manuscript of a Paper

Title – Concise (generally not exceeding 15 words) yet informative.

Authors – Only those who have *substantially* contributed and are prepared to take up public responsibility of the contents.

Keywords – About 5-6 for indexing purposes that could retrieve the paper from a database.

Abstract – Generally structured into Purpose, Background, Methods, Results, and Conclusion; lucid, stand alone, and containing all salient features of the study in not exceeding 300 words (consult the journals instructions).

Introduction – Rationale of the study and what new is expected to be achieved: research questions, objectives, and hypothesis.

Methods – Why the study was done in that particular manner including the comments on validity and reliability of results these methods are expected generate.

Results – Select data that focus on the stated objectives; make judicious use of tables and illustrations for precision and impact, respectively, without duplication.

and

Discussion – Implication of the results in the light of existing knowledge and resolution of conflict if any; conclusion based on evidence along with the limitations; keep opinions and comments separate from evidence-based results.

Acknowledgments – Thank those who contributed but not enough to qualify as author.

Key messages – Two or three messages in a box that highlight the achievements of the study.

References – Preferably in Vancouver format, and restrict the list to the minimum needed to substantiate the statements made in the text.

Appendix – Highly technical or specialised text not of much interest to the general reader.

13.1 PRELIMINARIES OF A MANUSCRIPT

Whether the target of the report (paper, thesis, or a full report) is a journal, of which there is a variety of hues from no takers to world-wide circulation, or the examiners that could be from local to international, preliminaries of a manuscript make biggest impact and determine its ability to attract attention.

13.1.1 TITLE

Title is probably the most important component of a paper. This is the first part of the manuscript seen by the editor and reviewer and provides first impression of the work. Although a report is referenced by the name of the authors but its utility in a particular context is evaluated by the title. It helps readers to find your work – thus it is important to include important keywords in the abstract. This is the first filter for the reader to decide its relevance for him. Thus, the title should be carefully worded: specific enough to describe the focus and lively enough to generate interest. It should be able to grab the attention of the reader and should be appealing. The title should be concise yet sufficiently informative for a reader to anticipate the contents. But do not try to sensationalise.

Specificity in Title

The title 'obesity and diabetes' is concise but fails to convey the subject matter. It is not informative. The title 'contribution of obesity to development of diabetes in post-menopausal women' describes the research adequately. As far as possible, keep the key words in front. Thus, 'sex differentials in obesity contribution to diabetes' is preferable than 'contribution of obesity to diabetes in males and females'.

It is a good idea to mention in the title itself that it is a randomized control trial, prospective study, case-control study, or what. This helps the reader to grasp the essential of the methodology you followed. Note that the locale of the study almost invariably appears in the title, particularly for an epidemiological study—sometimes even the year of the study is important, particularly when the conclusions are not generalizable to the other years. There is some confusion about specifying the locale of the study in the title. If a study is carried out on patients in one hospital in Delhi, can it be considered representative of the entire city? Some titles will say North India – others will even say India if published in a foreign journal. No firm guideline is available.

Long titles are boring, but do not sacrifice accuracy for brevity. Titles beginning with "A study of ..." are wastage of words. Avoid overly general title. Sometimes subtitle is a useful adjunct for increasing the specificity. Avoid abbreviations in title.

Title should also serve the interest of target audience. For example, for a general practitioner audience such as of Journal of Indian Medical Association and possibly British Medical Journal, the title should focus on applicability of your research whereas for super-speciality journal, the emphasis could be on technical aspects. The latter might need slightly longer titles to be able to describe the technical content of the research.

Types of Title of a Paper

Two types of titles are in vogue. First emphasises the investigation and second states the main result. The title 'A case-control study of influence of early life factors on adult morality in country ABC' states what has been investigated and how, without indicating the result. This provokes curiosity. In a question format, this can be stated as 'Do early life factors influence adult morality in country ABC?' You could be provocative if the research warrants but do not sensationalise the title. In an answer format, this could be worded as 'Childhood obesity in low-birth-weight babies reduces life expectancy: a case-control study in country ABC'. This is a positive statement and describes the main result of the study. No firm evidence is available to indicate which format makes biggest impact on readers. In our opinion, the last one—the answer format—is most informative and capable of enticing a person to read the article if he is interested in that topic. However, Lilleyman (1996) advises against conclusion-oriented title. Choose the format you consider most exciting for the target audience.

Thesis Title

The discussion in the preceding paragraph is focused on papers prepared for publication in a scientific journal. Title for **postgraduate thesis** or a **doctoral dissertation** is usually decided before the investigation in conducted, and certainly much before the results are available. And it cannot be changed at the time of writing. Thus, the title for these endeavours can never be in answer format. Precisely because no latitude is available, there is a tendency in some quarters to propose a nonspecific umbrella type of thesis topic that can incorporate variation in the investigation. An example is 'A study of occlusion of left main coronary artery'. Such nonspecification can occur for two reasons. One, to be able to incorporate various facets of the problem that emerge later, which indeed could be a legitimate reason for a doctoral dissertation, but the second reason could be lack of clarity about the specifics of the proposed investigation. Guard against the latter by following the advice enunciated in previous chapters. Examiners and other reviewers are smart enough to detect this lapse.

Title Page

In a thesis, title page contains your name and the name of your supervisors, possibly degrees (optional) and their affiliation regarding Unit or Department. In any case the name of the Department and the University comes at the bottom. A medical PG thesis title page also contains a phrase saying 'In partial fulfilment of the requirement of the degree of Doctor of Medicine/Master of Surgery'. Year of submission is also mentioned.

After the title page in a thesis comes the **Certificate** that says that the work is genuine and carried out by the student himself. This makes you accountable in case any fraud is discovered later. This must be signed by you. Some universities require that this be authenticated by the Chief Supervisor and even the head of the institution.

Then is the **Acknowledgement** page where you express gratitude to your supervisors and others whosoever helped in your endeavour including the patients and the laboratory/nursing staff. A thesis also contains a **Table of Contents** with page numbers for each chapter and each section. Examiners look at this critically to find where to go for a particular explanation.

For a paper for publication too, many journals require a title page with names and affiliation of all authors, address of the corresponding author (including email address), key words and possibly a running title. Full title is at the top in any case. Sometimes the word count is also required. Consult the Instructions to Authors of the journal to get a clear idea of what is required.

Authors should use standardised name for all their papers. Do not write Abhaya Indrayan in one paper and A. Indrayan in the other. If such different names are used, computer search and indexing services will count them separate.

13.1.2 KEY WORDS

Many medical journals require that 5-6 key words be identified for indexing purposes. The best resource for choosing key words is Medical Subject Heading (MeSH) list of MedLine. Think of words that the users would use to locate your research. Prefer popular words than sparingly used words. In any case, they must adequately describe the contents of the paper. Combination of two or more words is many times better variant than an orphaned word. 'Randomised controlled trial' is much better than 'Clinical trial' and 'Randomisation' separately.

13.1.3 ABSTRACT

Almost all medical journals require that an abstract not exceeding 300 words—sometimes only 150 words—is prepared that contains all salient features of the study. Thesis summary may be in 1000 words. In either case, it is an exercise in précis writing. Brevity and clarity are essential. Decide if it is easier to write abstract in the beginning before the full report. In some situations, this can crystalise thoughts and provide framework for the report. After writing the full paper, go back and improve the abstract if new thoughts emerge.

Abstract appears as such in indexing services such as PubMed and Excerpta Medica. Many evaluate the worth of a paper by the abstract. A good abstract helps in expediting the peer review by the journals and in evaluating the interest it would generate among its readers. Also, this serves as the gateway for the paper. This is the second-most-read part of your paper. The abstract itself is many times considered enough to provide the required information. It should accurately reflect the contents of your paper and should be written as a standalone text for independent reading. That is, it should make sense without reference to the main text. Only those readers who find from Abstract that the full paper could be useful would look for full paper. Thus, prepare an abstract in a manner that can persuade the reader to read the full paper. It does not mean to leave out holes. It only means that the abstract should indicate that it is a good research that needs to be studied greater detail.

Abstract contains the essence of the work in an intelligible, informative, and interesting manner. It should emphasise new and important aspect of the study. Where helpful, include hard data. But they should be in simplest of statistical terms. The tendency of most journals is to structure the abstract in Purpose, Background, Methods, Results, and Conclusions headings. Sometimes Limitations are also added. Each of these headings contains two or three sentences, and together should be able to describe the entire research in a coherent manner. These are concise statements of the details described in the next section under each of these headings. All parts of the Abstract must be consistent with the main text.

Do not repeat the title of study in the Abstract. If begins with rationale to justify the study. Then objectives or questions are precisely stated including a priori hypotheses. In the design, state for a trial that it is RCT or non-randomised controlled trial; placebo-controlled or controlled for existing treatment; any blinding, matching criteria; cross-over, before-after, up-and-down strategy; etc. For laboratory investigations, state any available gold, and how your testing compares with this gold. For observational study, specify that it is case-control, prospective or cross-sectional. For modelling, mention about training sample and validation sample. Specify that the study setting is community, primary care, referral centre, private clinic, ambulatory care, hospital clinic, admitted patients, etc. Briefly state the eligibility criteria for the subjects. State whether random sampling was adopted or consecutive, referred, volunteer or convenience sample was drawn. What exactly was intervention and how long did it continue. List the important outcome measures. State the confidence intervals, correlation, statistical significance, the difference you considered clinically important, number needed to treat, sensitivity/specificity and predictivity along with prevalence, etc. In the end, state both negative and positive conclusions with their practical implications. This list looks long but you will discover after some practice that precise and focused statements are not all that difficult to make. All these are the same as we will shortly discuss in detail for different sections of a thesis or a paper. Hardly ever, if at all, an abstract will contain any table or graph or references. It should not contain anything that is not included in the main body of the manuscript. Avoid abbreviations unless you are using the same term 3 or more times. Do not repeat yourself. and make sure that there are no contradictory statements.

Structured Abstract

Many journals require a structured abstract so that no vital information is missed. This may contain some or all the following headings.

Background – What is currently known and what are the gaps.

Aim and objectives – The gap you are trying to fill and the research question to be answered; include the broad aim and specify the objectives in measurable format.

Design – Laboratory experiment: one-way, two-way, repeated measures, etc. Clinical trial: randomised (cluster or simple), nonrandomised, blinded, cross-over, before-after. Observational study: record based, prospective, retrospective, or cross-sectional. Descriptive: clinical profile, demographic profile.

Setting – Hospital, clinic, multicentric, community, or any other.

Subjects – Inclusion-exclusion criteria, sampling method, sample size.

Intervention, if any – Intentionally introduced procedure or regimen to see its effect.

Measurements – Antecedent characteristics, confounders, and outcomes under study.

Results – Main findings of the study that answer the research question stated earlier; include key numerical results with confidence interval and *P*-values.

Limitations – Groups or situations where the results would not apply.

Conclusion – What this study adds despite the limitations.

Some journals may require less number of items – collapse as needed. For example, setting, subjects, intervention, measurements, and design can be merged under methods, and limitations can be a part of the conclusion.

13.2 MAIN BODY OF THE REPORT

As already stated, it is customary to prepare a medical research report in IMRaD format. This is a suitable format for publication is a scientific journal, and quite often used for postgraduate thesis also. For details of how to write a paper in IMRaD format, see PLoS Guidelines (2021). Review articles and methodological articles may have a different format.

13.2.1 INTRODUCTION

No problem arises in thin air. Begin the manuscript by describing how the problem arose: what was the context or the background? This could be extension of a previous work, difficulties faced in managing a public health problem, controversies appearing in the literature, unpleasant clinical experience of managing a specific type of patients, deficiency noted at the time of teaching, bottleneck observed in carrying out a research, or any such context. Separately identify the epistemic gaps due to universal lack of knowledge and uncertainties due to variation in the results. Include information about epidemiology, clinical relevance, and current practices regarding the topic and focus on local area without ignoring the international perspective. Emphasise if the research concerns a neglected topic.

Quote important literature if needed to expose any lacunae in knowledge, but do not include a full review. Prefer the recent and most relevant references. Reserve full review for Discussion section but ensure that up-to-date information is given. This should take the reader from what is known to what is not known. Involve the curiosity of the reader. Demonstrate that the work being reported is new, and it is needed. Explain its significance and rationale. Build a logical case and specify the conceptual framework. Then specify the questions under investigation clearly and concisely and explain their importance. For this, converting information needs to answerable questions may help. The problem should be clearly articulated. State the objectives in precise and evaluable terms. They should be worded in a very specific and focused manner. Identify the important antecedent and outcome variables, and the relationships under study. State any hypothesis under test. State also that this was a preplanned hypothesis or was formulated during or after collection of data. Specify the subjects of your study and describe the general research strategy but not the details. In short, the Introduction should contain a convincing statement about issues and should formulate the rationale for those issues. This should convince the reader that you have thought about the topic thoroughly well and have presented a tight case. A short introduction is preferred in a paper than a lengthy discourse because longer introduction tends to lose focus. Do not include much of general knowledge. But Introduction chapter in a thesis or dissertation can be long just as every other chapter.

Precisely define the target population to which your results are likely to apply. Mention about the intervention you propose to study (the details will be in Methods section) and specify the primary and secondary outcomes of interest. These should match with the objectives stated earlier.

It is sometimes helpful to give a preview of the principal results in Introduction that can guide the reader through the paper. In this case do not make sweeping claims. Do not give data or full result because that can dissuade him to read further.

In summary, the Introduction should include what is known, what is the gap, and what part of the gap you propose to fulfil. Also include objectives in a **SMART format** – Specific, Measurable, Achievable, Relevant and Timely. Introduction section should be structured in a manner that it leads naturally to the hypothesis to be investigated. The hypothesis should point to what the research is expected to achieve new for the world and should emanate from the objectives.

Do not be reluctant to use "I" or "We". This usage conveys the right message that it is your work, and you own it up, including any gaps and misses. This usage also helps in building up direct sentences instead of convoluted sentences.

If you find difficulty in starting with Introduction, try to write Results first and then come back to the Introduction.

13.2.2 METHODS

Credibility of a research depends to a great extent on the appropriate methodology. This impacts editorial assessment and reader's appreciation. This also is the backbone of transparency and replicability and describes the rigorousness with which the study was carried out. Describe it as accurately as possible: not the planned one but the one actually followed. Consult the protocol because that can provide substantial help in preparing the Methods section. The focus should be to describe why this study was done in that particular way. Do not try to gloss over the nonoptimal methods you had to use under local constraints, and state the actual methodology followed for the research. This is required for transparency and for replicability of the study. Specifically, include in this section the setting in which the study was carried out, the types of group of cases and controls studied, and the design adopted. Include justification of each. If your Methods section is long, divide it into subsections such as Subjects, Design, Measurements, Statistical Methods, etc.

Specify the setting. The setting could be a general community, a primary health centre, a referral or a general hospital (inpatients or outpatients), a private clinic, or any such facility. This helps readers to determine the applicability of the results to their own setting. If the source of data is records, specify that clearly. Also describe the steps taken to preserve the quality of the study. Talk about any poorly measured variables and how this deficiency was tackled. Use past tense except while describing the contents of the present paper.

As always, methods section should also be precise yet should provide enough details for anyone to repeat the investigation for confirmation. Imagine you are writing for replication and adoption in future but do not do methodological overkill. There is no need to mention basic methods that a reader is expected to know. Only new methods should be stated fully; for others just give reference. The reader should be convinced that the methodology is adequate to ensure reasonable reliability and validity of conclusions. Mention about ethical issues and the clearances you have obtained.

Also describe methodological constraints. Provide the flow diagram and check list where needed.

Subjects of the Study

Define your unit of study. This could be a patient of chronic kidney disease, a person undergoing a particular surgery, a child with bronchiolitis, a pregnant woman at primigravida, or a healthy person of age 65 years or more, or any such subject. Mention about inclusion and exclusion criteria and justify them.

Identify the broad group of cases (hospital admissions, OPD patients, patients detected in screening, a community, etc.) again and state how the eligible subjects were identified. If possible, give a count of the number of units in the 'population' and then come to the sample.

State the method you adopted to compute sample size with full justification of the minimum clinically relevant difference you want to detect or the aimed precision of the estimate you wish to generate. How these subjects were selected – any of the standard statistical random methods, or consecutive cases, or volunteers, etc. Provide the time frame of the study.

For analytical studies, describe all these in **PICO** format – Population, Intervention, (or Exposure), Comparative group and Outcome. Use **CONSORT** guidelines where appropriate, **STROBE** for observational studies, and **STARD** chart for diagnostic studies. For meta-analysis, use **MOOSE** (Meta-analysis of Observational Studies) or **QUOROM** (QUality Of Reporting Of Meta-analyses of clinical trials) guidelines. A brief of some of these appears later in this section.

Intervention and Instrumentation

Give full details of the intervention if any, including the dosage and the duration. For drugs and chemicals, include their generic name, route of administration, etc. If you must write commercial name, write it in parentheses. Explain ethical considerations. State the mechanism of follow-up and its duration, clearly specifying the censoring (incomplete observations because of the design) if any. The percentage of subjects who dropped out themselves should be stated separately from those who had to be withdrawn because of adverse effects. Any deviation from protocol and its reasons should be highlighted. Clearly mention about consents taken and how were they obtained.

Specify the instrumentation and provide references that describe them. Give details of any new or modified method or apparatus used including its testing. Justify the deviation, if any, you made from the standard practice. Give as much details as necessary for the reader to replicate the study. Demonstrate that your instrument is valid and reliable, and that you were able to use the instruments properly.

Design

All applicable elements of design as enumerated in Chapter 5 should be stated. State what specific groups were covered and why, and what was the period of recruitment. Establish that your design has adequate efficiency to track down the best evidence. State the statistical power and justify the difference you considered medically important. State whether the study is prospective, retrospective, or cross-sectional if observational; or therapeutic, prophylactic, diagnostic, or screening if a trial. Describe the design in detail. Justify the choice of controls and state the matching criteria if applicable. Lay out such as cross-over or repeated measures, and one-way, two-way, or factorial, etc., should be specified. Actual implementation of the intricacies such as randomisation, blinding and matching should be fully explained. In case the study involves medical predictions, describe about validation methods used. The reader should understand about all potential sources of bias and how were they controlled. Sometimes a diagram of flow of research helps to achieve clarity.

Data Collection and Collation

Clearly define antecedent and outcome measures including diagnostic criteria, and establish their relevance to the study objectives. Explain how you operationalised the research variables. State why you chose those indicators. Give sources of data and provide the method of assessment of each variable. Do not lose humility because there might be relevant data about which you were not aware or was not collected. Clearly state about the nonresponse, dropouts, recall bias, deficiency in the records, and the steps taken to minimize their impact on the results. These missed data may be as important as the ones collected, and the validity may suffer – the reviewers are quick to detect such instances. Comment on the rigorousness with which the data were collected to ensure accuracy. In case you have used categories such as mild, moderate, and serious, clearly specify how such categorization was derived. Categories are not desirable for continuous quantitative variables but if you have still used them for reasons such as easy interpretation, explain the rationale. If scores are used, give complete methodology or a reference to the source that describes it fully. Also comment on the validity and reliability of the scoring system. If your research is on developing a scoring system, provide details of its theoretical justification and state how you plan to assess its adequacy. State the time points when the information was elicited or recorded.

Identify the confounders and state how they were tackled. Limitations of the methods should be stated without inhibition including how these limitations might affect the results. Such a statement would tell the readers that you are aware of these gaps and would help them to evaluate the utility of results more realistically in the context of their own setting.

State also about the possibilities you envisioned of contamination in data and how did you clean up the data. This should include the remedial steps you took for handling missing data, if any. The second distinct possibility is error in measurement. This occurs all the time but must remain within tolerance limit. Your report must indicate to the reader that you were alive to such errors and were able to manage them with proper instrumentation and their adequate handling. In case multiple observers or raters are used, include how they were trained for standardised readings and how inter-rater reliability was assessed. For your own safety, raise a red flag at the time of drafting a report whenever you find possibility of sloppiness. Resolve them adequately in the final draft.

Statistical Methods

State the statistical methods you have used to analyse the data in sufficient detail to permit replication, particularly the specialised methods about which the readers, editors, reviewers, and examiners may not be aware. Explain how these methods are appropriate for the kind of data in hand, and how will they achieve the stated objectives of research. All statistical methods are based on certain set of assumptions and you must check that your data fulfils those assumptions. Gaussian pattern and linear relationship are among the assumptions where many researchers goof-up. Such requirements are ignored by the authors in the 'hope' that they will be fulfilled.

The procedures must conform to the research design, and the models and hypotheses you started with. Also state the methods you used to control confounding bias. Also describe methods you used to examine subgroups and interactions, and how any missing data were tackled. In case calculation was done for standardisation of values (such as z-score) for comparison or any such adjustment was made, state that also with reasons for such adjustments. Cite the reference if the method is not well-known and avoid giving the formula unless your paper is on methodology. Specify the computer package used. State the confidence level and the level of significance wherever applicable. Whereas 95 percent confidence and 5 percent level of significance tend to be accepted without question, any other level is expected to be accompanied by its justification. Describe how multiple *P*-values were adjusted to control the false positivity rate. Describe any validation method you used such as sensitivity analysis but do not include results in the methods section.

Ethical Considerations

Assure your readers, reviewers, and editors that you have followed all ethical guidelines in terms of informed consent and no harm was done to anybody. Also mention how adverse events, such as drug reactions, were handled and how the results were modified or not modified to adjust for such events. Include approval of the Institutional Ethics Committee.

In view of their importance, reporting ethics are discussed in detail in Chapter 15.

13.2.3 STROBE, CONSORT, STARD, PRISMA, QUOROM AND MOOSE STATEMENTS

Over the years, researchers have learnt and developed standardised systems for reporting methodology. These are available for at least five types of studies.

One is STrenghthening of Reporting of Observational studies in Epidemiology (STROBE). This was introduced in Chapter 5 in the context of observational studies such as prospective, retrospective (case-control) and cross-sectional studies. It is advisable to consult its latest version at *www.strobe-statement.org*. Much of what it states for methodology is already mentioned in the preceding paragraphs in this section. Additionally, it requires that you describe comparability of assessment methods if any variation occurred across groups. For prospective studies, give the method of follow-up, any variation in the follow-up duration from subject to subject, and how the loss to follow-up was addressed. For retrospective studies, give the rationale and how the cases and controls were chosen. In cross-sectional studies, if a method other than simple random was used for selection of subjects, describe the statistical methods in view of the sampling strategy.

Second is CONsolidated Standards Of Reporting of Trials (CONSORT). This applies to clinical trials and has been described in Chapter 5. We do not want to repeat it here. For its latest version, visit *www.consort-statement.org*.

The third is STAndards for Reporting of Diagnostic accuracy studies (STARD) statement for studies on validity of diagnostic tests. This was developed to improve the completeness and transparency of such studies and contains a list of essential items for reporting that can be used as a check list. The last update of this statement was done in 2015 and presented by Cohen et al. (2016).

The fourth is Preferred Reporting Items for Systematic reviews and Meta-Analyses (PRISMA). We have not discussed review studies in this book but mention about PRISMA here just in case you are interested in review studies. These studies review a large number of previously conducted studies on the same outcome and synthesize the results. Details of PRISMA are available at *www.prisma-statement.org*.

The fifth is QUality Of Reporting Of Meta-analyses (QUOROM). This describes a methodology for the consistent reporting of meta-analyses of Randomised Control Trials (RCTs). The corresponding guidelines for meta-analysis of observational studies is MOOSE. Both these include features such as the criteria for searching the articles, types of study designs considered, methods for assessing the study quality, etc. Since systematic reviews too are not subject matter of the present book, we are not giving further details.

EQUATOR (Enhancing the QUality and Transparency of health Research) network at *www.equator-network.org* has details of all these and much more at one place.

13.2.4 SAMPL GUIDELINES FOR REPORTING OF BASIC STATISTICAL METHODS

Many authors falter while reporting statistical methods and statistical results in their paper or thesis. For this, a comprehensive guideline has been prepared by Indrayan (2020). These are presented in Table 13-1.

FIGURE 13-1: Improved SAMPL guidelines for reporting basic statistical methods

Topic	No.	Item
Subjects under study	1	Identify the target population, state the method of selection of the sample, total sample size, stratification if any, and the groups under study.
Sample size	2a	State the sample size for each group and justify the size for the stated precision, alpha error, and/or power. For power, specify the smallest effect size considered medically important with reasons.
	2b	State the number of missing values, outliers and other exclusions with reasons, comment on the representativeness of the sample finally available for analysis, and describe possible biases with measures taken to control them.
Hypothesis	3a	State all the hypotheses keeping the study objectives in mind.
	3b	State the minimum effect size to be considered as medically important, if applicable, with its rationale (see Item 2a). For equivalence and non-inferiority studies, give the largest medically unimportant margin with reasons.
Variables under study	4a	State all the variables on which the data were collected and identify the ones on which the present analysis was done along with the rationale of the choice of variables. State the unit of measurement of each, and describe the validity of the methods of measurement for each variable.

Topic	No.	Item
	4b	Categorize continuous data for presentation of distribution if needed. If helpful, give histogram and comment on the distribution pattern, particularly of the outcome variables.
	4c	If dichotomous or polytomous categories have been used in analysis of continuous variables, explain the rationale of these categories in terms of clinical implication.
Antecedents and outcomes	5a	In the case of analytical studies, identify the antecedent factors under study, the outcomes of interest, and the covariates included.
	5b	Define the effect of interest in terms of the variables included in the study (the effect size can be difference between means or between proportions, odds ratio, correlation coefficient, phi coefficient, or any other measure).
Descriptive summaries	6	Summarize the data –Provide mean (SD) (and not mean ± SD) or median (IQR) of each continuous variable depending upon the Gaussian or (highly) skewed distribution, respectively (do not use SE here). For IQR, give the values of the first and third quartile. Do not give such summaries for groups with n ≤4; give the original values instead. For categorical data, state actual frequency in different categories and the percentage if n ≥20. All summaries should be with the appropriate degree of decimal accuracy as specified at the end of these guidelines*.
Modification of raw data	7	Describe transformation such as log and square-root, if any, with reasons and the method of calculation of scores, and rates and ratios, and fully specify the numerator, denominator and multiplier (per cent, per million, etc.) for each where applicable. For rates, specify the time period (per day, per year, etc.).
Baseline information	8	Summarize all important demographic and clinical features of the subjects in each group, particularly those that can affect the outcome (see Item 6).
Comparability of two or more groups	9	Before comparing two or more groups with respect to outcomes in terms of summaries such as means, proportions in different categories, and rates, confirm that the groups are comparable with regard to the baseline composition of the subjects for factors (such as the age distribution) that can affect the outcome. If not comparable, report the re-computed summaries after proper standardization. If standardization required but not done, state reasons and explain how the outcomes in various groups can still be compared.

Topic	No.	Item
Main method of analysis	10a	Describe the method for each analysis, confirm the validity of the underlying assumptions, and justify the parametric and non-parametric methods used for different variables. Provide reference or explain the methods not in common use. State the software used for analysis with version.
	10b	Identify post-hoc analysis if any, including sub-groups analysis, and interpret this as exploratory and not confirmatory.
Estimation	11	For descriptive part of the study, provide estimate of the mean, proportion, difference, etc. with 95% Confidence Interval (CI). Justify the Gaussian approximation in case this is used for computing the CI. In case any other confidence level is used, provide the rationale.
Tests of statistical hypothesis	12a	State the statistical hypothesis for each test. Give the name of each test and its exact P-value with df where relevant. For $P<0.001$, state with less than sign and for $P>0.999$ with more than sign. Indicate whether the test is one-tailed or two-tailed with the reasons thereof. Avoid the use of the term statistical significance and do not mention significance level (such as $\alpha = 0.05$) for your results. Mention about any adjustment made for multiple comparisons and for using multiple tests for any conclusion. Distinguish between family-wise error rate and experiment-wise error rate. Also mention the CI for the effect size such as mean difference between the groups.
	12b	Report all the results and not just those that have low P-value. Interpret larger P-value as inconclusive and not as negative result unless the power is high to detect a specified medically important effect. Distinguish between results with low P-value (conventional statistical significance) and medical significance of the results.
Robustness of results	13	Comment about the statistical limitations of the study in addition to the other limitations. Statistical limitations could be due to imprecision of the measurements, restricted analysis because of the nature of the data or size of sample in different groups, not fulfilling the underlying assumptions, lack of representativeness of the sample, compromised design, lack of internal or external validations, and such other deficiencies.

Topic	No.	Item
The following are needed if these methods have been used in your paper		
Correlation and cause-effect	14a	Report the value of the relevant correlation coefficient. If described as low, moderate or high, give the categories with their biological implications. Interpret conventional Pearson correlation coefficient for assessing linear relationship and not for any general relationship between continuous variables. For association between categorical variables, include the full contingency table and explain if any categories were merged for analysis purpose.
	14b	Distinguish between association/correlation and cause-effect. If cause-effect is implied, rule out all possible alternative explanations such as the role of confounders and biases.
	14c	Distinguish correlation/association from agreement.
Regression analysis	15a	Describe the purpose of the regression analysis (explanatory or predictive), identify the response (outcome) and regressor (antecedent) variables with the selection process if any, assess colinearity between independent variables, and provide medical and statistical rationale of the chosen model (linear/nonlinear, simple/multivariable). State the size of sample available for running each regression and comment on its adequacy. In case the model is being used for prediction of individual values, give prediction interval and not the CI for mean. Do not predict for values much beyond the values actually studied.
	15b	Report the regression equation with comments on its adequacy based on indicators such as coefficient of determination (η^2, whose linear component is R^2) for quantitative and generalized R^2 for logistic regression, and report exact P-value for each regression coefficient with the associated CI. For quantitative dependent in simple linear or curvilinear regression, plot the regression line or curve with scatter where helpful and comment on the randomness of the residuals. For logistic regression, specify the reference category for categorical regressors, give Odds Ratio (OR) and the CI for each variable – adjusted as well as unadjusted. For cohort studies, state the number of subjects with positive and negative outcomes, and the relative risk with their CI – again adjusted as well as unadjusted. In the case of multivariable regression, interpret regression coefficient as adjusted only for the other variables in the model and give plausible biological explanation of the model obtained.
	15c	Specify whether and how the model was validated, or why it could not be validated.

Topic	No.	Item
Survival analysis	16a	Describe the purpose of the survival analysis, identify the beginning- and the end-point for the duration under study, specify censoring, name the survival analysis method with the confirmation of the assumptions, plot the survival curve and report the median survival time with the CI, and discuss the points of inflexion in the survival curve, if relevant.
	16b	Where helpful, give the table with the estimated survival probability at each follow-up with the CI.
	16c	Specify the method used for comparing two or more survival curves if applicable and give exact P-value. Interpret it for overall survival pattern and not for specific time-points.

**Decimal accuracy (rounded) as follows:*

Percentages – One decimal place if n <100 and two decimal places for n ≥100;

Mean and SD (Median and IQR) – One decimal place more than the original values;

Correlation coefficient – Generally two decimal places;

Odds ratio, relative risk and hazard ratio – Generally two decimal places;

P-values – Exact P-values to three decimal places and not as P <0.05 or P ≥0.05 (For extremely small values, write P <0.001, and for extremely high values, write P >0.999).

13.2.5 RESULTS

Results section of the report states what has been found. It mirrors your research question. Always remember that results are not in your hand whereas objectives, design and other methods are products of your brain. No manipulation can be done with results although you can analyse the data in different ways. In fact, the method of analysis should also be specified in the protocol and the same should be followed – thus hardly any leeway is available. The results section should clearly establish the relevance of your methodology. Maintain integrity of the manuscript by stating the results in an upright manner. State not just the truth but the whole truth. For example, do not evade risks and side-effects of an intervention under test. Trust that scientific community is appreciative of frank statement about the negative result as much as positive result. All negative results are not failures – they save other workers to tread the same path. If there are failures, their frank admission elevates the confidence of the readers and increases the credence of results; it gives the impression that the authors are not trying to hide anything! Do not suppress findings that contradict or do not support your hypothesis. Results should include findings on everything that you stated in introduction.

Strive for clarity in describing the results. Coherence is the key word. Opinions based on hunches or preferences, anecdotes, experience, impressions, or conflicting evidence should be clearly identified, and should be stated separately from results. Comments also should be worded as comments and not mixed with results. All results must be evidence based: fully supported by data. Give an indication of how these results provide evidence for making decisions regarding health care of individuals or the society. Any inconsistency in findings based on diverse evidence must be explained. Use technical terms such as 'normal' and 'significant' with care.

All relevant analysis must be available before the Results section is finalised. Limit the results to the facts as revealed by the data. Do not try to extrapolate or generalise in the Results section. Do not discuss the results in this section. Do that in the Discussion section with proper explanation. Whilst the statement of the type that the difference between the treatment group and control group is statistically significant, or treatment gives significantly higher value than the other is appropriate for the Results section, the statement that treatment should be preferred should be part of the Discussion or Conclusion section.

First sentence of each paragraph of Results section should indicate the contents—the point addressed, or the question answered. With each paragraph, state the most important result first and then the less important ones. All the information within the paragraph must be related. Also, do not emphasize on data per se but on their interpretation. Start with descriptive results and move to the analytical results. But strive for continuity and flow. Results should narrate a story that makes sense without looking at the tables and graphs. This means that tables and graphs should be referred parenthetically that describes their interpretation. For example, do not write that 'comparison of treatment efficacy in different groups is in Figure X or Table Y' but write that 'treatment A was 10% more effective than treatment B (Figure X) and this difference is statistically significant ($P = 0.003$) (Table Y)'. Focus on take home message emanating from the results. Always give exact *P*-value but exceeding small *P*-values can be stated as $P < 0.001$. If you did re-analysis for any reason, mention that too. In case of adjustment, give adjusted *P*-values.

The trouble with most studies is that they end up with huge amount of data. You would probably analyse a wide range of data during the research and interpret it. They may all be interesting but describe in Results section only those that address the research question. Examine if some of your material is better placed in an appendix without interrupting the flow of text. The mantra is to provide a holistic picture by integrating various results and present them selectively. Do not ignore any serendipitous, unexpected, incidental, or accidental result. Use it to set the tone for future investigation. Such results can be important. Fleming's discovery of penicillin was based on an accidental result. Also see Example 13.1.

EXAMPLE 13.1: An accidental finding on possible role of Vitamin E in lowering prostate risk

Chase (2003) reports about a study designed to test beta-carotene for preventing lung tumours in Finnish smokers. The study found that the substance instead increased the risk of cancer. But it accidentally also revealed that vitamin E could lower the risk of prostate cancer and hyperplasia. Now trials are underway to test vitamin E and selenium as preventatives.

Conversely, sometimes a mass of good data is available but the time or expertise is not available to exploit it fully. This can particularly happen at the time of writing a postgraduate thesis for which sufficiently advanced action was not taken and it is to be submitted by a particular deadline. This is dangerous because hurrying up can lead to incomplete, even wrong conclusions.

Thesis, dissertation, and full report obviously will contain results in much more detail with explanation of nitty-gritty of the entire data. State also about the data collected but not analysed and give reasons for not doing so. Results in such reports should be comprehensive to cover all aspects of the problem. However, research papers for journals are considerably brief.

Since results are not by product of your brain, the quality of research should not depend on the type of results you obtain. Quality depends on how the problem was selected, how the objectives were determined, what methods were used, etc. Presentation of results conforming to the earlier premises and focussed discussion also determine the quality.

Tables and Figures

Tables and other illustrations are powerful tools. Text tells the story, but tables provide the evidence and graphs illustrate the results. Insert them as needed in an appropriate format and layout as explained in the next section. Exploit their potential to effectively convey the evidence on which the results are based. Use them either as complement to text or as a substitute. They must be self-contained for independent reading.

Describe the Subjects

Begin Results with the number of subjects actually studied at each stage of study – how many were potentially eligible, how many actually examined for eligibility, how many actually found eligible, how many were recruited for the study, how many dropped out and data were available on how many subjects, how many excluded from analysis for reasons such as outlying or wrong values and how many actually analysed in each group. A flow-diagram such as prescribed by CONSORT may be helpful. Give reasons for dropouts at each stage.

Next, describe the characteristics of subjects – their demographic (age, sex, rural/urban, etc.), social and clinical features, separately for cases and controls. Comment on their representativeness for the target population and explain how the results might get affected if not fully representative.

In the case of clinical trials and other experiments, demonstrate that the test and the control groups were comparable to begin with. Also say that not many dropped out of the study. If they did, show that the results are still unbiased. Include all the information on indications, dosage, route of administration, etc. Report the adverse effects of the intervention. Consider prognostic factors where relevant. Mention about any additional intervention that had to be done in some cases because of their condition and describe how it has not affected the validity of results. Substantive results should be sharply focussed on the objectives of the study. Ensure that all endpoints emanating from the primary and secondary objectives have been included but do not show any irrelevant data.

Statistical Results

The following guidelines are for the paper and not for thesis. Thesis will require much more detailed results. All mean values must be accompanied by the corresponding Standard Deviations (SDs). Do not give standard error because that can mask the actual inter-individual variation. Give confidence intervals where appropriate but remember while interpreting CIs that they apply to the group summaries such as mean and odds ratio, and not to the individual values. State the name of the statistical test at the time of giving *P*-value. Give exact *P*-values to 3 decimals but small *P*-values can be written as $P < 0.001$. There is no need to give values of chi-square, *t*, *F*, etc. Degrees of freedom also are not needed. The tests must have been mentioned in the Methods section. Intermediary quantities such as log-likelihood and sum of squares also are not needed but the final result, such as the value of R^2 estimates of the regression coefficients, or RR/OR that help in assessing the results should be included. While stating percentages, do not forget to mention the absolute number also. Percentages based on small *n* can be very deceptive. Give adequate number of decimals – as much as necessary to retrieve the original number. Follow the improved SAMPL guidelines (Indrayan 2020) as mentioned earlier that tell you what to report and how to report regarding various statistical aspects of your paper.

Do not use symbols, formulas, and equations in a medical paper unless absolutely necessary because they tend to make them complex for medical professionals. Some statistical results such as for ANCOVA and multiple comparisons in ANOVA can be difficult to communicate. Software outputs may be voluminous, and you may have to devote substantial time in filtering the results of substance. To put them into an intelligible table can be challenging. Thus, there is a tendency to report such results insufficiently. Even reviewers sometimes ignore this deficiency. Take help of a statistical facility in case you face difficulty. Keep the following points in mind.

1. Pay special attention to any sign of flawed data analysis. Appropriate method for the type of data should be used that gives the results exactly matching with the objective.
2. Do not confuse statistical significance with medical significance. First, statistical significance can be high (*P*-value really small) due to exceedingly large n even when the actual difference is small. Second, non-significance can be due to lack of power (small n). For statistically not significant difference, do not say that there is no difference – only that your study could not detect the difference.
3. Exercise caution in reporting results with marginal statistical significance such as with $P = 0.06$. Strict level 0.05 or relaxed—either way—looks like you are being unfair in the marginal cases.

Statistical reporting also depends on the design. For a case-control study, report the number found exposed in the two groups, Odds Ratio (OR), its Confidence Interval (CI) and statistical significance. Give both unadjusted and adjusted ORs for the exposure of interest as well as for all the covariates and confounders. For cohort studies, include the number with positive and negative outcomes, Relative Risk (RR) and CI – again unadjusted as well as adjusted. For trials, report about efficacy, use-effectiveness, side-effects, any unusual cases, etc.

In case you have investigated robustness of your results by validation sample, sensitivity or uncertainty analysis, provide the findings and explain the discrepancies, if any.

13.2.6 DISCUSSION

Discussion section is an intelligent exercise in logic, brevity, and clarity. It places findings in the context of clinical practice and health care, and illustrates your wisdom in integrating various facets of the results and the diverse results in the literature. This brings out the clinical significance of your results. Generally, this is the most useful part of a thesis or paper that helps readers to understand the implication of the findings. This elaborates how the results fit into the larger theory you initially proposed. Such a focus remains the core of the Discussion section. The language must be clear, precise, and unambiguous. It should have a clear link with the Introduction, else peer reviewers can be highly critical of your discussion

Clearly state what was known – its strength and weaknesses – and what exactly were the gaps (although this might be repetition of what you stated in the introduction section) and which part of the gap your results fulfilled, what remains. Compare and contrast various findings of different authors and give a critique of their methodology that could have affected these findings. Highlight their important findings that are relevant to your work.

Argumentation in Discussion can be exciting both for the authors as well as for the readers. To the readers, it allows to grasp the real relevance and utility of results in medical care, health policies, or evaluation programmes (Jenicek 2006a). To the authors, Discussion sometimes helps to rediscover the intricacies of the phenomenon that were possibly obscure earlier. Thus, an argumentative Discussion can be a useful exercise. See Jenicek (2006a) for details of how to write Discussion section in medical articles and what should it contain. The same principles apply to the thesis and bigger reports as well—just in more details.

Even the best evidence can be lost in poor argument. What argument is a good argument? Jenicek (2006b) suggests that this requires critical thinking which can be learnt. A cornerstone of critical appraisal is logic. A good argument contains a claim or proposition that must arise from infallible reasoning based on critically appraised evidence with qualifiers and exceptions. The qualifier must be convincing, and the argument should not look like a manoeuvre.

Discuss Your Results

Begin the discussion with medical context and then bring in significance of your findings in that context. Recapitulate the main findings without repeating the data. Emphasise the new or important findings without exaggerating. Discuss how your results support or do not support original hypothesis. Do not introduce new result that was not presented in the Results section. Explain how the statistical significance of your results might be real and not due to errors of measurements, confounding factors, or other biases. Discuss the statistically not significant results also if they are interesting. Explain what the results mean and how they are biologically plausible—what is their implication for the practice of medicine. Relate them to the objectives of the study. Include supportive evidence from the literature. Appraise the results critically and comment on their validity and reliability. Discuss how the results could be implemented and would benefit the medical science.

Do not be too assertive of your results because an element of uncertainty can never be ruled out. If the effect of your intervention is small, explain how this might still be valid. Comment on the statistical power of your study and establish reliability of new findings so that there is no suspicion. Discuss robustness of results to minor variation in the underlying procedures. Convince the reader that the results are trustworthy. Comment on the generalizability and practical significance, free from your own perception bias. The reader should be convinced that your discussion is balanced and not selective. Thus, say what you want to say about the results of your study but provide credible evidence. In case there is any accidental finding, explain how it may have arisen. Put forth a new hypothesis if it looks plausible since lateral thinking out of the box is always an asset. If the results do not provide a conclusive evidence, say that more work is needed.

Compare Your Results and Resolve Conflicts

Compare your results with those of other researchers, particularly of known or respectable groups working on that topic. Although the discussion sections is not supposed to have any table or figure but you can have one for comparing the finding with others. Analyse the literature critically without bias. (If you are reproducing whole or part of somebody else's figure or table, you may have to take permission.) Resolve any conflict by providing credible reasons and argue out why your results are convincing. Integrate them with the present knowledge. When relevant to your work, gently but firmly indicate the deficiencies in the work of others such as their faulty design, inadequate analysis, and wrong interpretation. Any rebuttal must be fully supported by evidence that makes it clear that you are not arrogant and respect other's work. Also, acknowledge the excellence of others when noticed.

Do not shy away from reporting discrepancies due to publication bias or methodological differences. If your results do not match and you are convinced that they are right, stick to them. The difficulty with other publications in that they are heavily biased towards positive results – negative results rarely see the light.

Limitations

Do not forget to mention the limitation of your study. No result has universal applicability. Rigorousness and transparency is your responsibility. Failure to report limitations suggests arrogance, or that the authors do not know about these limitations. Your report should not give an iota of inkling that there is any attempt to mislead the reader.

Uncertainties always remain and they can be easily acknowledged. More important in scientific research are methodological and data limitations such as nonresponse and not considering some of the known factors due to resource constraints or to avoid complexity. Reviewers and editors realize this, and the authors should not shy away from accepting such limitations. But make a convincing case that the results are still valid for whatever restricted segment of population. Mention the questions that this research has not been able to answer and discuss the potential for future research.

Conclusion

Distinguish between statistical result and scientific conclusion. The latter considers other evidence also – medical context, biological plausibility, present knowledge, clinical experience, etc. You should explain the mechanism how the conclusion emerged from the results and the collateral knowledge.

Produce a succinct conclusion and discuss its generalisability. It must be a warranted conclusion based on the evidence discussed earlier in the report. Link it to the objectives of the study. Justification of the conclusion should be fully articulated. Do not overinterpret the results and give full consideration to the multiplicity of analyses, findings of others and limitations of your study. State if the conclusion corroborates or contradicts the original hypothesis. Attach the appropriate degree of uncertainty about the final claim. Instead of restating the findings, emphasize on operative part of these findings. Very clearly state how does it add to the present knowledge, or how the results have contributed to the progress of science. Describe future perspective without being arrogant. For practical implication include recommendations where appropriate. For interventions, for example, the conclusion could be that it is sufficiently effective, or that it is promising but requires further investigation, or that the efficacy could not be established. The conclusion may also highlight the trade-offs between benefits and adverse effects. The benefits could be in terms of better efficacy or in terms of reduced cost or increased convenience. The adverse aspects could be side-effects, cost and inconvenience. Common errors in reaching conclusions are (i) interpreting lack of evidence for an effect as evidence of no effect, or not statistically significant as not different, (ii) ignoring warning signs of negative effect, (iii) reaching beyond the evidence by imputing own judgment, and (iv) stating that more research is needed without specifying what specific research is needed and why.

A conclusion is a take-home message. Remember that people, including scientists, resist change and they should be fully convinced before they use the new result. If you are refuting current practice, give almost infallible evidence. Miscues occur. Vaginal mesh for prolapse after childbirth was advocated but now found no more effective than standard care and observed to have severe complications in some cases.

Discussion in a Thesis

Discussion chapter in a **PG thesis** should be divided into sub-headings so that disparate ideas on different sub-topics are not mixed. In a big report or a dissertation, a chapter may be devoted to each subtopic. In that case, results and discussion on that topic would be together in that chapter. Since critical thinking is more important than data in a doctoral dissertation, discussion section has very special place in a dissertation. Use this section to demonstrate that concepts are getting precedence than results because that is what is expected in a dissertation.

Other Aspects of Discussion

Whether a small paper or a big report, never mix comments with the facts. Opinions should be clearly stated as opinions. Personal perspective is important but do not mix it with data-based results. If the result is on expected lines, explain the need to carry out the investigation in the first place.

Remember that statistical terms such as OR, CI, regression coefficients and *P*-values are not directly interpretable for application in medical practice. They need to be transformed to every day medical language that a practitioner can understand. Remember also that immediate uses of your research are the practitioners who deal with healthy and unhealthy people.

13.3 END FEATURES OF A REPORT

IMRaD is for the main body of a paper but there still remains substantial writing under the headings of Acknowledgements, Key Messages, and References. Guidelines on this segment are as follows.

13.3.1 ACKNOWLEDGMENT ETHICS

Primary medical research is essentially a team effort, but all members of the team may not qualify to be authors. They are thanked in the acknowledgement section for their contribution. People providing purely laboratory assistance, statistical assistance, data collection assistance, patient care assistance, editing help, clinical assistance, etc., outside their routine duty come in this category. Help of scientific advisers, persons who critically reviewed the manuscript, and departmental heads who provided general support should also be acknowledged. If you have received dataset from somebody, acknowledge this properly. All financial or material support must also be acknowledged including grant and contract numbers, and followships, if any. There is no need to be overenthusiastic about acknowledging help or acknowledging to serve vested interest. Example 13.2 illustrates what can go wrong even with this benign aspect of the paper.

EXAMPLE 13.2: Embarassing acknowledgement

Chatfield (2002) describes receiving a copy of an off print, acknowledging his statistical advice provided three years earlier on a trial that could not find significant difference between low-level laser therapy for rheumatoid arthritis of finger joints and the placebo. He had not seen the paper in either draft or final form. The paper had some inappropriate graphs. Perhaps the refereeing process also bypassed statistical content because the name of a (reputed) statistician appeared in the acknowledgements!

Instances of the type described in Example 13.2 are not uncommon. We have found ourselves in spot many times because of 'generosity' of authors in acknowledging our help without our knowledge. They misquoted our interpretation, even mentioned an out of context statistical procedure that was used for some other analysis. We now take an undertaking from our clients that they will not acknowledge our help without our approval. Many journals require that written permission be obtained from those acknowledged. Erstwhile Vancouver Group also endorses this requirement. If the acknowledged persons want to see the manuscript, show it to them so that they can check what you have written is right.

13.3.2 KEY MESSAGES

Information explosion has forced developments of new methods to keep abreast about new developments without devoting too much of time. Many journals are now switching to provide key messages in a box to summarise the salient features of the study in a few bulleted points. This certainly looks like a welcome development and seems very friendly not only to the readers but also to the reviewers and editors of journals who need to evaluate each paper for its technical worth and space in the journal. If you were clear about what you did and what was the main result, it would not be difficult to write key messages of your report.

Key message box would generally contain one bulleted sentence on each of (i) what is already known, (ii) what the research adds, (iii) what methodology was adopted, and (iv) what are the limitations. Each message should be complete in itself. The box containing key messages is not necessarily placed at the end in a printed paper, but it is customary at the time of writing to place it at the end of the manuscript. Considering importance and utility of these messages, it would not be surprising if over time they receive precedence even over abstract.

13.3.3 REFERENCES

"References may be the least noticed aspect of a scientific manuscript, but their proper use brings authority, credibility, and precision to scientific manuscripts. The reference section is an important part of a scientific manuscript because references acknowledge the work of other researchers that allowed you to formulate your hypothesis and enable readers of your article to locate those works. At some point, another researcher may reference your article, which allows the field to grow" (Foote 2007).

Selection of References

As stated earlier, the literature cited in your paper and thesis should preferably be recent and directly relevant to the work. If most citations are more than 10 years old, the study is not likely to be current or mainstream research. You can examine how many times an article has been cited by others. This is easily available on Google Scholar although restricted to the electronic media on the web. This excludes journals with printed version only or those early periods for whom electronic versions are not available.

The references should provide a balanced view in favour or against your results. Among these, if you have a choice, select the ones that are easily accessible to the reader such as free full text articles. Some critical readers of your work would like to see the work you have cited, and availability of free full text helps. At the other extreme are conference abstracts which are difficult to access. As much as possible, avoid citing such abstracts. Also, such abstracts generally contain rudimentary and insufficient information.

Originals of the reference material should have seen by at least one of the coauthors. Avoid citing papers under preparation or under communication, personal communications, and such other soft material. If you must, take written permission of the authors of such communications. Also, avoid references cited by others as they may be inaccurate. If you have to, state 'cited by .....'. Be careful about retracted papers. These can be searched by typing 'Retracted publication' [pt] in the search box of PubMed, where [pt] stands for publication type. Avoid citing references of newspapers, clippings, and magazines in a scientific communication.

Except for reviews and meta-analyses, it is not considered expedient to cite several references. In place of a comprehensive list, a few representative papers, possibly on different segments of population or from different areas, should be cited. Prefer references from the well-known peer reviewed journals or internationally acclaimed reports such as of the World Health Organization. The selection should be judicious. Also do not cite many references for a general statement. For example, saying that 'there are many studies on homocysteine level related to coronary heart disease (1-20)' does not impress anybody. Make it more specific such as 'ethnic groups in different countries with higher rate of myocardial infarction have been found with elevated level of homocysteine level (1-3)'. Also, there is no need to give references for well-known facts such as hypertension is related to obesity, and dietary factors are important precursors for colon cancer. Yet any statement that could be looked with suspicion should be accompanied by the reference (or the data) to provide it authenticity.

Technology has advanced and the references are not restricted these days to the print format only. Large number of medical journals are online with no print version.

In addition, you can also cite website of professional associations or other academic organizations. Use doi (digital object identifier) to cite such a reference. For this, mention the date of your last access because contents of websites can change quickly.

Format of References

Most journals require that references in the text be cited by consecutive numbers in the order they appear in text and listed at the end by these numbers. They must be cited immediately after the idea, in between the sentence if needed, and not necessarily at the end of the sentence. Increasing number of journals are switching to this format. The other format is to cite the reference in the text by the name of the authors (only the last name of the first author, followed by et al. if there are three or more) and the year of publication in parentheses as in this book. This format helps in remembering the citation and gives credit to the first author. Consult the Instruction for Authors of the journal to whom the manuscript is being sent for consideration and follow those instructions.

The style recommended by ICMJE for preparing the list of references is getting universal acceptance. Indexing services such as PubMed were already following nearly the same format. This format says that the authors' last name be written first followed by first letter of initial and middle name without full stop (.) sign and using comma in between the authors. Then write the title of the article. Next is the name of the journal with year of publication, followed by semicolon, volume number followed by colon, and first and last page number with a hyphen in between. There are slight changes for a citing a book, chapter in a book, proceedings of a conference, conference abstract, report, website, etc. See the ICMJE recommendations (2021) for details or follow the instructions of the journal concerned. It is customary to use PubMed abbreviations for name of journals. If the journal is not indexed, try to abbreviate according to the PubMed principles. If you are not confident, safe bet is to spell out the full name of the journal. For examples of references in this format, see the list at the end of this chapter.

Inaccuracies in references are common. You may like to check and recheck each reference for the spelling of the name of authors, any missed word in the title of the articles, year of publication, page numbers, etc.

To avoid errors, best is to use a software such as ProCite, Reference Manager and Biblioscape. Some of these are available free, open source. Next best thing to do is copy-paste the citation from PubMed and other electronic resources and rearrange with the desired format. The trend now is to provide the web-link also so that the reader can access the referenced article by a click.

Bibliography

Bibliography is different from the list of references. References are those that are cited in the text. You may have consulted other articles and material related to the topic but not cited in the manuscript. These might be of interest to the reader if he wishes to go into the depth of that topic. Most journals do not want bibliography—they restrict to the cited references only. But a bibliography could be useful adjunct to the theses, particularly to the Doctoral dissertations. For these, thesis supervisor is the best guide to suggest which publications to include in bibliography.

13.3.4 APPENDIX

Technical matter not of sufficient interest to the general audience of the report but of interest to specialists who want to know details go into the appendix. Medical journals tend to relegate mathematical content of a paper into appendix. Where needed, detailed tables can be provided in the appendix. These tables are given new numbers. In the case of thesis and dissertations, consent form, data collection form, etc., go into the appendix. When the study is small, the entire data set can be appended.

SUMMARY

Dissemination of results of your research may be the most exciting phase. Communication should be effective, and the objective should be reception by the audience and not transmission. It could be a written paper or a thesis, an oral presentation to an audience or a poster presentation in a conference but the present chapter is on writing.

A paper is written in brief whereas thesis in detail. None should have any duplication. Use tables and graphs to make your presentation crisp and easy to understand.

A thesis or a paper is effective when it is prepared with integrity. State the origin of the problem and describe the methodology actually followed. Discuss how all possible sources of bias were controlled and why the results are believable. State the results emphatically highlighting the achievement in terms of health improvement. Show robustness of results where feasible. Do not feel reluctant in describing the limitations. This enhances the credibility. Distinguish comments and opinions from evidence-based results. The presentation must be short but complete and should be robust to third party reviews.

Structure a report in established format such as IMRaD for a research paper and university guidelines for a Master's thesis and Doctoral dissertation. Authorship and acknowledgments should be according to acceptable ethics.

REFERENCES

Brand RA. Writing for clinical orthopedics and related research. Clin Orthop Rel Res 2003;413:1-7.

Chase M. Cancer prevention, at a price. The Wall Street Journal 2003 (June 24).

Chatfield C. Confession of a pragmatic statistician. The Statistician 2002;51 (Part 1):1-20.

Cohen JF, Korevaar DA, Altman DG, *et al.* STARD 2015 guidelines for reporting diagnostic accuracy studies: explanation and elaboration. BMJ Open 2016;**6:**e012799.

Foote M. Why references: giving credit and growing the field. Chest 2007;132:344-346.

Gladthorn AA. Writing the Winning Dissertation: A Step-by-Step Guide. Corwin Press, 1998.

ICMJE. Preparing a Manuscript for Submission to a Medical Journal. International Committee of Medical Journal Editors. http://www.icmje.org/recommendations/browse/manuscript-preparation/preparing-for-submission.html – accessed 8 March 2021

International Committee of Medical Journal Editors. Recommendations for the Conduct, Reporting, Editing, and Publication of Scholarly work in Medical Journals. *www.icmje.org*. - last accessed 19 January 2021.

Indrayan A. Reporting of basic statistical methods in biomedical journals: Improved SAMPL Guidelines. Indian Pediatr 2020 Jan 15;57(1):43-48.

Jenicek M. (a) How to read, understand, and write 'Discussion' section in medical articles: an exercise in critical thinking. Med Sci Monit 2006;12:SR28-SR36.

Jenicek M. (b) Towards evidence-based critical thinking medicine? Uses of best evidence in flawless argumentations. Med Sci Monit 2006;12:RA149-RA153.

Lilleyman JS. Titles, abstract, and authors, in, How to Write a Paper (Editor Hall GM). Byword Publishers, 1996.

Peh WCG, Ng KH. Effective Medical Writing: Pointers to getting your article published. Singapore Med J (i) Basic structure and type of scientific papers, 2008;49:522-524. (ii) Peh WCG, Ng KH. Title and title page, 2008;49:607-608. (iii) Ng KH, Peh WCG. Writing the materials and methods, 2008;49:856-858. (iv) Ng KH, Peh WCG. Writing the results, 2008;49:967-968. (v) Ng KH, Peh WCG. Preparing effective tables, 2009;50:117-118.

PLoS Guidelines. Welcome to the PLOS Writing Center: Your Resource for Scientific Writing and Publishing Essentials. https://plos.org/resources/writing-center/ - last accessed 8 January 2021

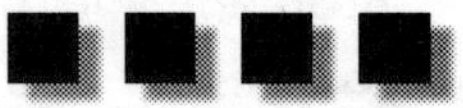

CHAPTER 14

How to Make Oral and Poster Presentations

KEY TERMS AND CONCEPTS

- ✓ Speaking
- ✓ Structure of the Talk
- ✓ PowerPoint Slides
- ✓ Dissertation Defence
- ✓ Layout of a Poster
- ✓ Poster Presentation

The objective of any presentation is communication. Remember that reception is more important in any communication than transmission. Mannerism is especially important to achieve this objective. An ideal communication passes clear message from the presenter to the audience without distraction. It is easily said than done. This section provides some tips for effective written and oral presentations.

Two full chapters are devoted to scientific writing because that is the dominant mode of communication of a research findings. However, oral presentation and poster presentation, such as in a conference, are also common. Whereas an established researcher is generally assigned to present his research in a plenary session, a new researcher such as a PG student, gets opportunity to present in a contributory session, particular as a poster. Either way, oral and poster presentations too require certain skills. These are discussed in this chapter. A summary is as follows.

Oral Presentation

- If you do not have natural talent to speak, it can be acquired by practice.
- Use conversational style – strike a chord with audience. Vary pitch and pace as needed to break monotony.
- Use anecdote or two particularly in the middle to regenerate interest.
- Accompany the talk by visual aids such as PowerPoint slides that help in retaining the focus and attracting the attention of the audience.
- Slides and transparencies should have only points (not verbatim text) and should not contain more than eight lines per slide in sufficiently large size font to be legible to those sitting on the back seats.

Poster Presentation

- Provides excellent opportunity of one-to-one interaction although it is rarely availed.
- Let the poster do the talking but be there by the poster to attend to any queries.
- Follow same rules as for an abstract but include one or two tables or graphs.

We discuss oral presentation first and then talk about poster presentation in the next section.

14.1 ORAL PRESENTATION

Oral presentation is different from written communication because it is a personal interface, and the audience had no chance to re-read if anything is not clear. Besides content, effectiveness of an oral presentation depends mostly on speaking style and, to some extent, on the visual aids such as transparencies and slides. These aids are discussed later in this section.

Oral presentation is generally from a podium and could be in the form of a **seminar,** which is more interactive with the audience or as a lecture where the audience is passive although questions can be asked. For research results, most oral presentations are made in a conference. This could be either a **plenary lecture** of 30 minutes to an hour before a big audience, an invited talk of 15 to 20 minutes to a medium-sized audience, or a **contributory paper** of nearly 10 minutes to a smaller audience. The other, now very popular, format of conference presentation is poster.

14.1.1 ESSENTIALS OF EFFECTIVE PRESENTATION

While research capabilities are important, communicating them in an effective manner is also important. Thus, presentation is one of those skills that a researcher must acquire. A presentation is a fast and potentially effective method for bringing people together to think, appreciate and review the results. It allows immediate interaction between all the participants and the presenter.

Remember that the objective of presentation is not transmission but reception. Thus audience is the focus. Your extremely good research may fail you if the audience do not capture its essence. Effective communication is the one whose message is understood and remembered.

Mind has segments to work as Cache, RAM, and hard disk of a computer where immediate, mid-term and long-term thoughts are stored. The presentation should be sharp to pierce the mental fog and to be able to hold attention of the audience long enough to be stored at a strategic location in their mind. A good presentation has not only content and structure but also packaging with human element to achieve this objective.

For some, speaking to an audience may top the worst fear. Your body can get into an over drive with release of adrenaline and cortisol, and notice butterflies in your stomach. They will easily fly away as you begin and provide words to your thought. Set the theme early in your presentation so that the audience knows what to expect. Think of what you would like in a presentation if you were in the audience. Establish the report by pretending one of them. Try to keep the audience engaged by phrases, small anecdotes, questions and inviting participation if that is allowed in the format of the organizers.

Remember that most audience are on your side. They want you to succeed. Translate this into reality by carefully delivering the talk. It should be packed with a punch that summarizes your research. Let it come unexpectedly so that the audience does not switch off even before your punch line and note how you influence the behaviour and attitude of the audience.

Best part is that all this can be acquired by practice. All you need is to pick up the finer nuances of making a good presentation, practice hard, learn from the feedback and practice more.

Read the right paper at right time (Greenhalgh 2019). Those working with COVID-19 pandemic know how quickly a study on the shape of the epidemic curve became outdated within a short period.

Speaking

Some people have natural talent, others can acquire speaking skills by following simple rules. Realise that a talk follows a much more informal format than a written paper. A conversational style in oral presentation can be very effective in communicating the ideas. Strike a chord with the audience by captivating them on the emotional front. Try to include an anecdote or two, that can infuse life in the presentation. For example, narrate story of an interesting patient (without his identification) that can keep the audience in good humour. If the presentation is on transfusions after liver transplantation, it may be interesting to add how a large number of transfusions in a case indicated the adverse outcome but survived. If you are not good at this, do some practice.

Keep an eye contact with the audience and throw words at them: only occasionally directing to the Chair and the Rapporteur; but never in the air nowhere. Avoid concentrating on the screen or computer although this has to be consulted off and on. Throw smile at different segments of audience at different times with eye contact as though they are with you. Audience will be staring at you and your facial expressions should convey that you are relaxed and comfortable. Your posture also conveys your thought process. Use it as a tool to reinforce support with the audience. Speak at slow pace, particularly if there are nonEnglish speaking persons in the audience but not at the cost of flow of delivery. Some 'ums' and 'errs' are not harmful but too many are distractors. Lower or raise your pitch according to the emphasis. A presentation at a uniform pitch can quickly put some at sleep. Use pauses and repeat critical information. Do not worry too much about syntax and the grammar so long as you are able to put across the ideas. If needed, pose questions and provide answers. Tailor the contents to the composition of the audience regarding the mix of expertise.

A good strategy for oral presentation is to repeat the key points: tell what you are going to tell (your plan of talk in brief), tell in detail according to available time what you want to say, and summarize what you said. The first part and the last part should match. Such repetition reinforces the essence of your research.

Practice does make perfect sense. Present the talk in your department before delivering it in a conference. In addition to practice, this will provide a feeling of the time needed for the presentation. A critical feedback from the friendly audience would help improve the talk.

Structure

It is obvious that a talk of 10 minutes cannot cover as much as a talk of 30 minutes. Do not try to pack too much in a short time: Just give gist of the work and encourage audience to read the full paper. Or prepare a handout for distribution. Omit the review of literature in an oral presentation except one or two references when essential. Abbreviate the methodology rather than results. Plan properly so that you do not overshoot your time. Remember to spare some time for question–answer session. This could be the most rewarding time for you to learn more about that topic. Audience loves to have a say. If there are no questions, provoke just one person. Others would follow.

An oral presentation is almost invariably more effective when accompanied by visual aids such as transparencies and slides. Some tips on how to prepare these are given next. Use illustrations to replace or supplement the text wherever appropriate. Diagrams, photographs, and cartoons can be very effective in oral presentation when sparingly used. Decide how you will fill interlude between slides so that continuity is maintained. Also establish link as you go from one idea to another. In the end, gratefully acknowledge the help received from the others.

Be prepared for tough questions. When a question is asked, repeat it for the entire audience. Ask the questioner if that is what he meant. Respect the questioner no matter how silly the question might look to you. Do not engage in prolonged arguments: instead, suggest a chat after the talk. If you do not know the answer, do not apologise but only offer to get back later, or suggest resources, or even ask audience for suggestions.

14.1.2 PRESENTATION AIDS

Major aid these days is PowerPoint presentation. This can be augmented by inserting voice but that is seldom done. Videos can also be presented as an additional feature to your oral presentation. Transparencies for overheads are becoming outdated but they have excellent feature that you can write and explain as on a blackboard.

Transparencies and Slides

Aids such as transparencies for overheads, and slides for projection serve two purposes. First, they keep the talk focused and coherent all though the presentation, and second, they attract attention of the audience who may otherwise distract. Simple rules for preparing these aids are given below. They are mentioned for slides but are equally applicable to transparencies as well. Use the following precautions in either case.

Remember that excellent design of slides cannot make up for deficiency in contents. Like a beautiful container, a good slide format can fool for once, but the lasting impression is provided by the thought process exhibited by the content. The purpose of slides is not so much to provide talking points to the presenter but to provide understanding to the audience of your research. Verbal and visual aids should be coherently integrated to provide a solid picture to the audience. Consider the following points.

1. Start preparing early and give yourself enough time to revise and improve the presentation. Rehearse it well.
2. Give a mock presentation within your institution/department, invite comments, and improve your slides.
3. Keep a back-up of your presentation in another pen-drive.
4. Visit the presentation room in advance and acquaint yourself with gadgets such as overhead projector, slide projector, LCD projector, computer, pointer, and projection screen. Apprise yourself about their operation particularly of those that you may have to handle as a speaker. Play your presentation and check that colour and symbols do not change. Sort all problems before presentation: never point out arrangement deficiencies in the talk.
5. Use slides only to reinforce a point. Depend mostly on your memory and knowledge to speak. Too many slides can spoil than help. Generally, not more than one slide per minute of presentation is recommended. Perhaps one slide per 2-minute is ideal. Maximum can be one slide per minute of talk. For a small 10-minute presentation, the distribution of slides can be as follows: Title – 1 slide, background – 1 slide, purpose/hypothesis – 1 slide, methods – 2 slides, results – 2 or 3 slides, conclusion – 1 slide.
6. Make sure you do not obstruct the view of the audience.
7. Make effective use of pointer while speaking. If pointer is not available, you can use mouse cursor to point to the text of interest.
8. Allow some lead time (a few seconds) between slides at the time of presentation for the audience to read the context.
9. Superimposition of one graph over the other can be very easily done with transparencies. Sometimes it is advisable to use transparencies as well as slides at the same time if facilities exist for such dual presentation.

Format of a Slide

- Never fill slides by verbatim sentences. They kill the interest and convey the message that you lack confidence. Only points or key words should be written but small sentences can be helpful in asserting a point.
- Write large: title in say 40-point font and text in 24-point. Do not include more than eight lines of text in one slide – preferably six lines or less. Cramming up too much of material in one slide reduces its intelligibility – consequently

compromises its effectiveness in communication. The slides should not be tiresome to read.

- Heading in each slide should be in bold letters and centred whereas the remaining text should be left aligned in upper-lower case as usual. Sans serif fonts such as Arial, Helvetica, and Tahoma may be preferable than serif fonts such as Times, Antiqua, and Courier. Avoid fancy fonts.
- Check slides for spellings and grammar. Proofread them with care after taking a printout. For hand-written transparencies, check for legibility.
- PowerPoint has special features for text formatting such as blink, fade, descend, spin, bounce, and float. They can be effectively used to place emphasis and to make the presentation interesting. But do not overdo it. Plain slides are generally preferred. For details of how to use PowerPoint see Gupta et al. (2002).
- When needed, use the format that divides the slide into two columns – one to carry table, photo, graph, etc., and the second to carry its text message. If the facility of simultaneous presentation of two slides is available, use it effectively for this purpose.
- Wherever possible, prefer graph over table. Table is difficult for the audience to decipher. If you must have a table, devote extra time for explaining its contents.
- Background and colour of text are debatable. Our experience suggests that plain white background with text in blue or black does a neat job.
- Contrast between colours of text and background must be maintained. Titles can be in colour such as scarlet. Use a uniform colour scheme and a consistent format.

Dissertation Defence

Most universities want public defence of a doctoral (Ph.D) dissertation. The audience generally would be faculty, and upcoming and outgoing students. There might be some other experts and examiners from other institutions and organisations. Generally, only those attend who are interested in the topic. It is an oral presentation by the candidate followed by gruelling question-answer session. Hopefully you have attended such defence yourself as a doctoral student and apprised yourself of the format.

Discuss your presentation with the colleagues and teachers in advance and get their feedback. Address their concern in the presentation. Opposing views may come up. Identify them and prepare in advance how they will be resolved.

Remember that your adviser is your ally. Although a dissertation is mostly the work of the student, adviser also has a stake. He is expected to keep the research on track. Thus, take his help in preparing the defence. Ensure his full support before, during, and after the presentation.

A good research empowers the science and not the candidate. Thus, do not emphasise lessons you learnt but emphasise the gains of your work to the science. Show that the research was planned and meticulously executed. Sometimes the process of research gets precedence over the utility of results. Thus, spend time in explaining the methodology. At any point of time, do not be defensive about your defence. A vigorous presentation with full preparation is the key to face the audience successfully.

14.2 POSTER PRESENTATION

A standard practice in conferences these days is to provide a space (e.g., boards) approximately of the size of 4′×5′ for contributors to display a poster on their work. The poster size is nearly 3′×4′. The presenter is expected to stand by it at specified timings and explain to who-so-ever cares to show interest. Despite steep increase in the number of conferences, only few get the opportunity to make oral presentation because of exponential increase in the presenters. Perhaps you will present most posters in your earlier career than oral presentations. A poster presentation provides a unique opportunity for one-to-one interaction with the audience.

Format of a poster depends much on the type of audience. The format would be different when the target group is specialists than if it is students. The primary purpose of a poster is not to present the details of your work but to attract attention so that the audience comes, and you can start a conversation and share the story.

The contents of a poster are slightly more than of an abstract but certainly much less than a full paper. Perhaps one or two tables or graphs can be included in the results section, and one or two reference can be cited. Such a facility is generally not available in an abstract. Otherwise the structure is the same as of an abstract and the same guidelines apply. Abstract contents were discussed in a previous chapter.

Although a poster can be prepared on, say, 6 pages of size A4 that are easy to carry in travel but there is an increasing tendency to prepare it as one big poster in literal sense. Modern technology allows printing of three feet wide paper to as much length as needed. The length of a poster is generally four feet. Real big size fonts can be used for titles and subtitles, and slightly smaller for text. Title should be readable from 3 meters so that anybody passing by can read and the text should be readable from a distance of one to two meters for those who stop by. Big size fonts also correctly forbid you to cramp up too much of information in a poster.

Since the poster audience is not captive as in oral presentation, it must have a format that can attract attention. Otherwise it will be ignored. It should be able to 'sell' just like an advertising billboard. One tool is the large font size as mentioned in the preceding paragraph. Second is layout. Try different layouts and select the one that looks most effective. A format that can do the 'talking' is preferred. Third is the choice of different fonts and colours. Do not overuse them. Consistency helps in retaining the attention. Perhaps two types of fonts (one for heading and the other for text) each in two colours (e.g., black and navy blue) on light brown or light grey background that contrasts are appropriate. You may like to try scarlet heading and black text in light grey boxes. Fourth is that the poster should be error free. Any error in content or spellings can be embarrassing because you are standing by the poster.

Some conferences organise competition and select best poster based on its structure, content, and attractiveness. This encourages presenters to make a poster that can communicate effectively.

Layout of a Poster

Title at the top should not be lengthy and should come in one line in big size font. Do not use exclusive capitals. Leave space on the side for institutional logo. A logo looks good, provides authenticity, and brings your institution into focus. Sometimes your institution attracts the attention of viewers.

Divide your poster into sections and clearly demarcate them by thick lines in light colour. These sections could be Purpose, Background, Methods, Results, Conclusion, Acknowledgements, and References. You may like to have any other structure. This structure should be recognisable from a distance. Bullet points do the trick very well.

Think of including a map showing location of your study, or one photograph of your hospital or the activity of the study. One or two graphs can be very attractive.

Be consistent in font size and colour so that the viewer knows that he is looking at similar things. For example, all sectional headings should be of same size and colour, and all graph headings should be of same size and colour but different from sectional headings. Tables and graphs can have light background. Use infographs in place of simple graphs. Font sizes should be proportionate to their importance and not unduly large or small. Use of underline should be rare, if at all, because this causes clutter.

Sufficient blank space helps viewers to get a balanced view. Cluttered posters are generally ignored by the viewers. One horizontal line should not generally contain more than 10 words for the viewers to remain focused.

Consider if you would like to have few copies of the poster or summary of your research in A4 size for handing out to anybody interested.

You may also want to include your address or e-mail address at the bottom for anyone to approach in case needed.

SUMMARY

Good speaking can be cultivated that can capture the audience. Use conversational style and add one or two anecdotes to make it interesting. Slides and posters should be prepared using established principles as enunciated in this chapter. Let the poster do the talking. For details of how to write a paper or thesis, see the previous chapter.

REFERENCES

Gupta P, Guglani L, Shah D. Exploring the power of PowerPoint. Indian Pediatr 2002;39:539-548.

Greenhalgh T. How to Read a Paper: The Basics of Evidence-based Medicine and Healthcare, 6th Edition. Wiley Blackwell, 2019

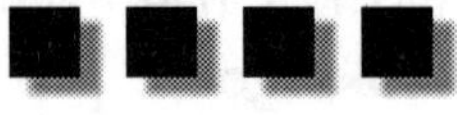

CHAPTER 15

What are the Reporting Ethics

KEY TERMS AND CONCEPTS

- ✓ Duplication
- ✓ Copyrights and Permissions
- ✓ Peer Review
- ✓ Misreporting
- ✓ Data Dredging
- ✓ Plagiarism
- ✓ Conflict of Interest
- ✓ Confidentiality
- ✓ Statistical Fallacies

Science progresses through work on new frontiers, the gateway of which is publication in a peer-reviewed journal. Such publications are also important for career advancement of the researcher and to succeed in an academic environment (Mathur et al. 2014). In the process, the ethical aspects of publication may be compromised.

Ethics is conforming to the standards of conduct. In the context of medical research, it has several facets. Concern for the welfare of the study subjects was expressed in Chapter 1. Research ethics is in terms of sufficient reasons to start a new investigation and using an appropriate design including adequate sample size so that the efforts do not go waste and there is no unnecessary exposure to the subjects. This was discussed in Chapter 5. Now we want to discuss about reporting ethics in this chapter although some of it too has already been discussed. For example, advice about truthful reporting of results without inhibition even if they are negative has already been given. Cheating by imputing fake data is denounced because this puts the reputation at stake not only of the person and the institution but of whole country. This risk is definitely not worth taking. (It is because of this that many researchers around the world suspect Indian medical research, and reviewers take extra care in reviewing any research by Indian workers). Acknowledging limitations and shortcomings of the investigation have also been emphasised. Also mentioned earlier is about unbiased review of literature not precluding opposite or variant view. After all this, some aspects of reporting ethics have still remained undiscussed. These include duplication and plagiarism, copyrights and permission, conflict of interest, peer review, statistical, fallacies, etc. In short, reporting ethics is about increasing the integrity of the report. A summary is given below.

Reporting Ethics Summary

- Duplicate publication based on already reported data is unethical unless it is a translation in another language or written for another audience with altered focus. In this case, acknowledge the original publication and give reference.
- Stealing the results or ideas of somebody else without acknowledgment is plagiarism. This is misconduct and deserves to be punished.
- Reproducing small part of a text, one figure, one table, etc., from a publication is allowed when the credit is cited, and a written permission is obtained.
- Clearly state about financial, personal, or professional conflict that has potential to influence your findings, even if they are not actually influenced.
- Respect peer review. Such a review is a standard practice in all scientific research.
- Do not misreport your findings and do not suppress inconvenient results. In other words, do not restrict your paper to the favourable results. Truthfully describe limitations of your research.
- Take abundant precaution to avoid statistical fallacies in your report. Some of these could be (i) using proportions where means should be used, (ii) calculating percentage when n is small, (iii) using too many decimals, (iv) analyzing before-after differences ignoring baseline values that could be relevant, (v) using inflated P-values, using hard cut-off even when the statistical significance is borderline, or not adjusting P-value when many analyses are done on same data, (vi) manipulating graphs for small difference to look large or vice-versa, (vii) reanalysis

of data after deleting some inconvenient values, and (viii) using black-box approach to the analysis.

Among many negative things talked about in this chapter about what not to do, we begin with a positive note on what to do. Ethics require that your paper when sent to the editor is accompanied by a proper covering letter. Hopefully you have selected a journal that has decent chance of accepting your paper.

Covering Letter

While sending a manuscript for publication, it is generally necessary that it is accompanied by a covering letter. Although a simple sentence saying that the enclosed manuscript be considered for publication works but the editors generally like to know what is this paper about and why have you chosen that journal. Thus, try writing a paragraph containing this information. Include information on your previous publications and presentations based on the same work, if any. Some journals would want to see a copy of this material to decide about suitability of the submitted papers. Also mention about the number of tables and illustrations enclosed. In case any of these is taken from another source, include permission to reproduce.

Some journals provide presubmission checklist that you need to complete. In case you have not been able to follow the journals instructions fully, give reasons why a particular instruction could not be followed. All this will help in expeditious processing. Some journals require signature of all the authors with specification of exact contribution of each author. The contribution sometimes goes into the body of the paper instead of the covering letter. If not included in the text, mention about conflict of interest in the covering letter. See later in this chapter for details of this conflict.

15.1 DUPLICATION

Distinguish between two kinds of duplication. First is duplication of own previous report, and second is copying others. The second is called plagiarism.

15.1.1 DUPLICATE PUBLICATION

Preparing three papers on different aspects of a work is not necessarily a duplication even if the data are the same. If the research has three distinct conclusions, each can be reported separately in a journal focused on that aspect. The expectation in this case though is that each paper will contain a reference of the previous or concurrent publications on that data. A full paper based on abstract or conference presentation earlier is also not considered duplication. Brief results reported in a clinical trial registry is also not duplication when full paper on this trial is cited. Two publications based on same data written in different languages or for different audience also is acceptable so long as the original publication is acknowledged, and the purpose of this new publication is clarified. A publication on assessing clinical agreement was first published in a statistical journal (Altman and Bland 1983) and repeated in Lancet (Bland and Altman 1986) with altered focus for medical professionals. This is not considered duplication. What then is a duplicate publication? Clear guidelines are yet to emerge, but the following discussion may help.

Two papers on the same aspect of same data possibly with differing titles in different journals is **duplication.** Sometimes cosmetic changes in presentation or in data contents (e.g., add one more variable to the five earlier analysed or add a few more subjects) are made to escape detection. Two papers with substantial overlap of results on the same or nearly the same data is also considered duplication. These occur mostly to falsely inflate the curriculum vita of the author. While working on pancreatic cancer, we detected two papers in PubMed database by Gold (1995) and Gold and Goldin (1998) with identical titles and substantially similar abstract. Both occupy 25 pages of the journal. Two articles by Patel et al. (2004) and by Patel et al. (2005) in different journals also have identical titles and essentially same abstract. We do not know what transpired but in such a case it is necessary to inform the editor about the previous publication. Preliminary reporting to media, other agencies, and a letter to the editor also come under this category. The Editor decides each case on its merit to publish or not. If previous publication is suppressed and this 'misconduct' is detected later, the journal may denounce publicly that can bring disrepute to the author and his institution or the funding agency. The Editor may also notify the institution or the funding agency regarding this misconduct that can jeopardise author's job. Never ever try to do this.

Instances of duplicate publication of the type mentioned in the preceding paragraph are rare but another misconduct of **redundant publication** goes on quite frequently. This occurs when the paper substantially overlaps with another paper. BMJ considers overlap more than 10% as threshold to be on guard and examine that both the papers before deciding on publication (BMJ 2013). Adding few cases or few more investigations or slightly different set of variables come in this category. Such papers unnecessary increase the load on the readers and journals. This should not be done. Journal editors are still grappling with the kind of response they should have against such redundant papers.

Publishing first on a website and then in print is also unethical. However, pre-prints or monographs do not fall in this category.

In the same vein, simultaneous submission of a paper to two or more journals is also unethical. The journals have right to penalise the author for this misconduct also. The penalty could be not considering any future paper from that author and informing the employer about this misconduct.

15.1.2 PLAGIARISM

Plagiarism is representing the results, ideas, and words of others as your own. This is cheating and abhorred more than the duplicate publication. All public documents such as publications in journals are for use by anyone, but the requirement is that the source must be acknowledged. Give the credit where due. Verbatim sentences of others should be in quotes with reference. If you want to avoid quotation marks, paraphrase in your words without changing the meaning and cite the source since the idea still belongs to somebody else. The whole idea is to respect other's intellectual property just as you would like yours to be respected. There is no need to cite reference for statements of common knowledge such as for saying that lack of exercise and high calorie intake contribute to obesity. Alarmingly, instances have been found where the 'experts' copy the idea of the articles they receive for review. This is dangerous. Many journals now use software such as *ithinticate* that detects common words and phrases in two documents. This helps to detect plagiarism immediately.

Another dangerous trend now catching up in India, particularly with PG theses, is the copy-paste 'technology'. Collect six previous theses on the topic similar to your research, identify sentences and paragraphs that you can incorporate, and copy-paste them in your thesis through a software. This certainly does not help your talent and a smart examiner will spot such handiwork. This may still get 'rewarded' if the examiner chooses to remain silent for ulterior motive but there is a chance to get punished too. In any case, this sets up terrible guilty feeling when you grow into a thesis supervisor and your students do the same.

15.1.3 COPYRIGHTS AND PERMISSIONS

Quoting a sentence or two, or borrowing ideas from a *cited* reference is one thing but reproducing a full paragraph or a figure or a photograph is another. The latter raises the issue of copyrights and permissions.

Almost all formal publications – journals, books, reports – are copyrighted these days. They clearly mention in the beginning that any kind of reproduction in full or in part is not allowed without written permission of the authority vesting copyright.

Otherwise a legal action can be taken. This however does not forbid anyone to make photocopies of a few pages for personal reading, but no part can be copied for commercial purposes.

Reproducing material from some other publication requires a written permission. Permission is indeed granted in scientific pursuits but many publishers charge a fee. This could be exorbitant for some authors to bear. Experience suggests that if it is a question of reproducing small part such as one figure or one table, and the inability to pay is shown, the publishers are benevolent for academic and scientific purposes and they may waive the fee in such cases. Do not hesitate to contact the publisher or the copyright owner for permission. The responsibility of obtaining the permission lies with the author.

Most journals want that copyright of the paper is transferred to the journal before it is published. Consider its implications such as in obtaining patents before the rights are transferred. If the patents are already obtained, inform the editor. A debate is going on regarding granting copyright to the publishers for the writing of the authors. Perhaps authors as individuals feel insecure to enforce copyrights whereas publishers have resources to protect the copyright. One view is that the authors should have right to distribute their work. Open access has loosened the hold of the publishers. In any case, realise that publishers have the copyright of the writing you did but the work or the result continues to be your own.

15.2 CONFLICTS AND REVIEWS

If attitude or behaviour of a research worker tends to get affected because of extraneous considerations, assume that there is some conflict of interest. Generally, self-interest is the cause of such conflicts. These arise mostly because of financial considerations but can arise due to personal or professional considerations as well. These conflicts can undermine public trust in medical research. In addition are issues such as misreporting and breach of confidentiality.

The second issue is of review of the submission by the editors and peers. Such reviews do not fall into classical 'conflict of interest' slot but we include them here because they too can lead to conflicting postures. The review is an exercise (i) for choosing more appropriate ones for publication among the large number submitted to a journal, and (ii) to try to improve the scientific content of the submissions. We discuss both these also in this section.

15.2.1 CONFLICT OF INTEREST

These can be categorised into financial conflicts and personal and professional conflicts.

Financial Conflicts

A funding agency naturally expects that the research sponsored by it will at least do it no harm if not further its interest. If the funding agency happens to be a company in the business of promoting a drug, device, or any intervention, and if the research findings go against that product, how to resolve this conflict? Integrity of the research is maintained by truthfully reporting what is found, and not be influenced by such extraneous considerations. The trend now is to rarely accept a research finding with potential conflict of interest even if it is not actually affected. Generally the research workers should not have any linkage with the company whose product is being researched, and certainly should not have stakes in that company. Accepting consultancy or honorarium from such a company is also considered as an adverse factor nor such 'inducements' should be accepted in near future after the research is over because that too can serve as a motivation to influence the findings. The influence can be indirect in designing, conducting the investigation, data analysis, and interpretation, and not just in reporting. Even when there are no financial interests, researchers do benefit when their hypothesis is validated. This can help in attracting more grants or may help in promotion. This, of course, in allowed.

Personal and Professional Conflicts

The results of a study can go against the results of your seniors or against a reputed research worker. To avoid conflict with them, you may delete certain part of the findings or try to modify them. Conflict can arise at the time of peer review also when reviewer happens to have connection with the company of the researched product. If the paper is from a competitor of a reviewer, the review could be biased. (See Peer review next.) Such conflicts can arise at the level of the editor also.

The author would not know about conflicts occurring at the level of reviewer or editor, but all other known or perceived conflicts should be disclosed at the time of submission of manuscript to a journal. Merely disclosing conflicts do not make them allowable. Explain how findings are not compromised because of any such extraneous consideration. The editor will decide that the integrity of research is maintained or not and publish accordingly. He may decide to publish conflict disclosures also for the benefit of the readers. Disclosing a conflict of interest does not necessarily reduce the worth of the report and it does not imply dishonesty either. On the other hand, this disclosure can enhance the credibility of the authors.

15.2.2 PEER REVIEW

As mentioned in a previous chapter, scepticism in science is a regular feature and fair criticism is welcome. Master's thesis is examined and graded according to its contents and presentation. Doctoral students may be asked to defend their dissertation in an open professional presentation where examiners also sit as audience. A question-answer session exposes the weaknesses and strengths of the work. A project report is also many times sent for review before being accepted. The reviewer may dislike the methodology or may question the validity of conclusion, and the author can steadfastly refuse to accept the suggestions. Arguments and explanations are the only way out to resolve these conflicts.

Review Process in Journals

Journals typically first do technical evaluation to confirm that the submission is according to their style and format. This is done by an administrative staff member at the journal office. If passed, the submission goes to the editor for review. The editor checks for its conformity to their policy and scope. The editor looks at the paper and may decide to reject it outright without sending it for review. Only those papers that look worthwhile in first reading are sent for review. If found suitable, it is sent to at least two subject matter experts for peer review.

All reputed professional journals, particularly in medical sciences, follow the system of peer review of articles submitted to them for publication. This process helps editors to decide the suitability for publishing the work. This is considered an important quality control measure and helps in improving accuracy and clarity of published research. Some journals approach three or four reviewers but the standard is two. Although this job requires considerable time of the reviewers, they are generally not paid. They are not part of the editorial staff either. Many do this thankless job willingly in the interest of science, possibly regarding this as a sign of recognition of their professional maturity. Perhaps it is a pleasure to review somebody else's work, and to comment on its strengths and weaknesses. When submitting a paper for publication, be prepared to receive comments, some of which may not be compliments. Shortcomings in the methods and flaws in the results can be highlighted. It is better to foresee them and prepare the manuscript accordingly. Peer review process can be very rewarding since it can increase the value of the report. There is another view, though. Little evidence exists of effectiveness of peer review, but considerable evidence exists of its deficiencies. This view arises from its failure in detecting some frauds (Smith 2006).

The dominant system earlier followed was masking of authors and institutions by deleting the first page of manuscript containing this information. This system is on decline. Perhaps the editors have found that most reviewers are unbiased, and knowledge of the name of the authors and institution does not affect the tone of review. Even when the authors and their affiliation are removed from the manuscript, the contents of the paper such as the topic, the source of objects, and the methodology can still provide hints about the identity of the authors. Thus, bias in some cases cannot be ruled out although this would be rare. Nevertheless, a review can be highly subjective and easily abused. Indian authors sometimes suffer because of the unfavourable perception built around the world due to misconduct of some so-called researchers in India.

Review of Theses

Almost all postgraduate (PG) theses are accepted with or without raising a question. That certainly has compromised quality of PG theses in India. Examiner may not be fully satisfied, may be even fully dissatisfied, but does not want to be perceived as a tough person or as the one trying to spoil the career of a student. Raising queries and rejecting a thesis involves a lot of work that many examiners want to avoid, and it involves threat to his examinership in future. Thus, the flaws in PG theses rarely come to the fore.

The situation with doctoral dissertations is not that easy although that also requires raising the present standard. Some examiners are strict and ask for revision. A caution is exercised both by the student and by the adviser to produce work that can be professionally defended.

Responding to the Reviews

Opposed to the theses, perhaps not more than 10 percent papers sent to good journals are accepted as submitted. Many are rejected for various reasons—mostly for not meeting the standard set by the journal. Most articles are referred back to the authors for revision, sometimes with inconvenient questions. Sometimes the revision suggested may be intractable. The authors in this case try out another journal using these suggestions to improve the quality of paper.

Sometimes a paper is rejected without assigning any reason. This could be painful, but a good manuscript can be rejected if it does not fit into the scope of the journal. It is for obviating this that we suggested that your covering letter should include why you selected that journal. Do not lose heart in case of rejection. There are instances when a paper was accepted after being rejected by 8 journals (Cummings and Rivara 2002). Many journals give reasons for rejection. Among the reasons could be that the research is only repetitive or just confirmatory with no new findings, or it has poor design, unclear hypothesis, poor presentation or any such gross deficiency. Brood over the reason coolly and examine what you can do to alleviate the deficiency. Remove the deficiency as much as possible and submit to another journal. If you have sincerely carried out a research, be assured that the paper will be accepted by one or the other journal. Many journals remain on hunt for suitable manuscripts.

Quite often the paper is returned with comments from one or two, even three reviewers that help you revise the manuscript. You must carefully read all the comments and prepare a detailed point-by-point reply. Do not ignore any comment even if it looks trivial because that can delay the acceptance. Some suggested changes may not be to your liking. Do not worry if your response is long. Explain the changes you have made in the manuscript in response to each comment, and also explain if you find that changes as per any comment will not be appropriate. For those comments that look appropriate to you, express gratitude to the reviewer for pointing out. Some journals require that changes in the manuscript be made in 'track changes' mode.

Experience suggests that it is expedient to comply with the comments of the reviewers and modify manuscript accordingly instead of raising a counter-argument. You may have to kowtow the editorial wishes. If you feel strongly about a comment, give a polite explanation why is it not appropriate, or cannot be complied. See if your writing lacks clarity that has led to this kind of comment. Cite supportive evidence. Merely giving explanation in reply to the comments is not enough: the text of the manuscript should also be accordingly changed so that it reflects the reply. Each comment must be individually attended. Get help from the other authors. Do not lose heart if the paper is not accepted even after complying with all the suggestions.

Some journals would not provide comments but only ask you to reduce the size of the paper. Almost all journals have space crunch although this is declining with online journals. You may have to think yourself which part of the text, which table and which figure to delete. Do so with discretion because the continuity and flow have to be maintained.

Sometimes there is a conflict in the comments themselves. One reviewer may ask you to delete some portion and the other may say that portion is good. One reviewer may also provide conflicting advice – for example to cut-short the paper and to add some explanation. You may have to make best out of such conflicts without raising a controversy.

Editors are not above the board either. They are perceived to be at tremendously advantageous position. Perhaps there is no author who has no grievances against one or the other editor. British and American journals are sometimes accused of being biased although they claim to bend backwards to accept quality papers from India. Some journals (e.g., Lancet) have appointed Ombudsman for redressal of grievances. You can file an appeal if you feel strongly about unfair rejection or any such occurrence.

15.3 CONFIDENTIALITY AND MISREPORTING

We have discussed ethics in conducting medical research earlier in Chapter 1 and the present chapter is on ethics to be followed in reporting of research findings. While confidentiality was discussed there, this requires to be re-emphasized in the context of reporting. Misreporting is in any case is a serious issue not just in the context of India but also globally.

15.3.1 CONFIDENTIALITY

In the context of publishing research, the question of confidentiality arises at least at two levels. First is the respect for privacy of the patients or subjects. No information should be part of your manuscript that can identify any individual. The names certainly cannot be revealed but things like photos and pedigrees should be sufficiently masked. Only in cases where necessary for scientific reasons, this identify can be revealed with full and expressed consent of the concerned person. This consent should be free of any duress or pressure.

The second is at the level of the authors and reviewers. All reviews must respect the confidentiality of the authors and the name of reviewers also are not disclosed. Authors have right to be not discussed for their work unless published. Reviewers cannot take advantage of their privilege of knowing the contents before publication. Nonetheless, the confidentiality of the authors can be breached in a rare case of fraud, when established, with respect to subjects, methods, statistical misappropriation, etc. This brings us to misreporting.

15.3.2 MISREPORTING

Scientific misconduct in terms of misreporting can go on unnoticed in subtle ways. This is manipulating the results and bogus research and includes cooking up the data, their alteration and image fabrication.

Result Manipulation

This can occur in one or more of the following ways.

1. Changing end point or outcome of interest from, say, death to complication or vice-versa when results for the planned outcome fail to come-up to the expectation of the investigator. This can also be in terms of looking at one-year outcome in place of two-year outcome originally planned, or any such variation.

2. Presenting the results groupwise instead of combined or vice-versa when such transposition helps to provide findings in support of the investigator's hypothesis.
3. Presenting results for a subgroup of patients pretending that other groups were not there.
4. Presenting univariate (unadjusted) results when the objective was to study the results adjusted for the confounders.
5. Presenting results for proportions when averages fail to serve the hypothesis of the investigator, or vice-versa; or using proportion where odds ratio (OR) should be used.
6. Arbitrary merging of categories to provide specific results.

These are few examples of many avenues that can be misused to cook up the results of your choice. Some will select part of the data to get 'evidence' in support of their hypothesis. There is a famous saying that if you look hard enough, part of the data can be located that would support almost any hypothesis. The difficulty is that such misreporting is hard to detect in a finished report, thus can go on unnoticed. It is for you to be true to yourself and the science, and report full facts. Correctly reported results replicate well and endeared while incorrectly reported results are soon forgotten. They may help your career resume but at a substantial cost to the science. You would never do this if you were a true doctor.

Having said all that, there might be valid reasons in rare cases to report part of the findings. These could be that you merged categories or groups as these had small numbers, you discovered interesting finding for a specific subgroup, you found that the data for a particular group is erroneous – not properly collected, etc. In such cases, explain what happened and why you are reporting part of the results.

Bogus Research

At the extreme is research based on fake data. No or very little data are collected, and the major part is imputed at will to get the desired results. This is fraud, to say the least.

You may have occasionally heard how a PG thesis was made up for 150 patients when only 15 were studied and how a fake researcher produced report on heart ailments in a community without doing much of a survey. This is equivalent to murdering a person for small pecuniary gain. Some kill their soul to report this kind of 'research'. This is easily detected, and the 'researcher' is trashed for ever.

15.4 STATISTICAL FALLACIES

Data analysis can always be geared to serve an ulterior motive but our concern in this chapter is with interpretation and particularly the reporting. Statistical fallacies in reporting are quite common. Although some of these occur inadvertently as clicking a wrong button but some could be deliberate. Show wisdom and avoid both. For details of the kind of statistical fallacies, see Indrayan and Malhotra (2018).

15.4.1 CHERRY-PICKING THE STATISTICAL INDICES

Statistical results can be manipulated by suitably picking the statistical indices. OR gives you different result than sample proportions. Following are the other rather simple examples.

Mean or Proportions

Depending upon the preference, the results can be provided in terms of mean of blood pressure (BP) levels or in terms of prevalence of hypertension, in terms of haemoglobin (Hb) level or in terms of anaemia, in terms of plasma glucose level or in terms of diabetes, etc. No such name is available for a measurement such as total lung capacity, but this can be categorized as low (<4.0 l), medium (4.0-5.9 l), and high (≥6.0 l). All quantitative measurements can be converted to qualities. The summary measure for quantities generally is mean and for qualities is proportion. Which one should be used in a research report? This must be decided at the time of writing the protocol and should be adhered to.

Means can lead to a conclusion different from the one reached by proportions. This provides a leeway to the investigator to try out both and report the one that suits a particular hypothesis. In addition, for anaemia, for example, various categories can be tried: <12 g/dl, <11 g/dl or <10 g/dl; and the one that looks 'favourable' can be adopted. Thus, the report may not truly reflect the findings. Our statistical advice is to stick to the original metric measurements and not convert them into categories. This is more exact and removes the subjectivity in devising categories. When categories are essential, state them before hand preferably at the time of writing the protocol and justify those categories. Do not change them later unless there are strong reason to do so.

Misuse of Percentages

If six patients out of eight respond to a new treatment, is it proper to say that the response rate is 75 percent? What about stating one out of two as 50 percent? Isn't preposterous to call zero out of one as nil and one out of one as complete? These are extreme examples but illustrate that percentages based on small n can be misleading. Generally no percentage should be stated when n is less than 30.

While assessing gestational age for 300 births, if 60 women do not know the date of last menstrual period, the percentage of births with gestation, say, 32-34 weeks should be calculated out of 240 and not 300. This is obvious yet many present percentages with a wrong denominator.

Linkage of hypertension with A, B, O blood groups has not been investigated much. If the distribution in a sample of hypertensives is A, 15%; B, 40%; AB, 25%; and O, 20%; it would be naive to conclude that hypertension is predominant in B group. These percentages should be compared with the blood group distribution in the target population for any such conclusion.

Summary measures such as mean and proportion, when based on the aggregated data, can be deceptive. They could mask or aggravate the variation present in subgroups. We illustrate this for percentages in Example 15.1.

EXAMPLE 15.1: Percentages based on aggregated data can mask subgroup variations

Consider case-fatality in cancer patients in a general hospital and a cancer hospital:

Stage of cancer	General Hospital			Cancer Hospital		
	n	Deaths	Case-fatality (%)	n	Deaths	Case-fatality (%)
Stages I & II	150	30	20	50	10	20
Stages III & IV	50	30	60	250	80	32
Total	200	60	30	300	90	30

Both the hospitals have same case-fatality in aggregate but actually the cancer hospital is receiving patients predominantly in advanced stages. In them, its performance is markedly better: 32 percent case-fatality in cancer hospital against 60 percent in a general hospital. If only the aggregate percentage is reported, this distinction is lost. It is for such discrepancies that standardisation is advocated.

Another fallacy occurs in stating too many decimal places. Percentage of 3 out of 35 can be stated to as many decimal places as one wishes to. The tendency in medical literature is to use excessive decimals. The rule is as follows. Use one decimal place if $n < 100$, two if $100 \geq n < 1000$, three if $1000 \leq n < 10,000$, etc. Mean and SD should be stated one decimal more than the accuracy of original values. This retains the accuracy without sounding too precarious. If uric acid is measured in mg/dl as 3.3,

4.5, etc., the mean and the SD should be stated with two decimals. For mean and SD of total lipids one decimal is enough since the measurement is in integers. Correlation coefficient is conventionally stated to two decimal places.

There are exceptions to these rules. Sometimes it is considered neat to state all results with same number of decimals, even when they are based on different *n*, or even when different measurements have different accuracies. Another concept is of **significant digits**. Zeroes immediately after decimal are not counted. Thus 0.0032 has two significant digits and 0.32 also has two significant digits. It would be unfair to state 0.0032 as 0.00 when the system of two decimal places is religiously followed for uniformity.

15.4.2 FALLACIOUS INTERPRETATION

Statistics is not everybody's cup of tea. While calculations can be done by a computer, interpretation of statistical results requires skill. Whereas many of examples of inadequate interpretation can be cited, the following illustrate what can go wrong.

Inadequate Interpretation

Many medical researchers are much too keen to look at the difference or gain in medical parameters after the treatment compared to values before treatment. In their keenness, they forget that a gain of 3 g/dl in Hb level over pretreatment value 8 g/dl has a different meaning than the same gain over the pretreatment value of 11 g/dl. It is relatively easy to affect a rise over lower Hb values than over higher values.

Another common misinterpretation is considering mere association or correlation as an evidence of cause-effect. Incidence of cardiovascular diseases in India is negatively correlated with birth rate but it has no causal implication. Such nonsense and spurious correlations were discussed in an earlier chapter. As another illustration, consider seeing 3 children wearing specs and watching TV for long hours. Can you conclude that wearing specs in children is associated with watching TV for long hours? The key is how many others watching TV for long hours do not wear specs. You will find many such instances in popular media, and many people believe them.

Misuse of *P*-values

Scientists debate about the validity of the conventional cut-off 0.05 for *P*-values. The opinion is growing to use confidence intervals instead of *P*-values. But there is no escape in some situations and a level has to be fixed to assess statistical significance. Certainly no magic happens at 0.05. A safe rule is to interpret *P* between 0.04 and 0.06

with caution and conclude that further work is needed. This is the same kind of precaution that is always taken for patients with borderline values. In any case, do not take *P*-values too seriously. They must be complemented by common sense. *P*-value is only the probability of Type I statistical error. Other statistical and nonstatistical errors cannot be ignored. Indrayan (2020) has given details how to strike a balance between *P*-values and the other corroborative or contradictory evidence for drawing valid conclusion.

Many examples can be cited from medical literature when more than one statistical test is done on the same data, each at level 0.05, without realising that this inflates the error rate. There are statistical methods such as Bonferroni and Tukey that should be used in such cases to control the chance of error to the specified level.

As stated earlier, statistical inferences are applicable only to random samples. The basic purpose is that the sample is representative of a defined target population and generalisability is intact. Many articles use tests of significance on nonrandom samples with ill-defined target population. Before extrapolating results to a larger group, ensure that the sample in the study is representative of that larger group. Implication of most medical findings is in managing future cases. Thus, examine how the conclusion will be applicable to the future cases and of what type. Write the discussion accordingly.

Misuse of Statistical Tools

Misuse of percentages and of *P*-values has already been discussed. Figure 15-1 (a and b) illustrate how a graph can be manipulated to show a small gradient as steep and vice-versa.

Most graphs do not fully represent the sample size. A mean or percentage based on $n = 3$ is shown the same way as the one based on $n = 50$. Even if n is stated in the graph, perhaps the perception and cognition received from the graph still remains the same.

Looking for linearity when the relationship is clearly nonlinear can damage the results. This was discussed in an earlier chapter. Ignoring assumptions such as Gaussian form of distribution, independence of observations, and uniform variance, can produce results of doubtful validity.

Statistical packages also are misused. Data are over analysed to investigate aspects that were not part of the protocol. Such analysis is not prohibited but a fallacy arises when they are packaged as original investigation and suppressing that these are incidental findings. The results of such analysis should be stated as tentative for the purpose of generating hypothesis rather than for testing it.

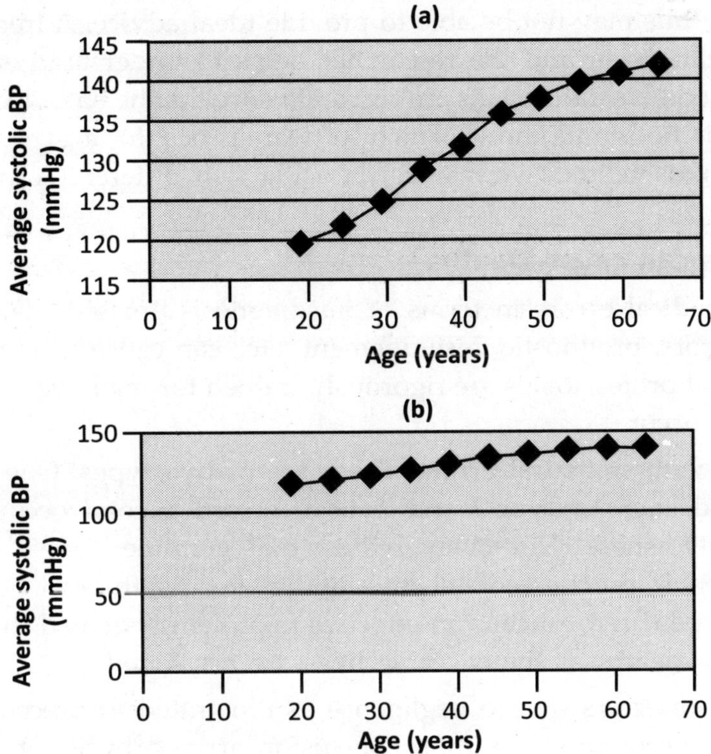

FIGURE 15-1: Same gradient shown as steep in Figure (a) and mild in Figure *(a)*

Data Dredging

All round availability of computers and software has made it easier to reanalyze the data after dropping some inconvenient observations. This misuse is called **data dredging**. Editors and reviewers would rarely be able to detect it because a finished report may not contain any such evidence.

Computer technology has surged ahead at a fast rate but the understanding of statistical methods among medical professionals has not kept that pace. As a result, some researchers use **black-box approach** to analyse the data. They just grind it through a statistical package without worrying about applicability of those methods to their data set. They may use regression where analysis of covariance is needed, use nonparametric methods where parametric methods are required, use nonlinear approach where linear is required, develop a model with eight variables where only four were enough, etc. Our advice is to involve a biostatistician right from the beginning and use his expertise where needed. He helps in improving both the design and analysis but cannot be expected to resurrect a badly designed study. Beware though that the biostatistician may not be able to fully comprehend the medical implications of the results and thus may not be able to provide ideal advice. A frequent interaction between the biostatistician and the researcher helps to understand each other better. Also realize that good biostatisticians are scarce. Ensure that he has adequate knowledge of the statistical methods and knows which software is best for a particular application. If time permits, cross-validate your analysis using two different software.

Statistical Errors can cause Deaths

You know that medical errors in terms of misdiagnosis, missed diagnosis, negligent care, treatment errors, prognostic misjudgement, etc., can cause misery and death. For this reason, medical professionals are rigorously trained for many years before licensed. Yet the errors do occur.

Compare this with statistical errors. These are of two types. One that are known and acknowledged such as Type I and Type II errors. Second occur due to lack of expertise and carelessness. Not many realize that genuine Type I error means an ineffective regimen is proclaimed effective and many deaths can occur due to this error. Similarly, Type II error means an effective treatment is denied to the patient, and this also can cause deaths as the saveable lives are not saved.

More serious are errors due to negligence as illustrated in preceding paragraphs. Uncounted deaths occur due to wrong conclusion arrived by inappropriate analysis and inaccurate data. These go unnoticed. This can happen with fully trained statistical professionals. But there are many researchers who have little or no expertise and training in statistical analysis. With the ready availability of statistical software, anybody and everybody think of him as statistical expert and do the analysis. Whereas medical professionals are trained for endless years in the business of saving lives and reducing suffering, neither statisticians nor medical researchers are trained with the same rigorousness. Medical biostatistics too is in the business of saving lives and reduce suffering although few realize this to be so. For details, see Indrayan (2018).

15.5 FINALLY YOURS

Medical researchers have a tall order of producing a worthwhile result when the uncertainties are galore, and many are insurmountable. The core of success lies in being able to identify the sources of uncertainties and using a methodology that can take care of most of them. Time spent in developing the proposal is well spent. Do not shy away from working hard at that stage. Constantly question about identification and management of medical uncertainties.

Credibility of research mostly depends on the sound methodology rather than on results. The objective is to reach to reliable and valid conclusions that are verifiable by repeating the investigation. Check that all known epistemic and aleatory uncertainties have been tackled, and the design has taken care of various sources of known biases. Those creep in despite the best design should be dealt with at the analysis stage. If this is achieved to the satisfaction of all concerned, consider that the research has attained high quality.

Do not succumb to the pressure of producing quantity at the expense of quality. A lengthy list of publications may give some mileage in the beginning but ultimately reputation cannot be built on shoddy research. Haste at the expense of care cannot pay. Most employments and promotions are based on, say, five best publications rather than the full list. In some instances, an extremely long list with low quality publications is disliked rather than appreciated. Thus, resist the temptation to publish or present a research that you know is substandard. Truth must be allowed to prevail by following ethical publication practices. A quality work gives immense satisfaction that a sloppy work cannot give.

In the end, we must emphasize that there is no alternative to common sense. Tools such as protocol, design, and statistical analyses are only aids to carry out research in a systematic manner. They must only complement the common sense and not replace it.

SUMMARY

Ethics is conforming to the standard of conduct. Much of medical research, particularly in India, lacks respect because of ethical deficiencies.

Your research report must contain not only truth but the whole truth. Do not delete inconvenient data or variables just to suit your hypothesis. Never ever try to make duplicate publication on the same data. This is easily detected even when cosmetic changes in the title or appearance are made.

Respect others' intellectual property as you would like yours. If you have to quote, cite reference and take permission for any reproduction.

Respect reviewers of the journals and try to accommodate their views as much as possible without sacrificing the integrity of your manuscript. Such reviews help to increase the quality of your paper.

Beware of statistical fallacies that can inadvertently enter your results. Whereas medical errors are known to cause misery and deaths, statistical errors too can cause deaths when inappropriate regimens are accepted, or appropriate regimens are denied for adoption.

REFERENCES

Altman DG, Bland JM. Measurement in medicine: the analysis of method comparison studies. The Statistician 1983;32:307-317.

Bland JM, Altman DG. Statistical methods for assessing agreement between two methods of clinical measurement. Lancet 1986;i:307-310.

BMJ. What we mean by "publication"? http://www.bmj.com/about_bmj/resources_authors/article-submission/what-we-mean-publication.

Cummings P, Rivara FP. Responding to reviewers' comments on submitted articles. Arch Pediatr Adolesc Med 2002;156:105-107.

Gold EB, Goldin SB. Epidemiology of and risk factors for pancreatic cancer. Surg Oncol Clin N Am 1998;7:67-91.

Gold EB. Epidemiology of and risk factors for pancreatic cancer. Surg Clin North Am 1995;75:819-843.

Hall GM (Editor). How to Write a Paper. Byword Publishers, 1996.

Indrayan A, Malhotra RK. Medical Biostatistics, 4th ed. CRC Press, 2018.

Indrayan A. Attack on statistical significance: A balanced approach for medical research. Indian J Med Res. 2020;151(4):275-278.

Indrayan A. Statistical fallacies & errors can also jeopardize life & health of many. Indian J Med Res. 2018;148(6):677-679.

Mathur VP, Sharma A, Dhillon JK, Kalra G. Moral philosophy of scholarly publications. Eur Sci Editing 2014;40:11-13

Patel SV, Hodge DO, Bourne WM. Corneal endothelium and posteoperative outcomes 15 years after penetrating keratoplasty. Trans Am Ophthalmol Soc 2004;102:57-65.

Patel SV, Hodge DO, Bouvne WM. Corneal endothelium and postoperative outcomes 15 years after penetrating keratoplasty. Am J Ophthalmol 2005;139:311-319.

Smith R. The Trouble with Medical Journals. Royal Society of Medicine Press, 2006.

Glossary of Methodological Terms

(Some of these terms have not occurred in the text)

In the explanation, the terms included in this Glossary are in italics. They can be referred within this Glossary. Some terms are explained in more detail and more succinctly here than in the text. For others, the explanation in the text is better.

Absolute risk — Same as *risk*. Contrast it with *relative risk*.

Absolute risk reduction — *Risk* difference between the control group and the intervention group.

Accuracy — Truthfulness or correctness of a particular value of a measurement to the reality. Age recorded as 7 years 4 months and 14 days is more accurate than recorded only as 7 years, although this additional accuracy may be redundant. Also BMI is more accurate measurement of overall obesity than ecto-, meso-, and endomorph categories.

Adaptive design – A research design that builds flexibility into itself at the time of designing. This flexibility could be adding or deleting a group, changing the outcome of interest, but most often, changing the sample size in each group when interim results indicate the need for doing so.

Addition rule (of probability) — The probability of occurrence of either of two or more *mutually exclusive events* is the sum of the probabilities of their individual occurrence.

Additive model — A model stating that combined effect of two or more factors is the sum total of their individual effects – valid when there is no *interaction.*

Adjusted correlation — Same as *partial correlation.*

Adjusted odds ratio — The odds ratio obtained after eliminating the effect of other *concomitant variables* that might be affecting the OR. This is generally obtained by including these concomitants in the *logistic regression.*

Adjusted rate — The net rate obtained after eliminating the effect of other *concomitants* that might be affecting the rate. This adjustment increases the comparability between rates in different segments of population.

Adjustment — A procedure by which the effect of structural differences in the two or more groups is minimised—thus, improving the comparability. Common methods of adjustment are *regression* and *standardisation*.

Aetiology diagram — A diagram that depicts the inter-relationship of various aetiological factors leading to the disease.

Aetiological factor — The characteristic that contributes to the occurrence of disease or a health condition. It may or may not be a causal factor.

Age-adjusted death rate — See *age standardisation*.

Age standardisation — A procedure of adjustment to remove the effect of differences in age composition of the groups to increase comparability. This adjustment is required when, for example, one group has older subjects than in the other and the outcomeof interest is death. For deaths, this is called age-adjusted death rate. This could be done by *direct standardisation* or *indirect standardisation*.

Age specific death rate — Number of deaths of specific age-group in one year per 1000 population of that age-group.

Agreement — When two procedures, two observers, or two sites, etc., tend to give the same result in each subject, they are said to be in agreement with one another. The extent of agreement is statistically measured by *Cohen's kappa*for qualitative data and by *limits of disagreement* for quantitative data.

Aleatory uncertainties — Uncertainties arising from variation in the factors internal to the system such as biological, psychological, and environmental. Contrast it with *epistemic uncertainties*.

Allocation bias — The systematic error in results arising from specific allocation of subjects to the test and control group, such as due to nonrandom allocation.

Alpha error — Same as *Type I error*.

Alpha error rate — The probability of *Type I error*.

Alpha level — Same as *significance level*.

Alternative hypothesis — A plausible hypothesis that is accepted when the *null hypothesis* is rejected.

Analysis — The process of going into the deep of a phenomenon, dataset, thought, etc., and looking at its various components.

Analysis bias (for data) — Gearing data analysis to support a particular hypothesis and ignoring aspects that contradict the hypothesis, e.g., using an inflated *P-value* for some statistical tests, using proportions when mean is appropriate, etc.

Analysis of Variance (ANOVA) — Breaking variance into its components such as within groups and between groups. This method is used in *regression analysis* and in various other situations but more commonly for comparing three or more means.

Analytical study — A study with the objective to identify the determinants or correlates of an outcome, such as *aetiological factors,* or to delineate their specific contribution to the outcome. See *observational study, experiment.*

ANCOVA — Acronym for ANalysisOfCOVAriance: a statistical procedure used when the dependent (or outcome) variable is quantitative, and the independent (or antecedents) variables are a mixture of quantitative and qualitative variables. This helps to adjust the result for confoundrs.

Anecdotal evidence — Incidental observation that lacks scientific scrutiny.

ANOVA — Acronym for *ANalysis Of VAriance:* A method for analysis of quantitative out-come when it is dependent on qualitative characteristics, particularly the groups of subjects.

Antagonism — The situation where combination of two or more factors depresses the intensity of outcome compared to the sum of their individual effects: a negative *interaction* effect.

Antecedent — A characteristic that precedes the outcome. It may or may not be (fully or partially) responsible for the outcome.

APACHEscore — Acronym for Acute Physiology and Chronic Health Evaluation: A scoring system that helps to assess the prognosis in case of critical condition of a patient. This is based on state of consciousness, reflexes, eye movements, blood pressure, etc.

Apgar score — Sum total of (0 to 2) scores assigned to each of heart rate, respiration, muscle tone, skin colour, and response to stimulation in a newborn. A low score such as less than 4 out of possible 10 is an indication of poor prognosis.

Area sampling — The method of sampling that uses geographical area as the unit. When the *sampling frame* of the *study units* is not available, area sampling can be used in a community-based study to select some areas by using a map, and then all the subjects in those selected areas can be included.

Area under the curve —The area under the *concentration curve* is used to assess the efficacy of a regimen and to compare the performance of two or more regimens.

Area under the ROC curve - The area from the *ROC curve* to the base: used as an indicator of the *validity* of a test in terms of *sensitivity* and *specificity* – can be used to compare performance of various medical tests.

Arithmetic mean — Same as *mean.*

Arm of a trial – The case (or test or intervention) group is one arm of a *trial* and the control group is the other arm. The test arm may have more than one regimen.

Ascertainment (or assessment) bias – Bias due to paying more attention to cases than controls in assessment, or giving more attention to specific outcomes of interest. Also when more accurate history is given by diseased then nondiseased, or when they are more cooperative than the others. Also when outcome of interest is morbidity but there are early deaths that no longer can contribute to morbidity. Assessment bias also occurs when the observer is able to establish more rapport with some respondents than others, e.g., due to cultural similarities. Diabetes and gallstone may appear to be associated because diabetics are regularly checked for gall stone and nondiabetics are not checked.

Association — The property of change in one qualitative factor being accompanied by the change in the other. This change can be causal, incidental, or due to a third intervening factor. The association can be full or partial of various degrees, and can be negative or positive.

Attack rate — New spells during a specified time interval (such as the period of an epidemic) as percentage of the total population at risk in the same interval. See *secondary attack rate.*

Attributable fraction (of risk) – The proportion of risk that can be validly assigned to a particular exposure.

Attributable risk – The additional *risk* that can be attributed to the presence of a risk factor. If risk of diabetes in those with both parents diabetics is 0.30 and in those with one parent diabetic is 0.25 (no other difference) then risk attributable to the diabetes in the second parent is 0.30 – 0.25 = 0.05.

Attribute – A qualitative characteristic.

Attrition – Loss of subjects during the course of the study. This can happen due to temporary unavailability, migration, refusal to participate, severe injury, or unrelated death.

Attrition bias – Systematic difference between the groups in the pattern of *attrition* of the subjects.

Auto-correlation – In a time series, the correlation of values with their preceding value. Auto-correlation of lag 2 is the correlation of values at time *t* with the values at time *t*–2. Correlation of monthly values such as of dengue cases with the cases 12 months ago will be auto-correlation of lag 12.

Balanced design – A design in which all groups have same number of subjects (equal *n*).

Bar diagram — A diagram appropriate for disjoint categories to show the number of subjects or mean or rates by bars of corresponding height.

Baseline data — The data that show the status of the subjects at the initial stage, generally at the time of beginning of the study. The baseline is used for evaluating whether any subsequent change is either due to intervention or some other factor.

Bayes' rule — The rule that converts probability of A given B to the inverse probability of B given A. Most common use of this in medicine is in obtaining the probability of disease given signs/symptoms by first obtaining the probability of signs/symptoms given disease, and in obtaining positive and negative *predictivities*on the basis of*sensitivity* and *specificity*. Both require some additional information.

Bed population ratio — Number of hospital beds per 1000 population or the number of people per bed in an area.

Before-after study — Assessing subjects before an intervention, and after the intervention to find changes—thus assessing the utility of the intervention without using a control group; also called a non-controlled trial. Part of the effect found in this study could be due to psychological factors (the placebo effect).

Bell-shaped distribution — Same as *Gaussian distribution.*

Berkson's bias — Occurs when the study is based on hospital cases but the exposure is such that increases the chance of admission. Thus hospital cases will have more exposure than hospital controls such as fracture in motor vehicle injury cases.

Beta error — Same as *Type II error.*

Beta error rate — The probability of *Type II error.*

Bias — A systematic error that can falsify or distort the results of a study. Contrast it with *random error*. Bias can arise due to a variety of sources:

(i) errors from faulty logic or incorrect premises;

(ii) nonrandom sample such as volunteers;

(iii) small sample that fails to represent the entire spectrum of subjects;

(iv) concomitant medication or concurrent disease that might seem unrelated;

(v) lack of matching in case and control groups;

(vi) unaccounted confounders;

(vii) wrong or blurred definitions that give room to assessor to use subjective interpretations;

(viii) errors in diagnostic or screening criteria;

(ix) insufficient instructions regarding what to do in unusual or unforeseen situations so that observers use their own discretion that can vary from observer to observer;

(x) more care in assessment of cases than controls;

(xi) differential recall of past events by cases and controls;

(xii) not being able to recall events of the past, or selective recall of serious events and not of mild events;

(xiii) differential compliance of regimen and instructions by cases and controls;

(xiv) suppression of information by patients because of stigma or otherwise;

(xv) premeditated response by a group after consulting each other;

(xvi) aberration in response due to unsuspecting event such as sudden illness or death in the family;

(xvii) deteriorated response in repeat testing due to fatigue in either observer or respondent, or improvement due to learning effect;

(xviii) some control subjects or some subjects in treatment group getting unaccounted therapy outside the study;

(xix) detection of some cases in early phase of the disease and some in the late phase;

(xx) prevalent cases could be more of those who survive for longer duration, and thus may be of better health;

(xxi) the study is based on hospital cases but the exposure is such that increases the chance of admission;

(xxii) observer able to establish rapport with some and not with other subjects due to cultural or other differences;

(xxiii) observer being more careful or attentive for specific type of subjects or special responses;

(xxiv) faulty instrument that gives erroneous readings;

(xxv) improper use of instrument;

(xxvi) systematic error in measurement, which could be either due to the instrument, or due to the observer;

(xxvii) subjects changing response just because they are being observed;

(xxviii) more accurate history by diseased than nondiseased or better cooperation by one group than the other;

(xxix) selective nonresponse;

(xxx) exclusion of some patients during mid-course if they develop an unrelated condition such as injury;

(xxxi) third party or natural introduction of unsuspecting new intervention among the respondents or their habitat that could alter the outcome;

(xxxii) contamination of controls by spill-over effect of cases when the two groups are not isolated;

(xxxiii) selective handling of outliers;

(xxxiv) digit preference;

(xxxv) gearing analysis to support a particular hypothesis;

(xxxvi) using differential *P*-values to support a particular view;

(xxxvii) lack of statistical power to detect medically important difference;

(xxxviii) incorrect interpretation of results;

(xxxix) preparing a report to support a particular view by suppressing some facts;

(xl) selective publication by journals; and

(xli) bias in presentation of results emphasizing one particular aspect and de-emphasizing the other.

The list is still not exhaustive. Some of these are explained in more detail in the text under the term for respective bias.

Bibliography — A list of *citations* of the related literature. This is different from the list of references because references are restricted to the literature actually cited in the text. Bibliography includes references to the other literature as well that are not cited but are related.

Bimodal distribution — A frequency distribution of a variable that has two modes; there will be two distinct peaks although one peak can be very small relative to the other. Age distribution of Hodgkin's disease has a smaller peak around 25 years and bigger peak at 55-60 years.

Binary variable — A characteristics that is assessed only in two categories such as ascites present or absent (or yes/no), or gender as male or female. A qualitative variable is mostly binary (in some cases could be *polytomous* and/or *ordinal*) but a quantitative variable can also be made binary by dividing into two categories such systolic blood pressure <140 and ≥ 140 mmHg.

Binomial distribution — The distribution that gives the probability of occurrence of x successes out of n where the probability for each is the same. If the chance of hypertension is the same 20% in all males of age 40-49 years, the probability that exactly 6 out of 10 coming to a clinic have hypertension is ${}^{10}C_6(0.20)^6(1 - 0.20)^{10-6}$ = 0.0055, by binomial distribution.

Bioequivalence — Similar course of the disease process in the two regimens under comparison: also evaluated in terms of comparable bioavailability of drug products, say, within 80% to 125% with respect to *area under the curve* and Cmax in the *concentration curve*. Also see *equivalence* and *therapeutic equivalence.*

Biological plausibility — Consistency with the present biological knowledge, which can be explained and not unknown.

BioSIS — The UK-based citation service that processes articles from a large number of journals, books, monographs, conference proceedings, etc., on all topics of biological sciences.

Biostatistics — The science dealing with medical uncertainties in a group of subjects—their identification, measurement, and control—leading to decision with less error.

Birth cohort — A cohort of people which is being followed since births – all births taking place at a specified time period.

Birth rate — Number of births in one year per 1000 population.

Biserial correlation — The correlation between a quantitative variable and a dichotomous variable such as between sex and creatinine level.

Bivariate analysis — A statistical analysis of data by considering two variables together, such as maternal haemoglobin level and birth-weight category, or alcohol intake and occurrence of liver cirrhosis. One or both variables can be either quantitative or qualitative.

Black box approach — Using computer to solve problems without understanding the implications of the underlying procedure.

Blinding — Keeping the experimental subject or the observer or both ignorant about which subject is in the case group and which in the control group in a trial.

Bonferroni procedure — When two or more comparisons or other statistical tests of hypothesis are done on the same set of data, the total probability of *alpha error* can increase much beyond the prefixed level such as 5%. In order to keep the error probability within the specified level α, the Bonferroni procedure is to do individual comparisons at α/k level of significance where k is the total number of comparisons. If $k = 4$ and $\alpha = 0.05$, each comparison is done at $0.05/4 = 0.0125$ level. This is a conservative procedure in the sense that the total level of significance is actually less than a.

Bootstrapping — A computer-based data resampling method that helps in estimating the sampling variance and other features — usually used when the features of the parent population are obscure or complex.

Box-and-whiskers plot — Same as *box plot*.

Box plot — A diagram that shows the median, the first and the third *quartile* (the difference between them giving an idea of dispersion, and the difference in distance from median on either side, of skewness), and the lowest and highest value after excluding outliers: a very effective method to present so many features of data in one diagram.

Bubble chart – A chart that depicts the varying quantity of a third variable with different values of two quantitative variable. How infant mortality (MR) changes as the time advances and income changes can be depicted by bubble chart where year can be on x-axis, income on y-axis and bubbles various sizes plotted as scatter: their size in proportion of the IMR.

Burden of disease – A composite measure of premature mortality from a disease and morbidity equated to mortality through a weighting system based on age, discounted duration, and severity of disease. Premature mortality is assessed in comparison to the mortality in the population with highest *life expectancy*.

Butterfly effect – An effect that blows out of proportion in course of time but starts from a minor effect. For example, a minor difference between two cancer patients at the time of detection may end up in quick proliferation in one and small changes in the other.

Capture-recapture method – A method to estimate the size of the population by the extent of overlap in two independent sources from the population. Under this method, one sample is taken and those with specified characteristics are marked. The entire sample is replaced back and allowed to randomly mix with the population. Now another sample is taken, and the number found with the mark are used to estimate the size of the population. This method is commonly used to estimate, say, tigers is the wild but is used in medicine to estimate the number of patients in a population when the patients go to two or more facilities for consultation.

Case – A person or unit of interest possessing a specified characteristic, such as a person with the disease or a family living in the conditions of interest.

Case-control study – Investigation of the antecedents in a group of cases and equivalent controls without introducing any intervention. The groups are defined on the basis of presence or absence of disease or any other outcome of interest. The logic of the design leads from effect to the cause. All case-control studies are inherently *retrospective*.

Case-fatality rate – The number of cases who die out of those who are suffering from a particular disease. This measures the *virulence* of the disease. Case-fatality in typhoid is low and high in tetanus. For chronic diseases such as cancers, the case-fatality may be 100% but measures such as 5-year death rate may be better indicators of the 'virulence' of such diseases.

Case group – The group of subjects that already has the disease or the condition under study.

Case-referent study – Same as *case-control study* but comparison is with some other disease and not placebo.

Caseseries — A specific group of patients with the disease of interest; generally consecutive cases reporting in a clinic or observed in a community. There is no control group in this set-up. Case series is one of the several methods of a *descriptive study*.

Case study — Study of one medically interesting individual, particularly regarding the *antecedent* and *outcome* factors as observed in that person.

Categorical data — All qualitative data are categorical. In addition, quantitative data are also summarized into categories. For example, for *smoking index* of 300 individuals, the table may have categories such as 0, 0.1-4.9, 5.0-9.9 and 10.0+. Sometimes such categories are used for analysis and inference purposes also.

Cause-effect relationship — *Statistically significant* dependence of an outcome on an antecedent so that any change in antecedent makes corresponding changes in the outcome when all confounders are absent. The relationship should also meet other criteria such as temporality, consistency and biological plausibility. See *necessary cause* and *sufficient cause.*

Cause-specific rate — The rate obtained when numerator is restricted to a particular cause (e.g., of morbidity or of mortality). Cause-specific death rate is the number of deaths due to a cause per thousand population. Sum of cause-specific death rates for all causes in the same as *crude death rate.*

Census — A *survey* of the entire population.

Centiles — Same as *percentiles*. See also *deciles, quartiles, tertiles.*

Central limit theorem — A statistical result that says that sum of a large number of values from any distribution tends to have a Gaussian distribution.

Central tendency — Among variations, there is still a tendency for a set of values to gather around a central value. Mean, median and mode are the popular measures of central tendency.

Chance — 1. Colloquial name for factors that are unknown or too complex to comprehend such as a collision occurring by chance.

2. Colloquial term for *probability.*

Chi-square test — A versatile statistical procedure that is used to test different types of hypothesis on proportions, such as equality, trend, and relationship.

Circular sampling — A systematic method of sampling that starts from any number and not necessarily from the beginning. Under this sampling, the (N + 1)th unit for selection is the first unit. This method removes some demerits of systematic sampling.

Citation — Identification data of a document containing the authors' name, title, publication name, volume, publication date, page numbers, etc.

Classification — Placing a unit to one of the two or more known classes or categories. Units within each category share some similarity among them, and units in different classes are dissimilar.

Clinical agreement — See *agreement*.

Clinical epidemiology — Application of principles of epidemiology to individual subjects, particularly to the patients.

Clinical equipoise — Genuine uncertainty among the experts about the relative merits of the regimens under trial: thus no research group is particularly disadvantaged.

Clinical significance — A situation where a result is capable of modifying the management of a patient.

Clinical thresholds (of normal range) — A range of values of a quantitative medical measurement in healthy subjects that has least overlap with the values found in diseased subjects so that the chance of misclassification is minimum. But the chance of error remains. For example, for blood pressure this is 140/90 mmHg.

Clinical trial — A medical experiment on human subjects, particularly in a clinic setup, such as to find *efficacy* and safety of a new therapeutic or diagnostic regimen.

Clinimetrics — Assigning scores to clinical entities for diagnostic or rating purposes—thus qualities are converted to quantities.

Close-ended question — A question for which list of possible answers is already provided and the respondent just ticks one or more of these answers.

Cluster — A group of subjects with some commonality—generally available in close proximity of time or space.

Cluster random sampling — Dividing the target population into *clusters* of specified size and selecting a few clusters by random method.

Cochrane Collaboration — An international organisation of producers and consumers of medical research that helps to clarify the research achievements, particularly health care interventions such as drugs, diet alteration and behaviour change. The focus is mostly on systematic reviews or correct *meta-analysis* of the relevant studies.

Cochrane Review — A review of trials, mostly based on *meta-analysis*, following specific guidelines of *Cochrane Collaboration*.

Coding — Assigning a numeric to a qualitative characteristic, such as code 1 for hypertension, code 2 for diabetes, code 3 for cancer, etc. Codes are not quantities, and care should be exercised that they are not used as quantities at the time of analysis. These are used only for convenience in data entry.

Coefficient of determination — The percentage of total variation in a variable explained by one or more of the others. In a *simple linear regression* setup, this is square of the correlation coefficient. In a *multiple linear regression* setup, this is square of the *multiple correlation coefficient*.

Coefficient of variation — Standard deviation divided by mean. This unit-free measure is used to compare dispersion of one variable with the other, such as dispersion of cholesterol level with dispersion of body temperature in a group of cases.

Cohen's kappa — For qualitative data, a measure of agreement in excess of chance between two or more observers, methods, sites, etc.

Cohort — A clearly defined person or a group of persons with some common feature, who are followed for an outcome in a specific period beginning from a defined common baseline: not necessarily beginning at the same time. A cohort of womentaking contraceptive pill may start from the day of first intake but it may include women starting in any chronological month of the year. See also *inception cohort*.

Cohort study — A prospective study of a *cohort* for a specified period, generally to observe the occurrence of an outcome of interest, and thereby determine the *incidence* and *risk*.

Collation of data — The process of rearranging the data into intelligible form so that either the conclusions can be drawn, or analysis can be done.

Community trial — Same as *field trial*.

Completely randomized design — A design under which the subjects are allocated completely at random to different groups with no consideration of any factor such as age and sex.

Compliance bias — Either higher noncompliance by treatment group relative to the control because of discomfort or poor intake of the drug, or better compliance by them because they are improving.

Concealment of allocation — The process of allocation of subjects to the groups that is impervious to any influence of the person making the allocation. Thus the group to which next subject will be allocated cannot be predicted. Among methods of such concealment are centralised randomisation without participation of the observer, coded and identically looking packing of the placebo and drug, and sequentially numbered opaque envelopes.

Concentration curve — Plot of quantitative response versus time such as of concentration of drug in body at different points of time after intake. This helps to find the *area under the curve* and the maximum concentration C_{max} and the time when the concentration is maximum T_{max}.

Conceptual bias — Errors arising from faulty logic or incorrect premises.

Concomitant variable — Same as *confounder*.

Concordance — Agreement or similarity between two individuals in a paired setup.

Concurrent validity — *Consistency* of response to two or more questions in the sense that they reflect the same pattern. For example, high calorie intake and low exercise together should correspond to greater obesity. Response to these three items should be consistent with one another.

Conditional probability — The probability of occurrence of an event such as disease when some a-priori information such as sign-symptoms are known: denoted by P(A/B) where after slash (/) sign is what is known a-priori.

Confidence bound — A one-sided *confidence interval.*

Confidence interval — The interval likely to contain the parameter value in repeated samples with a certain *confidence level.*

Confidence level — The degree of assurance that other studies of similar type will have the same result as obtained by the participants in the current study.

Conflict of interest — Personal, financial, or other interest of any investigator that could influence the finding or the interpretation.

Confidence limits — The upper and lower boundaries of a *confidence interval.*

Confounder — An extraneous factor that could be a full or partial explanation of the outcome of interest in addition to the factor under study so that its effect cannot be differentiated from the other: such as dietary factors when examining relationship between smoking and cervical cancer. Presence of unaccounted confounders decreases the *validity* of a study.

Confounder bias — Bias due to presence of one or more unaccounted *confounders.*

Consecutive sample — The sample of subjects where the enrolment is based on the sequence of their arrival, and none is excluded if eligible till the desired number is reached.

Consistency — Same as *reliability*.

CONSORT — Acronym for CONsolidated Standards Of Reporting of Trials: This provides guidelines on how a trial results should be reported.

Construct validity — The ability of a set of items or questions to assess a given theoretical concept. Suppose positive health is defined as the ability to withstand physical stress, and the intention is to measure it by excess in haemoglobin level, forced vital capacity, and pain bearing capacity. The ability to withstand stress is also separately measured by items such as lack of restriction in daily activity by injury or fever. The correspondence between these two assessments will indicate construct validity of the measurements. It is the agreement between the theoretical concept and the specific device used to measure that concept.

Content validity – Sufficiency or adequacy of the items or questions to measure a phenomenon. For example, spinal palpatory test may not have good content validity to identify spinal neuromusculoskeletal dysfunction. Content validity is judged by a panel of experts.

Contingency table – A table containing the number of subjects with different characteristics, which should be mutually exclusive and exhaustive, such as number of subjects with and without disease, and each with a positive or negative test. A contingency table is used to test if one characteristic is associated with the other.

Continuous variable – A variable that can theoretically have infinite number of possible values within a short range. Age is continuous since within 8 and 12, it can be 8.17, 10.874, 9.756 years, etc. Age can be measured in terms of days, hours and minutes, although practically there is no need to do this. Blood pressure is a continuous variable but measured in integers for convenience. Parity is not a continuous variable because there is no possibility of it being 2.75 or 1.6.

Control (group) – Used in two senses:

1. The group of subjects that do not receive the test regimen. They may receive placebo, or the existing standard regimen, or any other regimen that is appropriate for comparison.
2. The group without disease or without any other outcome of interest.

Control (programme) – A defined series of steps to reduce or eliminate a disease.

Control (statistical) – The statistical process of adjusting for any extraneous influence on the results.

Control (subject) – A person or unit of interest but not possessing the specified characteristic, such as a person not having the disease of interest, or a person being treated by regimen other than under test.

Controlled trial – A trial that compares intervention group to a control group: when not further qualified this generally indicates a trial with nonrandom or *quasi-random allocation* of subjects to the test and the control group.

Convenience sample – The group of subjects that are selected primarily because they were available at a convenient time or place. This is one of the several ways that a *purposive sample* can be drawn.

Convenience sampling– The selection of those subjects who are conveniently available.

Correlates – Factors that are related in some way to an outcome of interest. They may or may not be contributors to the outcome.

Correlation — The degree or strength of relationship between two quantitative variables. Loosely used for qualitative variables also. For *linear relationships,* it is measured by *Pearsonian correlation coefficient* that ranges from –1 to +1. A negative correlation means that increase in the value of one variable is accompanied by linear decrease in the other, and vice-versa. A positive correlation means that the two move together in the same direction. A correlation close to zero means that increase or decrease in one does not linearly affect the other. Correlation coefficient can be close to zero when a strong relationship is present but is nonlinear.

Correlation coefficient — See *Pearsonian correlation coefficient.* The other types of correlation are *Spearman's, multiple, partial,* etc.

Cost-benefit analysis — The assessment of benefit per unit of cost when both are measured in monetary units.

Cost-effectiveness analysis — The assessment of effectiveness (life saved, disability restricted, year of life gained, etc.) per unit of cost.

Covariance — A measure of how the product of two quantitative variables behave—used in calculating *correlation coefficient.*

Covariate — Same as *confounder*: generally used in a restrictive sense for quantitative variables only.

Cox regression — A type of *regression* that models logarithm of hazard ratio on the covariates that affect this ratio. Also see *proportional hazards model.*

Criterion standard — Same as *gold standard,* but a preferred term.

Criterion validity — Ability of a device to provide a measure that correlates or agrees with the criterion known to correctly measure the characteristic of interest.

Critical value (in the hypothesis testing) —The threshold value of the statistical test criterion such as c2, *t* and *F,* beyond which it is considered statistically significant.

Cross-over design — A design that stipulates that the same subjects will get the test and the control regimen after a washout period, but the sequence is randomised. Half the subjects get regimen A followed by B, and the other half B followed by A. Using same subjects for both the regimens reduces variability and thus also the level of uncertainty in the results.

Cross-product ratio — Same as *odds ratio.*

Cross-sectional study — An *analytical study* with a format that elicits information on the antecedents and the outcomes at the same time. Such a format is poor to investigate *cause-effect* type of relationship but is good to generate *hypothesis.*

Cross-tabulation — The process of obtaining the number of subjects of various types when divided by two characteristics simultaneously such as distribution of myocardial infarction cases by their lipoprotein(a) and homocysteine levels. In most cross-tabulations, these levels would be in categories such as 10.0–14.9, 15.0–19.9, etc.

c-statistic — A statistic that measures the area under an *ROC curve.*

Crude death rate — Total deaths in one year in a population divided by mid-year population.

Current Contents—The electronic database of table of contents and bibliographic citations from current issues of more than 7500 research journals in sciences, social sciences, arts, and humanities. This is updated every week.

Curve — Opposed to straight line, the curve depicts relationship that varies at different values of two variables. For example, one variable may increase for lower values of the other and then decrease for the higher values of the other. An example is the relationship between Glomerular Filtration Rate (GFR) in chronic renal failure cases and plasma creatinine level. As creatinine level reduces, GFR declines steeply in the beginning and then slowly.

Curvilinear relationship — A relationship that is depicted by a curve opposed to a line but can be converted to a line through some mathematical transformation.

Data — A set of observations, generally in numerical format but can be in text format also (plural of datum).

Database — A collection of items of data arranged in a predefined format, usually held on a computer.

Data cleaning — The process of correcting and deleting the incomplete or apparently wrong observations from the data set. Sometimes this may suggest a relook at the original source for finding the correct value.

Data dredging — Initially used for excessive analysis of data in search of new hypotheses, but now used for re-analysing data after deleting some inconvenient values so as to fit them into supporting a particular hypothesis—a very unfair practice that has now become so easy because of wide availability of computers.

Data editing — Same as *Data cleaning.*

Data Safety and Monitoring Board (DSMB) — An independent body of reputable persons who agree to monitor a research project regarding the integrity of data and adherence to protocol.

Death spectrum — Variety of causes of death: some people meet death slowly such as by cancer, and some sudden such as by myocardial infarction.

Deciles—Nine cut-points of values of a variable that divide the total number of subjects in ten equal parts: obtained after arranging the values in ascending order.

Decision analysis — The process of reaching to a decision after considering probabilities of various outcomes and value judgements regarding the *utility* of those outcomes. Decision analysis is considered a very effective method to take a valid decision under conditions of uncertainties.

Deduction method — The method of reaching to a conclusion for a particular individual on the basis of a known generalised result—from general to particular.

Degrees of freedom — The number of observations in a dataset that can freely vary once the parameters have been estimated. This concept is used in *chi-square, Student's t* and other statistical procedures since their distribution depends on degrees of freedom.

Definition bias — The bias due to

1. wrong or substandard definition such as of impotence on the basis of erectile dysfunction alone; or
2. blurred definition that gives room to assessor to use subjective interpretation such as blood pressure e"140/90 for hypertension without specifying what to do if systolic level is higher and diastolic is lower. Errors in diagnostic or screening criteria also come under this category.

Delphi method — A less scientific but quick method to arrive at a consensus among experts. In this method, the responses from a panel of experts are iteratively obtained that are progressively refined by reducing the options in successive rounds depending on what options are less preferred in the previous rounds.

Demography — The science that studies characteristics of a population such as age-sex distribution, urban-rural distribution, and trend over time.

Dependent variable — A variable that is sought to be explained by one or more of the other variables. The dependent variable is generally the *outcome* of interest whereas independent variables are the *antecedents*.

Descriptive analysis — Calculation of simple statistics such as mean, median, SD, number of subjects in different categories, etc.

Descriptive study — A study with the objective to delineate the distribution of disease or a health condition in a defined population, or to describe clinical features of specific kind of subjects. It also includes estimation of parameters such as mean and percentiles. This does not examine causality or aetiology. A descriptive study could be a *census*, a *sample survey* or a *case series*.

Design of experiments — See *experimental design*.

Design (of research) — The format of collection, compilation, and analysis of observations. See *descriptive study, analytical study*. Also see *sampling design*.

Design bias – A design of a study where the selection of subjects is not random, control group is not adequately matched, definitions of subjects of characteristics to be studied are loose, confounders are not properly accounted, etc.

Design effect – The effect on the *variance* of an estimate, and thus, on efficiency of a study, due to the *design* of the study, such as of *cluster random sampling* relative to the *simple random sampling*.

Determinant – A factor that is responsible, fully or partially, for an outcome.

Diagnostic score – A numerical score used as an aid in establishing diagnosis, such as thyroid scoring system to distinguish hypo-, eu- and hyperthyroidism based on the clinical assessment.

Diagnostic test – A criterion used for confirming the presence of disease or a condition. This should have high positive predictivity. The criterion could be a laboratory test, a radiological test, or a clinical observation.

Dichotomous variable – Same as *binary variable*.

Digit preference – Preference for certain digits such as 0 and 5. These digits become predominant in reporting and recording, and can affect the result.

Direct standardisation – A procedure of adjustment to bring the differential structure of two or more groups to a common (standard) base to increase their comparability: most commonly done for differential age structure that can easily affect mortality. In direct standardisation the observed subgroup specific rates are used on the standard group structure.

Disability-adjusted life expectancy – *Life expectancy* adjusted for equivalent life lost due to disability of varying degrees during the life time.

Disability-adjusted life years (DALYs) lost – The loss of years of life due to premature mortality compared to the population, with the highest *life expectancy* plus loss of equivalent years of life due to various disabilities of different severity and duration from morbidities or otherwise. This measures the *burden of disease* in a population. The disability arises from sickness from time to time.

Discrete variable – A variable that can take only finite, practically small, number of possible values. Parity for a woman is a discrete variable. Deaths in an area with population 200,000 is theoretically discrete but can be considered continuous for statistical purposes because it can take a large number of possible values.

Disease spectrum – Among many types of disease spectra, the one of special epidemiological interest is the proportion of population that is susceptible, proportion that has infection (apparent + inapparent), proportion that has disease, the proportion that has serious form of disease, and the proportion that die. Note that the subsequent proportion is nested in the preceding proportion. Disease spectrum helps to plan the research accordingly, and to take measures to control the disease.

Disease thresholds (of normal range) — The range of values of a quantitative measurement beyond which there is a considerable risk of presence of disease or occurrence of disease. The chance of *misclassification* remains in this threshold also as in any other such threshold.

Dispersion — The degree of variability or scatteredness of the values of a variable when measured for different subjects or at different times.

Dissertation — A detailed discourse or treatise on a particular topic providing it a new perspective: generally the written work submitted by a candidate for the award of a doctoral (PhD) degree.

Distal measures of health — The background characteristics that indirectly affect the health condition under consideration. Socioeconomic factors such as education, income and occupation make an impact on diet, hygiene and exercise that in turn affect the pathophysiological parameters, on the basis of which a condition is assessed. Thus socioeconomic are distal and pathophysiological parameters are *proximal measures*.

Distribution (statistical) — The pattern of values when obtained for a large number of subjects. For incubation period of AIDS, the distribution would tell us how many or what percentage of cases have incubation period between 5 and 6 years, what percentage between 6 and 7, 7 and 8, etc. Thus, the distribution tells what has been the dispersion and where has been the concentration of values. See *Gaussian distribution, skewed distribution*.

Dose-ranging trial — A *clinical trial* in which two or more doses of an agent are tested against each other to determine their relative *efficacy* and safety.

Dose-response relationship — Any kind of relationship between quantity of dose and the degree of response but generally indicating that higher the dose, higher the response, such as between smoking and lung cancer.

Double-blind trial — A *trial* in which neither the experimental subject nor the assessor knows that the subject has received the test regimen or the control regimen. This removes the possible bias in response and ascertainment.

Dropout — A subject who is initially enrolled for a study but whose subsequent measurements as required under the study protocol could not be obtained.

DSMB — Short for *Data Safety and Monitoring Board*.

Dunnett's test — A statistical test used to compare means in two or more test groups with the mean in the control group.

Ecological fallacy — The fallacy that arises from application of group-based result to individuals.

Ecological study — A study in which broad, between-population differences in patterns of exposure to a particular factor are compared with the incidence rates of the disease of interest in those populations.

Effectiveness — The extent to which a regimen is effective in meeting its objectives in actual field conditions or routine circumstances—generally measured in percentage. *Pragmatic trials, field trials* or *post-marketing surveillance* is used to evaluate effectiveness of drugs.

Effect size — Magnitude of effect of a factor on an outcome. This could be mean, proportion, difference, odds ratio, measure of association, etc. This could also be standardised mean difference between the test and control group obtained as the mean difference divided by its *standard error*.

Efficacy — The extent to which a regimen is effective in meeting its objectives in ideal conditions—generally measured in percentage. Generally *RCTs* are used to evaluate efficacy of a new regimen.

Efficiency — The frequency of desired outcome per unit of resource inputs such as time, money, and manpower. For example, coronary angiography using 4 French catheters may be more efficient procedure than 6 French catheters because of early ambulation without sacrificing the quality of images. Case-control studies are considered more efficient, particularly for rare outcomes, than prospective studies because of lower cost. Campaign against smoking may be more efficient for reducing deaths or for increasing life-years in a population than treatment of lung cancer patients.

Electronic resources — Resources available in electronic format such as patients' records in a hospital or other data on a computer. Compact Disk (CD), and particularly the world wide web (www). For literature, these include books, journals, reports, other documents, citation databases (e.g., PubMed) on internet, etc.

EMBase — Europe-based Excerpta Medica electronic dataset of more than 30 million records on medical and health research literature covering 9000 journals from more than 100 countries.

Empiricism — The process based on observations and evidence, opposed to theories.

Endogenous factor — A factor within the model under consideration. See also *exogenous factor.*

Endpoint — The outcome that a study is designed to assess. The examples are recovery, pain relief, duration of hospital stay, side-effects, disease progression, and death.

Epidemiology — The study of factors that affect distribution and determinants of disease or a health condition in a human population.

Epidemiologic consistency — The correspondence among the incidence, prevalence, duration of disease, mortality, etc., so that their underlying relationship is properly reflected.

Epistemic uncertainties — Uncertainties arising from limitation of knowledge and biases. Contrast it with *aleatory uncertainties*.

EQUATOR network — Acronym for Enhancing, QUality And Transparency Of health Research network that contains details of how various kinds of medical research should be reported.

Equipoise (subject) — Subjects are such that the outcome of test or control regimen is uncertain, i.e., the subjects are not chosen in a manner that they favour one regimen or the other—an ideal situation for conducting *RCTs* because either of the two regimens can be used without raising ethical issues, and the results would be more valid. Also see *clinical equipoise*.

Equipoise (clinical) — See *clinical equipoise*.

Equivalence — Difference between two or more groups or regimens by not more than a prespecified clinically irrelevant amount. Two regimens are considered *therapeutically equivalent* if their efficacy does not differ by more than a prespecified small amount. They are considered *bioequivalent* if the course of the disease or recovery in the two regimens is nearly the same. Therapeutic equivalence considers only the outcome whereas bioequivalence considers the entire course.

Equivalence trial – A clinical trial with the objective to examine the *equivalence* of two regimens.

ERMed– Short for Electronic Resources in Medicine: A database of literature (more than 1200 medical journals) being promoted by National Medical Library (India) for medical researchers in the country.

Error — See *bias, false positive, false negative, random error, Type I* and *Type II error.*

Error in research (honest, negligent and deliberate) — Honest error is absolutely unintentional that arises from limitation of knowledge, such as not taking care of unforeseen bias. Negligent error is gearing up investigations or findings to support a particular view neglecting the other evidence. Deliberate error is misconduct of plagiarism, reporting inflated sample size, cooking up the results, etc.

Ethics — See *medical ethics.*

Etiological factor — See *aetiological factor.*

Etiological diagram – A diagram that shows relationship between the antecedents and outcomes by arrows for direction of the effect. This generally includes the *distal* and *proximal* factors as well as *confounders.*

Evidence-based medicine – Using evidence as available in literature, in records, or in newly generated data, for managing patients after proper accounting of risks and benefits.

Evidence (levels of) – The strength or validity of evidence: a randomized double blind control trial is considered as the level-1 evidence as it is almost fool-proof when the trial is conducted with sufficient care. On the other hand, ecological studies provide evidence of poor qualify that can be easily refuted.

Exclusion criteria – The set of conditions presence of which will exclude an otherwise eligible subject from the study. Generally these conditions are indicative of severe form of disease or complications that render a subject unsuitable for that research. Exclusion criteria are part of the case definition that delineates the target population. The other part is *inclusion criteria.*

Exogenous factor – A factor that affects the outcome from outside and are not part of the model under consideration. See also *endogenous factor.*

Expectation of life – Same as *life expectancy*.

Experiment – A study of effect of intentionally introduced intervention or alteration of a factor, under controlled conditions. In medicine, the term is generally used for laboratory experiments. See *trial.*

Experimental design – The structure of an experiment in terms of inclusion and exclusion criteria for subjects, method of allocation of subjects to intervention or other groups, and number of subjects in various groups. Sometimes this also includes details of assessments, reliability and validity of tools and of measurements, etc.

Expert system (medical) – An intelligent computer aid to diagnosis, treatment, and prognosis. It is capable of storing all the information, and more importantly to selectively retrieve the relevant information as an aid to the physician, and is capable of suggesting a spectrum of diagnosis for the given set of complaints, examination results, laboratory findings, etc., and also suggests a possible line of treatment and the prognostic implications.

Explanatory model – A model that explains how an outcome might have occurred on the basis of other factors. The factors in this model must be biologically relevant. See also *predictive models.*

Explanatory trial – A trial done under near ideal conditions with practically no deviation. Contrast it with *pragmatic trial.*

Explanatory variable — Same as *independent variable* when used in an *explanatory model*.

Exploratory analysis — A method for examining the patterns and features of a dataset– generally based on graphical display.

Exploratory study — A small-scale study of relatively short duration, which is carried out to gain baseline knowledge about a problem for which little is known.

Exposure factors — The conditions to which a group is a suspected to have been exposed, which may alter the risk of the outcome of interest.

External validity — The generalisability of a result to those subjects that are not included in the study, i.e., the applicability of results to a larger population and not just to the study participants.

Face validity — The property of a measurement or an instrument to apparently look right or reasonable.

Factor — A characteristic that can, or suspected to, cause alteration in an outcome.

Factorial design — A design that includes all possible combinations of the *antecedent* factors under study. If there are three antecedent factors for visual acuity in adults—age in years as <40, 40–49 or 50+, gender as male or female, and haemoglobin level in g/dl as <10.0, 10.0–12.9, 13.0–14.9 or 15.0+ then a total of 3×2×4 = 24 combinations are required to be studied in a factorial experiment, and each combination must be tried on at least some subjects by design.

Fallacies — See *statistical fallacies*.

False negative — A person with disease classified as without disease. In place of disease, false negativity can be for any other *attribute*.

False positive — A person without disease classified as with disease. In place of disease, false positivity can be for any other *attribute*.

Field trial — An *experiment* on human subjects in a community, such as vitamin A supplementation to children less than 3 years for examining improvement in their nutrition status.

File-drawer effect — When a draft of a research paper is kept in a drawer for long time, many deficiencies are noted when taken out. These deficiencies occur either because of new learning about the topic or the language, or because of change in attitude towards the problem.

Fisher's exact test — A statistical test used for 2×2 contingency table to find statistically significant difference when the number of subjects is small. When the number is large, this is approximated by *chi-square*.

Fixed effects model — A statistical model that stipulates that the levels of factors under study are the only ones of interest. Contrast it with *random effects model.*

Focus group discussion — A popular method of qualitative studies in which a cross-section of informed group of people is encouraged to discuss a specific problem. When properly guided and annotated, such a discussion may lead to an effective solution.

Follow-up study — Same as *prospective study*.

Food-frequency questionnaire — A form which includes a list of 100-150 commonly consumed foods and provides space to fill-in how often each food is eaten. It may also include information on serving-size, variation by season, etc.

Force of mortality — *Hazard* of death at an instantaneous point of time. In an air accident, the force of mortality is exceedingly high. In home it is extremely low. The force of mortality in leukaemia is high relative to breast cancer.

Four-fold table — A *contingency table* with two rows and two columns so that the total number of cells is four (excluding the totals).

Frequency — Used in two senses:

1. Frequency of occurrence per unit of time (per month, per year, etc.).
2. Number of subjects with a particular characteristic or with values in a particular interval, such as how many cardiac patients have homocysteine level between 10 and 14 mmol/l.

Frequency curve — A graphical representation of the *frequency distribution* by a smooth curve.

Frequency distribution — A statistical distribution of subjects that displays the number of subjects with different levels of measurement, e.g., how many have diastolic blood pressure <70 mmHg, how many between 70–74, 75–79, etc.

Frequency matching — Same as *group matching*. See also *matching*.

Frequency polygon — A graphical representation of the *frequency distribution* by a polygon shape.

***F*-test** — A statistical procedure for *test of hypothesis* on equality of three or more means, and for other setups such as *regression*.

Gantt chart — A chart that shows *timeline* of a project: the duration and dates of beginning and ending its various phases.

Garbage-in, garbage-out syndrome — The tendency of getting poor output or poor outcome when the inputs or efforts are poor.

Gaussian distribution — Distribution of values of a quantitative variable such that they are symmetric with respect to a middle value with same mean, median and mode, and the frequencies taper-off rapidly in a particular manner on both sides—a bell-shaped distribution.

General linear model — A model that describes a *dependent variable* as a linear combination of a set of *independent variables* with two important features:

1. the variables could be qualitative or quantitative or mixture, and
2. the variables could be square, cube, logarithm, or any such function of the original variable.

ANOVA, ANCOVA and *regression* are special cases of general linear model.

Geometric mean — *n*th root of multiplication of *n* positive values.

g-index — A measure of quality of a researcher based on the papers cited by others. A g-index = 15 means that top cited 15 papers of a researcher have been cited at least 152 = 225 times. Also see *h-index*.

Gold standard — In medical assessment, a method, procedure, or a measurement with almost 100% sensitivity/specificity or 100% predictivity: an extremely difficult proposition to achieve. As a compromise, the best available is considered "gold", against which the newer tests are compared. Thus the better term is criterion standard. This need not be a single or simple procedure but could include follow-up of subjects or their surgery for presence of a disease.

Goodness of fit — How well the actual observations fit into a specified pattern. The goodness of fit is statistically tested mostly by *chi-square* method.

Group matching — See *matching*.

Group sequential design — A research design under which pre-decided number of cases are sequentially added in groups when so required to get convincing evidence of efficacy of the regimen or of its futility.

Grouped data — Quantitative values in categories such as age into 0–4, 5–9, 10–14, etc.

Guttman scale — A binary (yes/no) set of questions are on Guttman scale when they follow a hierarchy so that "yes" to any item implies that the answer is yes to all the subsequent (or preceding) items. Visual acuity follows Guttman scale since if one can read font size 24 from a distance of 14 inch this implies that she/he can read any bigger font size from the same distance.

Half-life - The duration at which time-dependent outcome or response is 50%. Half life of a drug could be few hours when its availability in the body is one-half of what was ingested.

Haphazard sampling — A mixture of *convenience, volunteer, snowball sampling,* etc., that does not follow any specific procedure.

Harmonic mean – Reciprocal of the mean of reciprocals.

Hawthorne effect – The tendency of subjects changing their response when they know that they are being observed. This can happen with the test group as well as the control group.

Hazard – The force of occurrence of an event at a (instantaneous) point of time, such as force of mortality or of morbidity when measured per unit of time. This could exceed one.

Hazard rate – The risk of occurrence of an event per unit of time. *Risk* by itself is not per unit of time.

Hazard ratio – The ratio of hazard rate of occurrence of an event per unit of time in one condition relative to another condition, such as hazard ratio of developing diabetes in obese to nonobese per year.

Health situation analysis – An exercise to assess the health condition of the people in an area, availability and utilization of health infrastructure, expenditure on health, etc.

Healthy life expectancy – The remaining portion of life at any age that would be spent without any morbidity. Life expectancy at age 40 may be 36 years but healthy life expectancy would be only 30 years if 6 years on average are spent in nonhealthy states as per the current pattern of morbidities.

Helsinki Declaration – A set of ethical rules to plan, conduct, and report a study on human subjects.

Herd immunity – When a large percentage of susceptibles such as more than 90% is immunized, the infection feels strangulated, as it is not able to find susceptibles in its proximity. Thus the infection fails to spread.

Heterogeneity – Variability or differentials among measurements, subjects, specimen, results, estimates, etc. Contrast it with *homogeneity*.

***h*-index** – A measure of quality of research of a person based on the citations of his work. An *h*-index = 12 means that his 12 papers have received at least 12 citations each. See also, *g-index*.

Histogram – A diagram showing the number or percentage of subjects with values in different intervals by means of contiguous bars: used only for quantitative variables.

Historical cohort – A *cohort* whose common baseline is in the past, and mostly outcomes too have already occurred. But the format of investigation still is from antecedent to outcome. The past is reconstructed mostly on the basis of records or recall.

Historical control — A *control group* or a subject for which information was collected earlier than the group being currently studied. This information can be biased because of changes over time in risk pattern, techniques, concepts, etc.

Homogeneity — Similarity among measurements, subjects, specimen, results, estimates, etc. Contrast it with *heterogeneity*.

Homoscedasticity — Equality of variance of values in different groups.

Hypothesis — A statement of belief that is made before the investigation regarding the status of parameters under study, including those that measure relationship. See *null hypothesis, alternative hypothesis*.

ICD — Short for *International Classification of Diseases*.

Iceberg phenomenon — When there are a large number of undetected cases for each detected case, such as in the case of HIV infection. Also, when one clinical case means many infected but inapparent cases such as for COVID-19.

Impact factor (of a journal) — The average number of times articles from a journal are cited by others in preceding two years — a service of the Institute for Scientific Information for journals covered by Citation Index.

Imputation — The process of filling in of plausible values for missing data.

IMRaD format — A format for writing research articles—Introduction, Material and Methods, Results, and Discussion.

Inception cohort — A cohort assembled at the beginning phase of disease or any other condition, which is followed up to examine its course or outcome.

Incidence — The number of cases newly occurring or arising over a defined period of time.

Incidence density — Same as *incidence* but now number of new spells are counted instead of persons newly affected. One person can have more than one spell of diseases such as diarrhoea and angina in a defined period.

Incidence rate — Incidence per unit of time and per unit of population. If incidence of benign prostatic hyperplasia in a population of 1,00,000 adults in six months is 16 cases, the incidence rate is 0.32 per 1000 adults per year. This can also be calculated per *person-year* or per 100 person-years, etc.

Incident cases — Same as *incidence*.

Inclusion criteria — The set of characteristics such as age, disease, and severity, which are necessary in a subject to be considered eligible for inclusion in the study. Some of these subjects may become ineligible when *exclusion criteria* are imposed. The inclusion and exclusion criteria together define the study subject and the *target population*.

Independent events — If occurrence of one event does not affect the occurrence of the other, they are called independent. Body temperature is generally independent of blood pressure levels but not of heart rate. Occurrence of typhoid is independent of colour blindness—none affects the other. Although, weight does not affect height in adults but they are not independent since height affects weight. Independence is both ways.

Independent variable — A variable that is used as an explanation of another variable. Independent variables are mostly the *antecedent factors* that affect or suspected to affect the (dependent) outcome. Some of these variables can be manipulated by the medical community to alter the outcome.

Index — A composite of two or more indicators, such as body mass index (BMI) for obesity that combines height and weight, and Indrayan's *smoking index* for a combination of age at initiation, duration, quantity and type of smoking, and the time elapsed since quitting by exsmokers.

Index case — An affected person who might affect others also. In the case of infection, the infected person is an index case who can spread the disease. When a new person is infected, he can be an index case for other susceptibles.

Indicator — A single measurement that indicates the existence or magnitude of a condition. Signs-symptoms are indicators of a disease, smoking an indicator of lung cancer risk, and Infant Mortality Rate (IMR) is an indicator of mortality in infancy. Contrast it with an *index*, which is obtained by combining two or more indicators.

Indirect standardisation — Removing the effect of differential structure of the group by using standard subgroup specific rates on two or more groups.

Indirectly standardised death rate — For age, same age-specific death rates are used on the observed age-structure of two or more groups to recalculate the death rate. These (called, standard) age-specific death rates are chosen by the researcher. Age is the most frequent factor for standardisation but similar standardisation can be done for any factor. Indirect standardization is used when observed specific rates are unreliable due to small numbers, or are not available.

Indrayan's smoking index — A summary measure of the burden of smoking in a person taking several aspects into consideration: (i) age at start, (ii) number of cigarettes/bidi/cigars smoked per day and duration of each, (iii) active and passive smoking, and (iv) time elapsed since cessation of smoking if stopped.

Induction — The method of reaching to a generalized conclusion after compiling the individual cases—from particular to general.

Infectiousness — The property of a disease to be able to infect *susceptibles* on exposure: but generally used to measure how many can be infected. COVID-19 is a highly infectious disease since an exposed susceptible is very likely to catch the infection.

Infectivity — The proportion actually infected out of those exposed.

Infographics — Representation of multiple graphs and related text into one panel.

Information bias — Suppression of some information by some subjects because of stigma or any other reason. Also loosely used for any type of bias in the data.

Informed consent — Agreement by a subject to participate in a research or some such endeavour after he is fully explained the favourable and adverse implications of participation.

Instruction bias — Use of varying individual discretion to resolve doubtful and unforeseen situations when the instructions are not complete, or not properly understood.

Instrument bias — A systematic error in an instrument to consistently give either lower or higher values than actual. Presence of air bubble in mercury column of a sphygmomanometer makes the instrument biased. Improper use of an instrument can also cause this bias.

Intention-to-treat analysis — Analysis that includes *dropouts* or other subjects with incomplete data or those who had to be changed from one therapy to the other due to developing a medical complication assuming worst or average scenario for them: all subjects continue to be considered in the group to which they were originally assigned.

Interaction — Simultaneous presence of two or more antecedent factors affecting the outcome either negatively or positively so that the net effect is not the same as the sum of their individual effects. It is called *antagonism* when the interaction effect is negative and called *synergism* when this is positive. But there could be other interactions that are not classifiable into any of these two categories.

Internal consistency — Mostly, consistency within the set of actual observations. One observation should be consistent with the other, or one variable should be consistent with the other. If systolic blood pressure of a person is 110 mmHg and the diastolic blood pressure is 95 mmHg then they are inconsistent unless there are specific reasons for such disparate readings. At the group level, HIV prevalence should be higher among those practicing multipartner sex. If the prevalence in this group is lower than those with single partner then this is inconsistent, and raises doubts about internal validity of data. If a study shows lower morbidity after exposure to a risk factor but lower mortality without the risk then this also may be internally inconsistent.

Internal validity (of a study) — When the biases are sufficiently under control so that the difference in the outcomes among groups can be legitimately ascribed to the hypothesized factor under investigation. Thus the results hold true at least for the subjects included in the study. An internally valid study may or may not be externally valid. There are situations when a sample provides excellent results for itself but fails when used on another sample from the same *target population*.

International Classification of Diseases (ICD) — A system of classification of diseases, injuries and causes of death into relevant groups, and assigning code to each condition, so as to promote uniformity and comparability across health care establishments in various countries. The ICD is revised every 10 years by the World Health Organisation to incorporate new diseases and new understandings.

Interpretation bias — Incorrect interpretation of results, either knowingly to support a particular hypothesis, or unknowingly due to carelessness.

Interval estimation — The process of assigning a range of values to a parameter within which it is expected to lie in repeated studies of that type.

Intervention study — A study of the impact of an intentionally introduced intervention on a predefined outcome. *Experiments* and *trials* are intervention studies.

Interviewer bias — Greater attention paid by interviewers to certain type of subjects or certain responses, relative to the others—thus introducing bias in the recorded responses.

Inter-observer variability — The variation between observers that occurs when the same measurement on the same subject is taken by different observers. A high inter-observer variability indicates poor *reliability* of the measurement.

Intra-class correlation — The *correlation* among same quantitative measurements within the same subjects or such other units at different times, by different observers, by different methods, etc.

Intra-observer variability — The variation that occurs when a measurement is taken repeatedly by the same observer. This indicates poor *reliability* of that observer.

Inter-rater reliability— The extent of agreement between the measurements obtained by different raters when they use the same measuring device on the same group of subjects.

Inverse probability — The conditional probability P(B/A) compared to P(A/B): often used to find predictivities P(D+/T+) and P(D–/T–) using sensitivity P(T+/D+) and specificity P(T–/D–) of a test, where D and T are for disease and test, respectively.

Item analysis — A set of techniques for assessing the efficiency of items of a test for properly discriminating between the good and not-so-good outcomes.

Kaplan-Meir method — The method of *survival analysis* that is used when the exact survival duration is assessed—thus these durations are not fixed time intervals.

Kappa — A measure of agreement in excess of chance in qualitative data; used for assessing *inter-rater reliability* and for other such agreements.

Keywords — The set of words that describes the essential features of a study. These words are used for indexing purposes so that the article is quickly retrieved for that category.

Kuskal-Wallis test — A *nonparametric test* for comparing *central tendency* in three or more groups.

Lead-time bias — Can occur when some subjects under study are enrolled in early phase of the disease and some in late phase of the disease. This may apparently show that early detected cases have higher duration of survival without any real prolongation of life.

Left-skewed distribution — See *skewed distribution*.

Length bias — The bias due to inclusion of disproportionately more cases with longer survival time in one group than the other: thus cases that show rapid progression of disease are not well represented.

Level of significance — The maximum tolerable probability of *Type I error* that is fixed in advance, such as 5%: denoted by a. In statistical terms, this is the agreed tolerated threshold of probability of wrongly rejecting a true null hypothesis.

Life expectancy — The average number of years a person is expected to live as per the current pattern of mortality. It can be calculated 'at birth' or at any other age. A life expectancy of 36 years at age 40 means that the average life span after the age 40 years is 36 years in that community. In this population, life expectancy at birth could be only 71 years. Life expectancy is a mortality indicator measured in terms of survival duration.

Life table — A summary of the death and survival pattern of a group of people at different ages—generally for the entire population of an area but can be used for patients of a particular disease also.

Life table method — The method of *survival analysis* that is used when the survival is assessed at fixed time intervals, such as weeks, months, or years. The time intervals are fixed in advance.

Likelihood ratio — Ratio of positivity of a test in the cases with disease and the positivity in those without disease. Positive likelihood ratio measures the increase in odds of disease when the test result is positive, and negative likelihood ratio measures the decrease in odds of disease when the test result is negative.

Likert scale — A system for obtaining the response to a question by the extent of agreement with a declarative statement. For example, the statement could be "I am happy with the nursing services in this hospital" and the choices are strongly disagree, disagree, indifferent, agree and strongly agree.

Limits of disagreement — A procedure for measuring extent of disagreement between two quantitative measurements obtained by two methods, two laboratories, two sites, etc., on the same subjects. These limits are obtained as (mean of differences) ± 2(SD of differences). If these limits are far too wide that can change clinical assessment, the disagreement is considered beyond clinical tolerance.

Line diagram — A diagram showing the trend by lines.

Linear regression — See *linear relationship*.

Linear relationship — A relationship that moves in a line with either positive or negative slope. The essential feature of a linear relationship is that one variable changes exactly by same amount when the other changes by one unit. If systolic blood pressure rises by ½ mmHg per year of age over the entire adult age from 20 to 59 years, the relationship is linear in this age-interval. Linearity can also include many variables. See *multiple linear regression,* also *curvilinear relationship*.

Logarithmic scale — A scale that compresses large and extremely large values to relatively small values: log 10 is 1, log 100 is 2, log 1000 is 3, etc.

Logistic regression — The regression where the dependent variable is the *odds* of occurrence of an event. The independent variables may be qualitative or quantitative. This regression is based on a specific mathematical form, called logistic model.

Longitudinal study — A study where the same set of individuals is periodically assessed for one or more defined outcomes.

Mann-Whitney test — A *nonparametric test* for comparing *central tendency* in two groups: analogous to *t-test* for Gaussian data. Gives exactly the same result as *Wilcoxon test*.

Mantel-Haenszel procedure — A statistical procedure for *stratified analysis* of qualitative data that combines evidence from two or more inter-related *contingency tables*.

Masking — Whereas the term blinding is used for the subjects and investigators, masking is for the regimen and the procedures. They are packaged or administered in a manner that they look similar.

Master chart — An arrangement of data that prepares one record for each subject: thus data available in several pages of questionnaire/schedule are converted to one line in, say, Excel software. This helps to get full view of the data in one shot.

Matching — Deliberate selection of control subjects with the same characteristics as the cases except for the disease or the condition under study. This increases the comparability. In practice only a few characteristics can be matched. Mostly it is one-to-one matching, which is called pair-matching, but sometimes can be group matching also. In the former, each control is matched with one case, and in the latter one group is matched with the other on average or for the pattern on the whole.

Mathematical model — An equation that expresses an outcome in terms of set of antecedents. This necessarily is a simple representation of a complex process. See also *model.*

McNemar test — A chi-square test used for paired qualitative data, e.g., same subjects tested by histology and Polymerase Chain Reaction (PCR) for extrapulmonary tuberculosis. McNemar test will reveal whether histology and PCR significantly disagree or not.

Mean — The average.

Measurement bias — Systematic error in measurement. This could be either due to faulty instrument, or due to carelessness of the observer.

Measures of association — The parameters that quantify the degree of association between two or more qualitative factors. Chi-square based measures are (i) phi coefficient, (ii) Cramer's V, and (iii) contingency coefficient. More useful measures are (i) proportional reduction in error, and (ii) relative risk or odds ratio. For data on *ordinal scale,* these are Kendall is tau, Somer's*d* and Goodman-Kruskal gamma.

Median — The most middle value obtained after arranging values in increasing or decreasing order. Median seeks to divide the group in two equal halves, each with $n/2$ individuals. Sometimes in practice exactly equal halves are not possible, and they are divided into nearly equal halves.

Mediators and moderators — Those extraneous factors that can alter the nature and extent of a relationship. Mediators are those that emerge after the cause starts to operate and moderators are those that are present before the cause starts to operate.

Medical decision process — The process of taking decisions regarding diagnosis, treating or not treating a patient, what treatment to prescribe, when to stop, etc., after considering the chances of success of various alternatives and their respective utility in terms of likely outcome.

Medical ethics — The discipline that considers individual patient's welfare above everything else—thus puts restrictions on how research involving human subjects should be done. Sometimes animal experimentation is also included in its domain. See *Helsinki Declaration.*

Medically significant — A result that is capable of modifying the management of any aspect of health or disease.

Medical uncertainties — Uncertainties in medical measurements and outcomes due to various sources of variation, and other factors such as lack of knowledge, poor compliance, incomplete information on the patient, etc. These can be diagnostic, treatment, prognostic, predictive, or other types of uncertainties. See *aleatory uncertainties, epistemic uncertainties.*

MedLine — An electronic database of citations from more than 5000 medical journals published in different languages in different parts of the world. This is the most useful resource of medical research literature, and the dominant part of PubMed.

Memory lapse — See *recall bias.*

MeSH — Medical Subject Heading: an important resource to search articles in *MedLine*. This reduces problems arising from, e.g., British and American spellings, and has a tree structure that branches off into a series of progressively narrower terms.

Meta-analysis — A procedure of combining evidence in different reports on the same aspect. If different trials on the same regimen report varying efficacy, they can be combined to come to a unified conclusion, which may command substantially more confidence than result of any one of the individual trials.

Metric scale — Measurement in terms of numerics such as blood glucose and cholesterol level. Contrast it with measurement in terms of attributes such as gender and signs-symptoms. Metric scale gives rise to quantitative data.

Mid-course bias — The bias arising during the course of the study. Some patients who develop conditions unrelated to the one under investigation, such as injury, and have to be excluded. Some may have to be excluded because of related but serious condition requiring special care. In a field trial, this bias can occur when a new health facility or a new health problem starts in the study area that was not visualised earlier, and has potential to affect the results.

Misclassification — Classifying diseased as healthy (or nondiseased) or nondiseased as diseased. The first could be called *missed diagnosis* and the second as *misdiagnosis*. In place of healthy/diseased this could be any other categorization.

Misdiagnosis — Diagnosing a person as suffering from a particular disease when he does not have that disease (the person can have any other disease).

Missed diagnosis — Not being able to detect a particular disease in a person when it is present.

Mode — The most commonly occurring value, i.e., a value seen in highest number of subjects.

Model — A simplified version of a complex process. A model could be mathematical, graphical, structural, etc.

MOOSE statement — Guidelines for reporting of meta-analysis and systematic reviews of observational studies.

Morbidity — Any aberration in health—can be measured in a person by frequency, severity, and duration of illness, and in a community by incidence, prevalence, severity pattern, and duration distribution.

Multicentric study — A study conducted at different locations with a common *protocol*.

Multicolinearity— Existence of high correlation between two or more *independent variables* in a *regression analysis* setup.

Multifactorial aetiology — Occurrence of disease depending on multiple factors: hypertension is a univariate disease because the diagnosis depends entirely on blood pressure level, but it has multifactorial aetiology since its occurrence depends on heredity factors, life stress, diet, obesity, etc. Malaria has one-factor aetiology.

Multiple comparisons — Several comparisons based on the same data. If each comparison is statistically done with 0.05 *level of significance*, the total probability of *Type I error* can be enormously large. To keep this within the specified level, statistical procedures such as *Tukey*, *Bonferroni* and *Dunnett* are used for comparison of group means.

Multiple controls — More than one control subject for each case. In a case-control setup, sometimes it is easier to enrol controls than cases. The reliability of the results can be increased in this situation by enrolling 2 or 3 or even 4 controls per case.

Multiple correlation coefficient — The degree of *linear relationship* of one quantitative variable with two or more simultaneously considered *quantitative variables*.

Multiple linear regression — A *regression* in which a *dependent variable* is sought to be explained by linear combination of more than one *independent variables*: such as regression of systolic blood pressure on age, obesity, and socio-economic status. For one dependent and one independent variable, see *simple linear regression*.

Multiple regression — A *regression* that expresses the nature of relationship of one (dependent) variable on two or more of the other (independent) variables. This could be linear or nonlinear.

Multiple responses — More than one response to one question or one item, such as two or more complaints of a patient at the same time, or listing of two or more sources of infection when asked about HIV.

Multiplication rule (of probability) — The probability of joint occurrence of two or more *independent events* is the multiplication of their individual probabilities.

Multistage random sampling — The process of sampling where a subset is chosen at *random* from units at different stages. First stage units can be cities, second stage hospitals (within chosen cities), third stage wards (within chosen hospitals) and fourth stage patients (within chosen wards).

Multivariate analysis — A set of statistical procedures that considers several variables together for drawing a conclusion. If the variables are inter-related, as they would in most situations, the results of multivariate analysis could be very different from separate *univariate analyses*.

Multivariate diagnosis — The diagnosis that depends on a multitude of measurements. The diagnosis of liver cirrhosis depends on oedema, ascites, spider naevi on the chest, oesophageal varices, gastric ulcer, liver function test results, etc., whereas the diagnosis of diabetes mellitus depends only on blood glucose level. The former is a multivariate diagnosis and the latter is univariate.

Multivariate setup — A situation where several variables are considered simultaneously.

Mutually exclusive and exhaustive events — The set of events wherein only one can occur at a point of time. Blood group of a patient would either be O, or A, or B or AB. These are mutually exclusive. Signs-symptoms such as pain, diarrhoea and vomiting are not mutually exclusive—they can occur together in a patient. Exhaustive means that one of these events must occur and nothing is left out. Blood groups O, A, B, and AB are exhaustive also as the blood group cannot be other than these.

Natural experiments — Intervention by nature opposed to interventions by humans, earthquakes, iodine deficiency in water and climate are the examples that can modify the outcome.

Necessary cause — A cause that must be present to change the outcome. Exposure to an infection such as coronavirus is necessary for it to produce that particular disease but not sufficient since in some cases infection can remain subclinical and may not produce the disease. Hypertension is not a necessary cause of stroke (neither it is sufficient). See *sufficient cause*.

Negative association — Presence of one factor associated with absence of the other, and vice-versa, in more subjects than expected by chance.

Negative correlation — Higher values of one variable generally accompanied by lower values of the other, and vice-versa, i.e., the two variables tend to move in quantitatively reverse direction such as age and visual acuity.

Negative predictivity - Short for 'predictive value of a negative test'. This is the probability that a person with negative test really turns out to be free from the disease. Since a test is used only on suspected cases, the predictivity should be evaluated on the basis of suspected cases only.

Negative trial – A *trial* that reports that difference between the test and control regimens is not statistically significant, i.e., the test regimen is not found effective.

Nested case-control study – A *case-control study* where cases are identified through a *prospective study.* Controls may or may not be from the prospective study.

N-of-1 trial – A trial on one patient who undergoes repeated pairs of treatment periods such that he gets experimental treatment one period and the control therapy the other period. The sequence can be randomised. The patient and the physician can be blinded regarding the sequence. Treatment periods are replicated until a result one way or the other is obtained.

Nominal scale – Assessment of a characteristic in terms of names only. Blood group is on a nominal scale since O, A, B and AB are just names with no order or no grading among them. The other type of scale for qualitative variable is *ordinal* where grading is present such as hypotensive, normotensive, probably hypertensive and definitely hypertensive.

Nomogram – A collection of inter-related lines or curves such that the corresponding values can be read by using straight-edged ruler put across those lines or curves.

Noninferiority trial – A *trial* to examine if one regimen is not inferior to the standard regimen by more than clinically unimportant margin.

Nonlinear relationship – A relationship that is characterised by a curve instead of a line. Oestrogen level in a woman has a cyclic variation over menstrual periods, and thus the relationship is nonlinear. Many organisms multiply exponentially as the days after exposure pass, and not linearly. COVID-19cases in different countries increased in a nonlinear fashion.

Nonparametric test – A statistical *test of hypothesis* that does not focus on a parameter such as mean. This does not require *Gaussian* or any other specific form of distribution of the variable. The usual tests such as *t* and *F* require Gaussianity but *chi-square* is nonparametric. Other popular nonparametric tests are *Mann-Whitney* (or *Wilcoxon*), *Kruskal-Wallis*, and *Friedman*. These are generally based on ranks rather than the exact values.

Nonrandom sample – Same as *purposive sample.* Can include volunteers, referred cases, case series, convenience sample, etc.

Nonrandomised control trial – A trial in which the subjects are assigned to the case group and the control group as per the convenience. Contrast it with *RCT*.

Nonresponse – Not being to able to collect full or partial information on subjects once they are included in a study. This can happen due to unrelated death, injury, moving out of the area, left against medical advice, refusal to cooperate, etc.

Nonsampling errors — Opposed to *sampling errors*, nonsampling errors arise mostly due to lack of planning or due to lack of knowledge. The examples are presence of *confounders, nonresponse*, partial compliance, biased sample, inadequate measurement, etc.

Nonsense correlation — A correlation between two variables that incidentally occurs because each is related to a third irrelevant variable. Such correlation has no biological plausibility. For example, there might be a correlation between births in India and temperature in Boston, both of which rise in the months of August and September each year.

Normal deviate — The difference of a value from its mean when expressed in SD units, such as LDL cholesterol in a patient being more than 1.25*SD away from the mean in healthy subjects. Normal deviate is 1.25 in this example. Compared to the absolute difference, this deviate gives a more realistic assessment of how far the value is from mean. Generally, the same as *z-score*.

Normal distribution — Same as *Gaussian distribution*.

Normalisation (of variables) — Standardisation of values to (0,1) scale with minimum getting a zero value and the maximum getting a value one. The others get proportional values.

Normal level — A level generally seen in healthy individuals. This is not necessarily ideal or optimal. Normal level may be different for children than for adults, or different for males than for females, etc.

Normal range — The range of values (of a quantitative medical measurement), which is generally seen in healthy individuals in a population or its specified segment.

Nuisance variable — A variable not of interest but interfering and spoiling the picture.

Null hypothesis — A *hypothesis* that says that there is no or specified difference, or that asserts the existing knowledge, and is tested for refutation by the study.

Number Needed to Treat (NNT) — The average number of subjects that must be treated to get one favourable outcome or to prevent one adverse outcome. If improved blood pressure control of 15 subjects is required for 10 years to prevent one death from myocardial infarction, then NNT for this outcome is 15 subjects for 10 years. Mathematically, this is reciprocal of *absolute risk reduction.*

Observational study — A study based on observation of the natural occurrences (no intervention). See *case-control study, cross-sectional study, prospective study,*

Observer bias — Observer being more careful or attentive to specific type of patients or particular responses.

Odds — The chance or frequency of occurrence or presence of a characteristic relative to its non-occurrence or absence. If the chance of occurrence is 75%, the odds are 3:1. Generally calculated for presence of antecedent factors.

Odds ratio — The ratio of *odds* in one group to the odds in the other (generally the control group).

One-sided alternative — A directional alternative hypothesis in the sense of asserting that the value can be only either more than the null value or less than the null value. Contrast it with the *two-sided alternative.*

One-tailed test — While testing equality of two groups, it is sometimes not known beforehand that which group could be better (or worse). For example, this happens when a test regimen is being compared with the existing regimen. This requires a two-tailed test. However, while comparing a test regimen with placebo, if there is an assurance that test regimen cannot be worse than placebo, one-tailed test is used.

One-to-one matching — See *matching*.

One-way classification — The division of subjects of interest by only one characteristic, such as dividing cases of bronchial asthma by their smoking status only.

One-way design — A study that is planned to investigate the effect of levels of only one factor. The levels could be two such as presence and absence, or more than two such as none, mild, moderate, and serious.

Open-ended question — A question whose answer is allowed to be recorded in verbatim as given by the respondent. Contrast it with a *close-ended question* that provides a list of possible answers.

Open trial — Nonblind trial where the participants and the assessors know what treatment was given to whom.

Ordinal association – Association between two ordinal characteristics such as severity of disease and socio-economic status. This is measured by Kendall's tau, Somer'*sd* or Goodman-Kruskal gamma.

Ordinal scale — A scale that measures a *polytomous* characteristic in a defined order, such as severity of disease into mild, moderate, serious, and critical. The 'distance' between mild and moderate is undefined. Division of blood group into O, A, B, and AB is polytomous but not ordinal since these blood groups do not have any order—none is better or worse than the other.

Outcome — A disease or a health condition of interest including any change in health status that may occur after exposure to antecedents or interventions. It may or may not be a result of the antecedents.

Outlier – A value that is far away from the other values. If duration of hospital stay after a cholecystectomy is 2, 3 or 4 days for most patients but happens to be 14 days for one patient because of complications, this value of 14 days is an outlier.

Outlier bias – Differential management of different *outliers*: e.g., considering some extreme value as outlier and not others, or not ignoring outliers if they support a particular hypothesis.

Over matching – Matching for confounders that affect both the outcome as well as the risk factors. Such matching can produce biased results.

Pair-matching – See *matching*.

Paradigm – A system, a pattern of thought, or a model regarding a phenomenon.

Parallel control group – Opposed to the treatment group that receives regimen under test, parallel control group is another group of subjects that receives either placebo or an existing regimen. Contrast it with before-after study where there is no separate (parallel) control group.

Parameter – A summary measure for any characteristic in the *target population*, such as percentage of cirrhosis patients with high aspartate aminotransferase, or rate of increase of systolic blood pressure in healthy subjects per year of age. The parameter pertains to the entire population of interest and not to the sample.

Parsimonious model – A *model* containing small number of factors yet providing adequate explanation.

Partial correlation – The *correlation* between two quantitative measurements when third or other measurements affecting them are considered fixed, and thus their effect is eliminated. Generally considers only the linear relationship.

Pathogenicity – The ability to produce the clinical manifestation of disease in an infected person. Measles is not only infectious but also highly pathogenic—the disease appears in most susceptibles when infected. Generally measured by the percentage of infected who develop the disease. Tuberculosis is not a highly pathogenic disease.

Pearsonian correlation coefficient – A measure of the degree of *linear relationship* between two quantitative variables. This ranges from –1 to +1 with zero in between indicating no linear relationship. A negative correlation means that increase in one is accompanied by decrease in the other or vice-versa, whereas a positive correlation means that both increase or decrease together at least to some extent.

Peer review – A refereeing process of a research proposal, article, thesis, etc., by expert colleagues for technical merit.

Percentiles – Ninetynine cut-points of a quantitative variable that divide a group of subjects into one hundred segments after arranging in ascending order such that each segment has the same or nearly the same number (n/100) of subjects.

Person-years — The sum total of years observed for different individuals. If one person is followed-up for 3 years, second for 1½ years and third for 2 years, then the person-years of follow-up is 3 + 1½ + 2 = 6½ years. Similarly there could be person-weeks or person-months.

Phases of a trial — In phase I, the maximum tolerated dose and pharmacological properties including toxicity and safety are determined by a trial on a group of volunteers, usually without controls. The objectives of phase II are to investigate clinical efficacy, incidence of side-effects, identify a dose schedule, and to collect further pharmacological data. Most phase II trials have a control group. Phase III is an RCT that is done after achieving success in the first two phases to firmly establish efficacy and safety. *Post-marketing surveillance* is sometimes called phase IV.

PICO method — A method to divide the research question into its components so that nothing is missed. P: problem, population, patients; I: intervention or exposure, indicator; C: control, comparator; O: outcome.

Pie diagram — A diagram showing the proportions of subjects in different groups or with different *mutually exclusive and exhaustive* characteristics by means of segments of a circular pie.

Pilot study — A small-scale forerunner study to learn about the situation and the variables.

Placebo — An inert substance or a procedure that is neither harmful nor beneficial. The objective of placebo is that the subject gets the perception that he is receiving treatment—thus removing perception bias in trials.

Placebo-controlled trial — Study of efficacy and safety of a regimen in comparison to a group that receives *placebo*. Contrast it with trials in which the comparison group receives existing (active) regimen.

Placebo effect — The psychological effect on a patient of the perception that he is receiving a treatment although the treatment is dummy, and the person generally does not know that it is dummy. This is the main reason for conducting placebo-controlled trials. Also see *Hawthorne effect*.

Plagiarism — Unauthorized use of someone else's language and thoughts and projecting them as your own.

Point estimation — The process of finding a single value of a parameter as an estimate based on the study sample.

Polytomous variable — A characteristics divided into three or more exclusive categories, such as severity of disease into mild, moderate, serious and critical, or liver disease as cirrhosis, hepatitis, and malignancy. A quantitative measurement such as cholesterol level can be made polytomous when divided into small number of categories such as -99, 100-179, 180-249 and 250+ mg/dl.

Population — The totality of individuals or units of interest. There could be a 'population' of blood samples collected in a year. If the interest is restricted to only suspected cases of liver diseases, the population comprises blood samples of such cases only. If the interest is further restricted to the cases attending OPD in a group of hospitals, the population is also accordingly restricted.

Population attributable risk — The risk in the total population minus the risk in unexposed subjects. In the population, some are exposed but most are unexposed. This measures the impact on the population of eliminating that exposure.

Positive association — Presence of one factor associated with the presence of the other, and absence with absence, in more subjects than expected by chance.

Positive correlation — Higher values of one quantitative variable generally accompanied by higher values of the other and the lower values with lower, i.e., they tend to move in the same direction.

Positive predictivity — Short for 'predictive value of a positive test'. This is the probability that a person with positive test really turns out to be suffering from the disease. Depends heavily on the prevalence of the disease. Since a test is used only on suspected cases, the predictivity should be evaluated on the basis of suspected cases only.

Posterior probability — See *prior probability.*

Posthoc comparison — The comparison of groups for their initial equivalence after collection of data.

Post-marketing surveillance — Keeping a tab on outcome and side-effects of a formulation after it is introduced into the market: sometimes called phase IV of a *clinical trial.*

Post-test probability — The probability of occurrence or presence of an event such as disease after the test results are available. See *prior probability.*

Power — The probability that a study or a trial will be able to detect a specified effect when present. This is calculated as (1 – Probability of *Type II error*)—i.e., the probability of correctly concluding that the specified effect exists when it is indeed present. This measures the ability to demonstrate an effect when one really exists and depends primarily on the number of subjects in a study and the magnitude of the effect to be detected.

PowerPoint — A software of Microsoft Corporation that helps to make slides, which can be directly projected from the electronic format. This software has several features regarding designing the slide. The presentation of research to an audience can be very effective with the help of PowerPoint slides.

Pragmatic trial — A trial done under standard clinical practice so that accepted variation such as during drug intake are allowed. Contrast it with *explanatory trial* done under near-ideal conditions with practically no deviation.

Precision — Same as *reliability* but measured statistically as inverse of the *variance.*

Prediction error — The difference between an observed value and a predicted value based on models or based on other considerations.

Predictive model — A model that predicts the outcome on the basics of antecedents. A predictive model focuses on correct prediction and does not worry about the biological process or relevance of the predictors. Choice of predictors is not important. Two different models can be equally good in prediction.

Predictive validity (of a test) — The average of the *positive predictivity* and *negative predictivity* of a test. This can be used as a combined measure of the two types of predictivities when both are equally important for the outcome of interest.

Predictivity (of a test) — See *positive predictivity* and *negative predictivity.*

Prevention trial — A human experiment for a preventive strategy such as exercise and diet changes or a regimen involving vitamins, to prevent occurrence or recurrence of a disease, or any other adverse condition.

Pretest probability — The probability of occurrence or presence of an event such as disease before the test results are available: generally the same as prevalence rate in the specified group. Contrast it with *post-test probability*. See also *prior probability.*

Pretesting — Checking the workability, adequacy, reliability, etc., of a tool before using it for actual study. The tool could be an instrument, a laboratory procedure, a questionnaire, or any other.

Prevalence — The number of cases of interest present or existing at any specific time, usually at the time of the survey.

Prevalence rate — *Prevalence* per unit of population or per unit of susceptibles, such as percent, per thousand and per million. Note that prevalence rate is not a 'rate' as it does not signify frequency of occurrence per unit of time—it is only a proportion. Conventionally, but wrongly, it is called a rate.

Prevalence ratio — Ratio of *prevalence rate* in one group to the other.

Prevalent cases — Same as *prevalence.*

Primary data — Data that are directly collected from the respondents. Contrast it with *secondary data* that already exist in databases, records, reports, articles, etc.

Primordial factors — Factors that work behind the scene, are precursors, or are those that give rise to risk factors. Life style is a primordial factor that can give rise to risk factors such as obesity and smoking.

Prior probability — The chance of occurrence or presence of an event such as disease or death in a patient when nothing is known about the condition of the patient. Once something, such as signs-symptoms-measurements, is known, the diagnosis becomes substantially more focused and the probability changes. The latter is called the *posterior probability*. When further information becomes available, this posterior becomes prior probability and the new probability based on the fresh information becomes posterior.

PRISMA – Acronym for Preferred Reporting Items for Systematic Reviews and Meta Analyses: A checklist of 27 items and a flow diagram of how the studies for reviews were selected and processed for joint conclusion.

Probability — A measure of belief in occurrence of an event or presence of a characteristic. This can be obtained either on the basis of theoretical considerations such as 1/6 for each of the 6 faces of a dice, on the basis of experience, or on the basis of frequency of occurrence when total occurrences are very large. Probability is the degree of certainty of occurrence of an event on a 0 to 1 scale. Probability of death is 1 for all individuals but the probability of death of a pancreatic cancer case within 5 years of detection could be 0.6.

ProCite— The software that manages bibliographic citations; can be used in conjunction with *MedLine*.

Proforma — A prototype or a sample of a format on which the observations are to be recorded.

Prognostic factor — A characteristic that can help in prediction of the eventual development of an outcome such as recovery, complication, and death. This does not necessarily imply a *cause-effect relationship*.

Prognostic stratification — A *stratification* done after examining the pattern of observations, such as categorising patients as mild, moderate, serious on the basis of new criteria developed after the patients are seen. In the usual *stratification,* the criteria are decided before seeing the patients.

Prophylactic trial — An experiment on a prophylactic measure such as amnioinfusion for meconium-stained amniotic fluid at the time of childbirth, or in the community such as iron supplementation to adolescent girls.

Proportion — The measure of how big the part of is of the whole. The whole is considered as one. If 20% of a population have blood group A, the proportion is 0.20 or 1/5.

Proportional hazards model — A model that works when ratio of logarithm of hazard in test group to control group remains same all through the period of observation. This is an important prerequisite for the validity of Cox model.

Proportional reduction in error — The reduction in error in prediction of the outcome when a particular antecedent is used for prediction relative to when it is not used.

Prospective study — A study that investigates outcomes for known antecedents. The follow-up of subjects is inherent in this kind of study since the occurrence of outcome can take time.

Protocol — A comprehensive statement regarding steps to be taken and followed for conducting a study. See *research protocol.*

Proximal measures — Measurements directly on *outcome*, contrasted with *distal measures*. Impact of vitamin A supplementation to children below three years can be measured proximally by rise in retinol level. In contrast, distally, the impact can be measured by growth pattern. Research results many times depend on appropriate choice of proximal measures for the outcome of interest.

PubMed — An extension of *MedLine* database of articles published in selected journals.

Publication bias — Publication of one type of articles more often than the other types, such as more frequent publication of positive results than negative results.

Purposive sampling — Nonrandom sampling the includes subjects to serve the specific purpose, such as volunteers in phase I of *clinical trials*. See *convenience sampling, haphazard sampling, snowball sampling, volunteer studies.* All these are methods of purposive sampling.

Putative factors — The risk factors popularly believed to be the causes of an outcome – they may not be the actual operational factors.

***P*-value** — The probability of *Type I error*, i.e., the chance that an effect is concluded when actually there is none: the chance that the result could have been produced by random sampling fluctuations rather than being actual. This is the probability of false positive result due to sampling.

Qualitative data — A set of observations on qualitative characteristics of individuals such as signs and symptoms. These can be *nominal* or *ordinal*. The only real summary measure for qualitative data is proportion of subjects with a specified characteristic, although for some ordinal data, scores can be assigned that can be treated as numerics.

Qualitative variable — A characteristic that is assessed in terms of attributes such as gender and degree of severity of disease: a variable that yields *qualitative data*.

Quality of life — Comfort and functionality of persons, generally as perceived by the person himself.

Quality of life trial — A trial for a regimen that could improve quality of life of people in ill-health, particularly those with chronic diseases or degenerative conditions.

Quantiles — Cut-points of values of a variable that divide the total number of subjects into desired number of equal groups. Examples are *percentiles, deciles, quartiles* and*tertiles.*

Quantitative data — Collection of observations on characteristics that could be numerically expressed for an individual such as haemoglobin level, blood pressure, and blood glucose level. Most common summary measures for quantitative data are *mean* and *Standard Deviation (SD).*

Quantitative variable — A characteristic that is measured in terms of numerics, such as creatinine level and parity of a woman: a variable that yields quantitative data. See also *continuous variable, discrete variable.*

Quartiles — Three cut-points of values of a variable that divide a group in four equal parts with regard to number of subjects, after the values are arranged in ascending order.

Quasi-random allocation — Allocation of subjects to test and control group by following apparently random method such as alternation (such as odd/even) and based on birth data that are not strictly random.

Questionnaire — A survey instrument that contains a predetermined series of questions that are supposed to be put in verbatim to the respondents or can be self-administered. It contains space for recording responses also.

Quota sampling — Purposive selection of pre-specified number (quota) of subjects from each segment of population without using random method.

QUOROM - QUality Of Reporting Of Meta-analysis. This was updated and revised into *PRISMA* in 2009.

Random — Unpredictable, like lottery.

Random allocation — Same as *randomisation.*

Random effects model — A statistical model that stipulates that the levels of factors under study are random samples of the possible levels. Contrast it with *fixed effects model.*

Random error — An error that has no bias, and which is natural to occur in observations because of biological or other variation beyond control. These errors are small, and some are positive some negative so that the long-term average is close to zero. Most random errors are small and few are large. This gives rise to Gaussian distribution of such errors.

Random sampling — Sampling in a manner that the selection cannot be predicted. The chance of selection of various units can be equal or unequal. The popular methods of random sampling are *simple, systematic, stratified, cluster,* and *multistage.*

Randomisation — Allocation of subjects to different groups in a random manner with equal chance. The objective is that unaccounted factors are almost equally distributed among groups, and there is no bias on this count. Randomisation could be open so that the participants or the observers know which subject is in which group, or it could be blind.

Randomised clinical trial — An experiment on human beings where the subjects are randomly allocated to various *arms of a trial.* These arms may be various treatments or different dosage groups. When one arm is the control group, this becomes *randomised controlled trial.*

Randomised controlled trial — A *trial* where there is a control group (in addition to the test group) and the allocation of subjects to the control and test groups is by random method. This is considered to be the ideal methodology to evaluate efficacy of a new regimen (preventive, therapeutic or diagnostic) particularly when it is *double-blind.*

Rasch analysis — The process of recalibration of a test (such as a questionnaire) so as to increase the chance of higher correct answers to more difficult questions by more able persons.

Rate — The frequency with which events occur per unit of time, such as deaths per year or new cases per month. Time is a necessary ingredient of a rate. Generally measured per unit of population such as percent, per thousand and per million.

Ratio — Strength or magnitude or number of one quantity relative to the other, such as male-female ratio and albumin-globulin ratio.

RCT — Short for *randomised controlled trial.*

Recall bias — Not being able to recall events occurring far away in the past with the same frequency as those occurring recently. This introduces *bias* in favour of recent occurrences. Also occurs when diseased cases are able to recall because of their suffering but controls fail to recall as much. Also when serious episodes are easily recalled and mild episodes tend to be forgotten.

Receiving operating characteristic curve — Same as *ROC curve.*

Record linkage — The process of linking different records of one person at different facilities to make one comprehensive record.

Reference population — Same as *target population.*

Reference values — Same as *normal levels.*

Referred sample – A group of subjects that are referred for specialised handling. A study can be carried out on a referred sample although the results cannot be generalised.

Regression analysis – The statistical procedure to find a *regression equation.*

Regression equation – The nature of relationship of one variable with one or more of others, generally expressed as a mathematical equation that best fits the data. Also called a *regression model.*

Regression coefficient – The quantity that delineates the change in a dependent variable for one unit change in the independent variable. If regression coefficient of birthweight (in gm) on maternal haemoglobin level is +60, it means that birthweight increases on average by 60 gm for each 1g/dl increase in maternal haemoglobin level.

Regression line – Graphical presentation of *linear regression.*

Regression model – Same as *regression equation.*

Regressor – Same as *independent variable* in a *regression equation.*

Relationship – The property of change in one variable when the other changes. This change can be causal, incidental, or due to a third intervening variable. Mathematically this could be linear, quadratic, logarithmic, etc.

Relative risk – *Risk* of occurrence of an outcome in the presence of one factor (exposure) relative to the risk in the presence of another (generally control) factor.

Relative risk reduction – Reduction in *absolute risk* after an intervention as percentage of the risk in exposed group before intervention.

Reliability – Ability to repeat the performance. The performance could be poor but same performance every time means good reliability. Statistically, this means smaller *variance* in repeated measurements.

Repeatability – Same as *reproducibility.*

Repeated measures – When the same subject is observed repeatedly after specified time gaps, such as monitoring blood pressure and heart rate at 1, 5, 10, 15 and 30 minutes after a administering anaesthesia.

Replication – Trying the same regimen on more than one equivalent group so as to get an idea of the repeatability. Replications, when yielding similar results, increase the reliability of the results.

Reporting bias – Highlighting findings in a report that support a particular view at the cost of the other.

Reproducibility – The ability to give similar result when another study is conducted in identical conditions.

Reproduction number (of infection) — The rate at which an *index case* infects others in the entire transmission phase. If the reproduction rate is one or more, the infection sustains itself and spreads in the population, like COVID-19 did in many countries. If the reproduction rate is less than one, the infection will die down or will stabilize at a low level. Basic reproduction number (R_0) is the number infected when there is no barrier, and all contacts are susceptible. In case some people develop immunity or there is some nonpharmacological intervention (mask, social distancing), the reproduction number at time t (R_t) would be much less than R_0.

Research — Discovery of new facts, enunciation of new principles, or fresh interpretation of the known facts or principles.

Research design — Same as *design* for a research study.

Research protocol — Statement on planned steps of research, including background information and rationale, objectives and hypotheses, review of literature, methodology, ethics, statistical evaluation, and references.

Response bias — (i) Not giving proper history due to stigma such as in STDs or for any other reason, and (ii) selective nonresponse, i.e., persons who are not seriously ill do not fully cooperate.

Retrospective cohort — Same as *historical cohort.*

Retrospective follow-up study — A study based on a *historical cohort.*

Retrospective study — A study that investigates antecedents for known outcomes. The recruitment of cases can be prospective spanning a duration such as all cases reporting in one year period. But the investigation is from effect to the cause.

Reverse causation — Also called retro causation or backward causation, reverse causation refers to a situation where apparently the outcome precedes the cause. For example, the studies might indicate that obese people are more depressed while actually depression may change diet preferences and cause obesity.

Right-skewed distribution — See *skewed distribution.*

Risk — The chance of occurrence of an *outcome* of interest. It is not necessary that the outcome is adverse to health. See *attributable risk, population attributable risk,* and *relative risk.*

Risk difference — The difference in risk of occurrence of a condition in two setups, such as risk of glaucoma in vegetarians vs. risk in nonvegetarians. Same as *attributable risk.*

Risk factor — A characteristic that is suspected to affect the outcome, such as obesity for hypertension. Risk factor could be an aspect of personal behaviour or life-style, an environmental exposure, an inherited or in-born characteristic, or any other.

Risk ratio – Same as *relative risk.*

Robust method – A method that is not much affected by minor variation in its applicability conditions.

ROC curve – A curve that depicts the relationship between sensitivity of a quantitative test for different thresholds and the corresponding (1–specificity), such as for different T4 values for diagnosis of hyperthyroidism. This curve helps to evaluate the applicability of a test and helps to compare performance of one test with the other, such as of T4 with T3, or T4 with TSH.

Sample – A part of the *target population,* which is actually studied.

Sample size – The number of subjects or units in a sample.

Sample survey – A cross-sectional study of antecedents and outcomes on a sample of subjects from a defined population. Generally, this is a large-scale survey covering a full state or full country.

Sampling – Choosing a part from the whole, such as choosing 300 child births out of 5000 in a hospital in one year for studying the intrauterine growth retardation. See *random sampling, purposive sampling.*

Sampling bias – The bias due to (i) *nonrandom sample* such as volunteers that do not represent the *target population,* and (ii) small sample that fails to represent the entire spectrum of subjects.

Sampling design – The method of selection of *sample* out of the *population* of subjects.

Sampling error – The tendency of one sample giving a different result than the other sample, and neither possibly giving exactly the same result as in the *population.* This is not an error in conventional sense but is a natural fluctuation.

Sampling fluctuation – The tendency of different samples giving different results, even if drawn from the same *target population.* This happens because different samples contain individuals who are different from those in other samples.

Sampling fraction – The extent of sampling such as one out of eight, or one out of twenty.

Sampling frame – A list of units in the *target population* from which sample is drawn.

Sampling method – The procedure to choose or select a fraction out of the *target population.*

Sampling unit – The unit used for sampling. In a *multistage sampling,* there is a separate sampling unit for each stage.

Sampling variation – Same as *sampling fluctuation.*

Scales of measurement — The system of differentiating one type of observation from the other. When names are used (opposed to grades) for differentiation, the scale is called nominal. Signs and symptoms are generally measured on *nominal scale*. Textual grades such as mild, moderate, serious, are measurements on *ordinal scale*. Numeric measurements such as body mass index are on *metric scale*.

Scatter diagram — A diagram displaying values of one quantitative variable for different values of the other variable by plotting points. This is also called the (x, y) plot.

Schedule — A form that contains a set of items on which information is to be obtained. It contains space also to record the responses.

SciSearch — The software of the Institute for Scientific Information for searching citations in Science Citation Index and Current Contents.

Score — Quantification of a set of (mostly) qualitative measurements, such as APACHE score. Scores in medicine are used either to grade severity of a condition, as an aid to reach to a diagnosis, or to assess prognosis.

Screening test — A criterion used to locate possible positives that can be later confirmed by stricter criterion. A screening criterion should have high negative predictivity. The criterion could be a laboratory test, a radiological test, or a clinical observation.

Screening trial — A trial for evaluating *efficacy* and safety of a *screening test* or the one to detect risk factors.

SD — Short for *standard deviation*.

Secondary attack rate — The number of people who get sick within the incubation period after exposure to an infective person. This infective person is called the *index case*.

Secondary data — The data that are already lying somewhere as in records or literature. Contrast it with *primary data*.

Selection bias — The bias occurring due to selection of nonrepresentative group of subjects—thus affecting the generalisability of the findings. This can occur either because the selection is done with a purpose, such as of volunteers, or unwittingly due to selection of surviving subjects (if the disease under study is rapidly fatal), due to selection of younger subjects who have survived (many of the older ones may have died), etc. Lack of matching in case and control groups can also be called selection bias. All these can affect the *validity* of results.

Sensitivity — Ability to identify known positives as positives. If CPK ≥120 IU is present in 60% known cases of myocardial infarction, then sensitivity of this cut-off is 60%. Sensitivity is not a *valid* indicator of diagnostic value of the test. It only measures the intrinsic ability of a test to detect a disease when it is already known to be present.

Sensitivity analysis — The analysis to assess the impact of changes in assumptions and other conditions on the outcome. Because of limitation of knowledge, various assumptions are made in a study. For example, it is generally assumed that cure rate depends linearly on treatment regimen, host characteristics and compliance. Two kinds of *epistemic uncertainties* arise—one what happens if the dependence is not linear but is quadratic or any other type, and second, what happens if this is assumed to depend also on physical strength and mental toughness of the patients. Answers to such questions are obtained by sensitivity analysis. This analysis assesses the robustness of the results.

Sequential sampling — Serial sampling of subjects, one by one, to be stopped when scientifically acceptable result either way is available.

Severity score — A *score* used to grade severity of a condition such as *Apgar score* and *APACHE score.*

Sign test — A *nonparametric test* based on sign (negative or positive) of differences between two sets of observations. This test is used to compare two groups for their *central tendency.*

Significance — See *statistical significance* and *medical significance.*

Significance level — Same as *level of significance.*

Simple linear regression — A *regression* in which a dependent variable is sought to be explained linearly by only one independent variable, such as regression of systolic blood pressure on age. Other correlates are ignored in this setup, and the relationship format is limited to linear.

Simple random sampling — Sampling in a manner that all individuals have same chance of being selected.

Simple regression — Relationship between one independent and one dependent variable. It could be *linear* or *nonlinear.*

Simpson's paradox — In some cases the tendency of aggregated data showing a result very different from the results from disaggregated (stratified) data. This can happen due to *interaction* effect of the stratifying variable.

Simulation — Generation of data based on certain *model.*

Single blind trial — The subject is not informed that he is receiving test regimen or the control regimen in a *trial* but the investigator is aware of the allocation.

Skewed distribution — Opposed to symmetric such as *Gaussian,* generally a distribution is considered skewed when values on one side of *mode* vary much more than on the other side. It is right-skewed when values more than mode have more variation, and left-skewed when values less than mode have more variation.

SMART objectives — The desirable format of the objectives of research: Specific, Measurable, Achievable, Relevant, and Timely.

Smoking index — A measure of the burden of smoking since birth with weightage for age at initiation, quantity of smoking, duration of smoking, type of smoking (filter/ nonfilter/ bidi/ cigar, active/passive), and duration elapsed since quitting by exsmokers.

Snowball sampling — One eligible person, such as a client of sex-worker, is asked to list others known to him and eligible that can be included in the sample, and those in turn are asked to identify others, so on.

Spearman's correlation — A measure of strength of relationship between two quantitative variables when they are converted to ranks.

Specificity — Ability to identify known negatives as negatives. If AFB is negative in 95% of the healthy subjects, its specificity is 95%. In practice, a test is rarely used on healthy subjects. It is used on suspected cases. In them, the specificity may be very different.

Spectrum of disease — The distribution of subjects by affected and not affected, and among affected by severity of affliction.

Spurious association — A false *association* that could arise due to presence of *confounders, bias,* or merely a *chance*.

Spurious correlation — A false *correlation* that could arise due to presence of *confounders, bias,* or merely a *chance*.

Standard deviation (SD) — Most common and generally most appropriate measure of dispersion obtained as positive square root of *variance*.

Standard error (SE) — The measure for sample-to-sample variability in a summary measure such as *mean* and *median*. Just as the measurements such as haemoglobin level differ from person to person, so do the sample summaries from sample to sample. Mean haemoglobin level in one sample would be different from another sample even when both are drawn from the same *target population*. The extent of variability in such summaries is measured by their respective standard errors. Actually, this is the *standard deviation* of mean or median or any other summary measure as the case may be.

Standardisation (of groups) — The procedure that makes two different groups comparable by bringing them on to a common base or a common standard, such as *age-standardization*.

Standardisation (of variables) — Subtracting mean from the variable and dividing by the standard deviation (SD): thus standardisation makes mean = 0 and SD = 1.

Standardised death rate (directly standardised) — Recalculated death rate when one or more factors affecting deaths (such as age structure) are brought at par with the comparison group, or both brought to a common base. This substantially increases comparability that crude death rate lacks when one group is young and the other is old. Common base structure (called, standard) of population is chosen by the researcher.

Standardised mortality ratio — Ratio of actually observed deaths to expected deaths based on standard death rates. If this ratio is more than one, the *force of mortality* is higher in the study group compared to the standard group.

Standard treatment — An approved or widely accepted treatment modality for an ailment.

STARD statement — Acronym for STAndard for Reporting of Diagnostic accuracy studies: guidelines for reporting of results of studies on diagnostic validity of medical tools.

Statistic — A summary measure for any characteristic in the sample or the group actually studied, such as mean, median or standard deviation of a sample, or proportion of subjects found affected in a sample.

Statistical analysis — Subjecting data to the rigours of statistical methods so that the uncertainty levels are either quantified or minimized, or both.

Statistical fallacies — Many fallacies can occur in the results because of improper use of statistical methods. Some of these are due to (i) use of improper denominator for computing rate or percentage, (ii) not accounting for variable periods of exposure that could affect the rate of outcome, (iii) considering mixture of two groups as one, (iv) misuse of percentages such as 2 out 4 being stated as 50%, (v) using means for emphasising a point without considering the standard deviation, (vi) inappropriate scales in the graphs, (vii) looking at linearity when in fact the relationship is *nonlinear*, (viii) ignoring important prerequisites such as randomness, independence, equality of variances and *Gaussian* form of distribution, (ix) using means where proportions are adequate, or vice-versa, (x) ignoring baseline values, (xi) using too many *statistical tests* on the same set of data without adjusting *P-values* (xii) quantitative analysis of codes, (xiii) jumping to *cause-effect relationship* without sufficient examination of data, and (xiv) multivariate conclusions on the basis of several *univariate analyses*.

Statistical power — Same as *power*.

Statistical significance — A result is statistically significant if the chance of wrongly rejecting *null hypothesis* is less than the prefixed level such as 5%. The implication is that chance differences in samples would produce that kind of result in less than

5 times out of 100—thus chance is not a likely explanation for that result and could be real.

Statistical test — A procedure to find *P-value* corresponding to a *null hypothesis* on the basis of the given data. Depending upon the type of data and the type of hypothesis, a large number of statistical tests are available. Most popular of these are *Student's t-test* and *chi-square test.*

Statistical threshold (of normal range) — Mean ± 2SD where mean and standard deviation (SD) are obtained from measurements in a large number of healthy individuals. There is a chance of classifying nearly 5% healthy individuals with extreme values as sick when this range is used as normal.

Statistics — A science that helps to manage uncertainties in the data. Also, plural of *statistic.*

Stopping rules — Rules for stopping a clinical trial while it is still continuing. Stopping can be done either for futility when it is found on interim assessment that there is practically no chance of concluding the desired efficacy, or can be stopped for efficacy when the interim data analysis finds convincing evidence of the desired efficacy.

Strata — The divisions obtained after *stratification* (the singular is stratum).

Stratification — Division of subjects into relevant groups.

Stratified analysis — A statistical procedure to adjust for the effect of *confounders* or other correlates by studying different *strata.*

Stratified random sampling — Separate *simple random sampling* from each group after *stratification.*

Strength of relationship — The consistency of change in one factor when the other changes. If one unit change in one factor results in nearly the same change in the other in most of the subjects, the strength is high. Note that the strength is not related to the magnitude of change. Small change, if consistent, would mean high degree of relationship.

STROBE – Acronym for STrengthening the Reporting of OBservational studies in Epidemiology: A checklist of items for reporting results of an *observational study.*

Structured questionnaire – A *questionnaire* where question have list of possible answers. The respondent has just to tick the correct response for himself.

Student's *t*-test — Same as *t-test.*

Study design — Same as *design.*

Study setting — The environment in which the study is conducted. The setting could be a general hospital, a referral centre, private practice, ambulatory care, community, etc.

Sufficient cause — A cause that by itself is sufficient to change the outcome. Exposure to measles virus in a susceptible is sufficient to produce the disease. In fact this cause is both necessary and sufficient. Hanging by rope is sufficient to cause death but is not necessary as a cause for death.

Superiority trial – A *clinical trial* that has objective to examine if the regimen under test is better by at least a predefined clinically important margin.

Surrogate outcome — Outcomes that are not of direct interest but reflect the outcome of direct interest, such as pallor for nutritional level. Surrogates are generally easy to assess and do not require long follow-up.

Surrogate variable — A makeshift substitute variable that is used when the actually required variable cannot be measured. If the respondents are shy of revealing income, surrogates such as size of house, car, telephone and television can be used to assess the level of income. Since they are surrogate, they may or may not reveal the true status.

Survey — A *descriptive study* done generally on scientifically selected subjects. Another descriptive study methodology is *case series.*

Survival analysis — Analysis of survival durations. Survival duration is generic—it can be duration between any specified events such as between end of operation and beginning of consciousness, between beginning of treatment and time at complete recovery, etc. Two popular methods of survival analysis are *life table method* and *Kaplan-Meir method.*

Survival curve — A graph that depicts survival pattern of the subjects over the observed period of time. It begins at 100% (all alive) and shows gradual or rapid decline as the time passes depending on the disease under study.

Survival function — A mathematical expression for *survival curve.*

Susceptibility — Proneness to catch an infection or a disease. A person who is effectively immunised against tetanus is not susceptible to tetanus, and a child is not susceptible to the usual sexually transmitted diseases.

Synergism — A situation where two factors when present together accentuate the outcome more than their individual capacities. Iron and folic acid are synergistic for increasing the haemoglobin level.

Synthesis (of research) — The process of combining diverse evidence from different researches to come to a holistic conclusion.

Systematic error — Same as *bias.*

Systematic random sampling — Selection of first individual at random and others automatically at regular spacing depending on *sampling fraction.*

Target population — Same as *population*. Also called the reference population.

Tertiles — Two cut-points of values of a variable that divide a group into three equal parts (each part with same number of subjects) after arranging in ascending order.

Test group — The group of subjects that is receiving or has received the regimen under test.

Test of hypothesis — The procedure used to test whether sufficient evidence exists against a *null hypothesis*: mostly a statistical procedure.

Test of significance — A statistical procedure to test whether or not the observations fall into a specified pattern, such as equal means of two or more groups, or following a linear trend. If they do not, the result is called statistically significant. This requires prior fixing of the *level of significance* that specifies the maximum tolerable probability of *Type I error*.

Test-retest reliability — Agreement between responses when the same instrument such as a questionnaire is administered to the same set of people again; stability of the responses in repeated use of the instrument.

Therapeutic equivalence — Comparable safety and efficacy of two or more treatment modalities when administered under the conditions specified for each modality. These conditions could be different for different modalities. Also see *equivalence*.

Therapeutic trial — A *clinical trial* on a therapeutic agent or regimen to evaluate its *efficacy* and safety.

Thesis — A proposal or hypothesis forwarded after a careful investigation accompanied by full details: generally the written work submitted by a candidate in fulfilment of partial requirement for the award of Master's degree. See also *dissertation*.

Time-line — A chart or a table that states the durations and dates of beginning and ending various phases of a project, some of which can overlap.

Training sample – The sample of subjects which is used to develop a model. This model is subsequently tested on *validation sample*.

Transformation — When the data pattern is far from Gaussian, transformation is applied such as log and inverse ($1/x$) so that the values tend to follow Gaussian pattern. Transformation is also done to achieve *homoscedasticity*.

Translational research – The *research* that tries to bridge the gap between discoveries and their application to actual life situations.

Transmissibility — Used in two senses:

1. The ability to transmit (infection or disease) from one to the other. HIV is transmissible through several modes such as blood transfusion. Cancer is not transmissible.

2. The force of transmission: when exposed what percentage of susceptibles get the infection or disease. HIV is more transmissible from male to female than from female to male.

Trial — An experiment on human subjects. See *clinical trial, field trial, prophylactic trial, therapeutic trial* and *vaccine trial.*

***T*-Score** — *T*-score of $x = \frac{x - \theta}{s}$ where s is the sample SD and θ is the optimal value so that *T*-score tells how far away a value is from its optimal in SD units. This is quite commonly used for assessing bone mineral density.

***t*-test** — A statistical procedure to test hypothesis of equality of two *means,* and for certain other hypotheses relating to parameters such as *regression coefficient* under the assumption of Gaussianity.

Tukey's test — A statistical test for pairwise comparisons of means when there are three or more groups. This test keeps the probability of the total *Type I error* within the specified *level of significance,* but this level could actually be lower than specified.

Twin studies — Studies of twins, particularly identical twins, to find the effect of differential environment on their health since genetic makeup of both is the same.

Two-sided alternative — An *alternative hypothesis* that stipulates that the *parameter* value can be higher or lower than the null value. Both directions are admissible. This type of alternative is setup when it is not known that the value is going to be higher or lower than the specified value.

Two-tailed test — See *One-tailed test.*

Two-way classification — Division of subjects by two characteristics simultaneously, such as dividing cases of diabetes mellitus by their obesity category and smoking category.

Two-way design — A study that is planned to investigate the effect of levels of two antecedent factors, such as effect of obesity (BMI<20.0, 20.0-24.9, 25.0-29.9 or 30.0+) and smoking (none, mild, moderate or heavy) on blood glucose level. Their *interaction* can also be investigated in this kind of *design.*

Type I error — The error of rejecting a true *null hypothesis,* i.e., concluding that there is a difference when actually there is none. The sample or data might be such that this lead to such a wrong conclusion. This error leads to false positive result.

Type II error — The error of wrongly concluding that there is no difference when actually some difference is present. This error leads to false negative result.

Type III error — This occurs when the researchers investigate wrong direction of effect. For example, if the population value of the parameter under test is actually more than the null value, the sample might give a value so much below that the researcher rejects the null and concludes that the population value is also below the null value. Also used for the right answer to a wrong question.

Unbalanced design — A *design* with unequal number of subjects in different groups.

Uncertainty analysis — The analysis that delineates the effect of change in the value of the *parameter* under assessment on the conclusion. One component of this is the *sampling fluctuation* in the estimate of the parameters, and the other is the plausible change in the values themselves that can affect the outcome.

Uncertainty principle (in a clinical trial) — The principle that says that the outcome of various arms of trial should be a-priori uncertain. One specific uncertainty situation is that the a-priori chances of each regimen being successful are nearly equal—called *clinical equipoise.*

Unit of study — The unit (individual, patient, blood sample, biopsy, etc.) that is used to obtain the required information.

Univariate analysis — The analysis regarding one variable at a time. The combined result of several univariate analyses may be very different from the result obtained by simultaneous consideration of these variables. See also *multivariate analysis.*

Universe — The broad group of subjects for which the findings could be generalised or implicated. Statistically this is broader than the *target population* and can include future subjects.

Up-and-down trial — A trial where a start is made with an assumed average dose and it is increased or decreased by predetermined step in subsequent subjects depending upon the dose is not effective or effective, respectively.

Vaccine trial — An experiment on human population to evaluate potency, efficacy, and safety of a vaccine.

Validation sample — A sample used to validate the results of the study. It could be a subsample of the original sample that is kept aside for this purpose, or could be a new sample of subjects.

Validity (of a measurement) — Ability to hit the target (or around it): ability to assess what is really intended to be assessed. Weight by itself is not a valid indicator of obesity in adults but body mass index that uses height also is. For a medical test, validity is measured by *sensitivity, specificity* and *predictivities* (positive and negative).

Validity (of a study) — The ability of a study to provide correct conclusion, considering the representativeness and size of sample, *validity of measurements,* and the soundness of methods. See also *internal validity* and *external validity.*

Validity (of a survey instrument or a test) — Ability of an instrument (such as a questionnaire or a schedule) or of a test to provide the information that matches with the objectives of the study. For its varieties, see *concurrent validity, content validity, construct validity, criterion validity, face validity,* and *predictive validity.*

Vancouver style (or format) – A style of writing research papers agreed by editors of more than 500 medical journals published around the world. It includes instructions on who could and should be authors, what help must be acknowledged, how to structure the text, and how to cite references. The system of citing references matches closely with the system followed by *MedLine*.

Variable – A characteristic that varies from person to person, or from situation to situation. Platelet count in different persons is variable but number of eyes or number of fingers is rarely a variable. See *quantitative variable, qualitative variable, discrete variable, continuous variable, dependent variable,* and *independent variable.*

Variance – A measure of dispersion or scatteredness of quantitative data obtained as average of the squared deviations from mean.

Virulence – The ability to produce severe form of disease that can threaten life. Rabies is a highly virulent disease and cholera is not–measured as percentage of cases who go into severe form. See *infectivity, pathogenicity.*

Volunteer studies – A study done on volunteers, opposed to randomly selected subjects. Results from such studies can be used to identify tolerated dose and some side-effects of a test regimen but cannot be used to estimate efficacy.

Waist-height ratio – The ratio of waist circumference to height. This ratio realizes that people with more height can have more waist circumference without being obese.

Waist-hip ratio – The ratio of waist circumference to hip measurement: sometimes considered a more valid measure of obesity than *body mass index*. Waist-hip ratio measures only central obesity, whereas body mass index is for overall obesity including central obesity.

Washout period – In a *cross-over trial,* the period elapsed between withdrawal of first treatment, and start of the second treatment. This period allows time for any effect of the first treatment to vanish before the second is started.

Wilcoxon test – Another method to do *Mann-Whitney test* for comparing central tendency of two groups. Both give exactly same result, and they are algebraically equivalent.

Zelen design – Under this design, the patients in a clinical trial randomized to a group are asked for consent to be in that group. If consent is not given, the patient goes to another group. This is considered more ethical but no blinding can done and the analysis of data is difficult.

z-score – Same as *normal deviate* but sometimes measured from median instead of mean, particularly in assessing growth: difference of a value from group mean in terms of how many times of SD.

z-test – A statistical *test of hypothesis* based on Gaussian distribution, generally used to compare two means or two proportions.

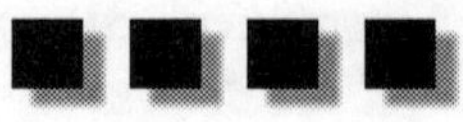

Index

D

E

F

G

H

I

K

L

N

O

P

Q

R

S

T

U

V

W

Z

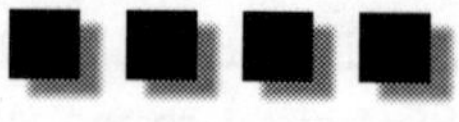

Notes 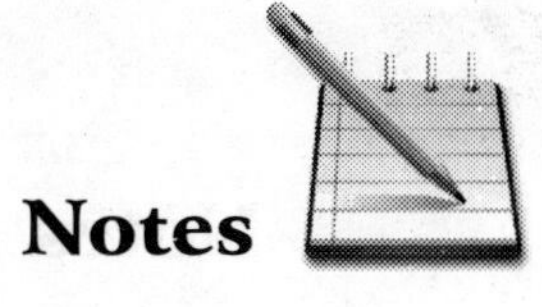

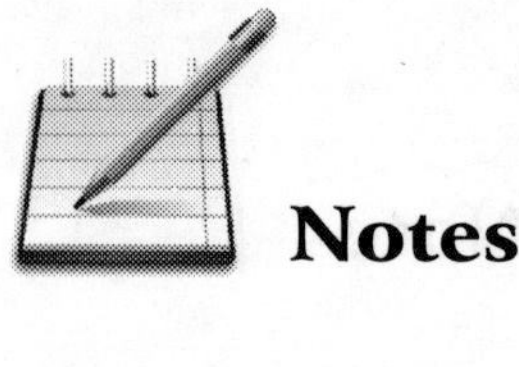

Notes

Notes 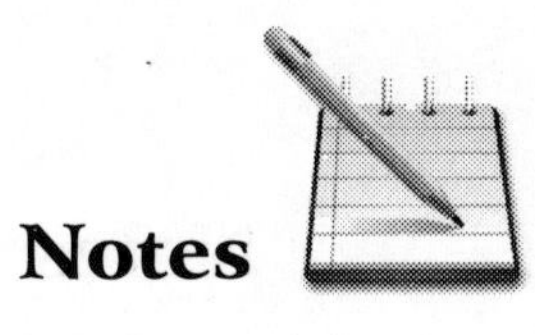

Notes